LIVE LONGER LIVE BETTER

READER'S DIGEST

LIVE LONGER LIVE BETTER

Adding Years to Your Life

And Life to Your Years

Reader's Digest

THE READER'S DIGEST ASSOCIATION, INC., PLEASANTVILLE, NEW YORK / MONTREAL

STAFF

Project Editor
SUZANNE E. WEISS

Project Art Editor
PERRI DeFINO

Senior Research Editor
EILEEN EINFRANK

Senior Associate Editors
ELISABETH JAKAB, NANCY SHUKER

Research Associate
DEIRDRE VAN DYK

Editorial Assistant
VITA GARDNER

◼

READER'S DIGEST GENERAL BOOKS
Editor-in-Chief: JOHN A. POPE, JR.
General Books Editor, U.S.: SUSAN WERNERT LEWIS
Affinity Directors: WILL BRADBURY, JIM DWYER,
KAARI WARD
Art Director: EVELYN BAUER
Editorial Director: JANE POLLEY
Research Director: LAUREL A. GILBRIDE
Group Art Editors: ROBERT M. GRANT,
JOEL MUSLER
Copy Chief: EDWARD W. ATKINSON
Picture Editor: MARION BODINE
Head Librarian: JO MANNING

CONTRIBUTORS

Designer
DIANE LEMONIDES

Art Associate
BARBARA LAPIC

Picture Researcher
MARION PAONE

Editors
MICHELE C. FISHER, PH.D., R.D.,
DENSIE WEBB, PH.D., R.D.,
PATRICIA BARNETT, LEE FOWLER

Copy Editor
VIRGINIA CROFT

Research Associate
MARTHA PROCTOR

Recipe Developer
SANDRA ROSE GLUCK

Food Stylist
DELORES CUSTER

Indexer
SYDNEY WOLFE COHEN

◼

Chief Writers
GORDON BAKOULIS, JEAN CALLAHAN,
SERENA STOCKWELL, CAROL WEEG

Writers
KATHARINE COLTON, GERRY SCHREMP,
CARL PROUJAN, ROLLENE W. SAAL,
PAM LAMBERT, MARY LYN MAISCOTT,
MICHAEL S. SANDERS, GUY A. LESTER,
MARJORIE ANNE FLORY

◼

ARTISTS
Photography
COLIN COOKE, JAN COBB,
MARC ROSENTHAL

Medical Illustration
KEITH KASNOT, C.M.I.

Airbrush
JOHN EDWARDS

Chart Graphics
GRAPHIC CHART & MAP CO., INC.,
ARNE HURTY

Silhouettes
RAY SKIBINSKI

Fashion Illustration
DONNA MAHALKO

CHIEF CONSULTANT
ARTHUR W. FEINBERG, M.D.
MEDICAL DIRECTOR, CENTER FOR EXTENDED
CARE AND REHABILITATION
CHIEF, DIVISION OF GERIATRIC MEDICINE
NORTH SHORE UNIVERSITY HOSPITAL
PROFESSOR OF CLINICAL MEDICINE
CORNELL UNIVERSITY MEDICAL COLLEGE

CHAPTER CONSULTANTS
Chapter 1
BRUCE E. HIRSCH, M.D.
ASSISTANT PROFESSOR OF MEDICINE
CORNELL UNIVERSITY MEDICAL COLLEGE
SENIOR ASSISTANT ATTENDING PHYSICIAN IN THE
DIVISION OF INFECTIOUS DISEASES—NORTH
SHORE UNIVERSITY HOSPITAL

Chapter 2
MARION NESTLE, PH.D., M.P.H.
PROFESSOR AND CHAIR
DEPARTMENT OF NUTRITION, FOOD, AND HOTEL
MANAGEMENT
NEW YORK UNIVERSITY

Chapter 3
RONALD S. FEINGOLD, PH.D.
PROFESSOR AND CHAIR
DEPARTMENT OF HEALTH, PHYSICAL EDUCATION
& HUMAN PERFORMANCE SCIENCE
ADELPHI UNIVERSITY

Chapter 4
STANLEY DARROW, D.D.S., F.A.C.D., F.A.G.D.
ATTENDING DENTIST
FLUSHING HOSPITAL & MEDICAL CENTER

W. PETER MCCABE, M.D.
SECTION CHIEF, PLASTIC AND HAND SURGERY
SAINT JOHN'S HOSPITAL
CLINICAL ASSISTANT PROFESSOR OF SURGERY
WAYNE STATE UNIVERSITY

VICTOR J. SELMANOWITZ, M.D.
DERMATOLOGIST, NEW YORK, NEW YORK

Chapter 5
HERBERT HARRIS KRAUSS, PH.D.
PROFESSOR OF PSYCHOLOGY AND CHAIR
DEPARTMENT OF PSYCHOLOGY
HUNTER COLLEGE, CITY UNIVERSITY OF NEW YORK

Chapter 6
JOANNE GOTTRIDGE, M.D.
CHIEF, DIVISION OF AMBULATORY MEDICINE
NORTH SHORE UNIVERSITY HOSPITAL
ASSOCIATE PROFESSOR OF CLINICAL MEDICINE
CORNELL UNIVERSITY MEDICAL COLLEGE

Chapter 7
ROBERT H. BROWN, M.D.
ATTENDING SURGEON
MANHATTAN EYE & EAR HOSPITAL

B. ROBERT MEYER, M.D.
DIRECTOR, DEPARTMENT OF MEDICINE
BRONX MUNICIPAL HOSPITAL CENTER
ASSOCIATE PROFESSOR OF MEDICINE
ALBERT EINSTEIN COLLEGE OF MEDICINE

Chapter 8
SUSAN C. HIRSCH, M.D.
PERSONNEL HEALTH PHYSICIAN
NORTH SHORE UNIVERSITY HOSPITAL
CLINICAL INSTRUCTOR IN MEDICINE
CORNELL UNIVERSITY MEDICAL COLLEGE

Library of Congress Cataloging in Publication Data
Live longer, live better: adding years to your life and life to your
years.
   p.   cm.
  Includes index.
  ISBN 0-89577-578-6
  1. Longevity. 2. Health I. Reader's Digest Association.
RA776.75.L584 1995
613—dc20
                                              93-31829

ABOUT THIS BOOK

. . . .

What more could you wish for yourself or for someone you love than a long, healthy life? Doctors and other scientists who study aging now believe that you can do more than just wish for such a gift (see Chapter 1). A healthy lifestyle has a major impact on your longevity and well-being. LIVE LONGER, LIVE BETTER shows you how you can establish and maintain such a lifestyle. The foods you eat, for example, provide more than nourishment and energy; the right diet can help you prevent and fight disease (see Chapter 2). Regular exercise is also crucial to your good health; you don't have to become a skilled athlete, however, to enjoy the benefits of physical fitness (see Chapter 3).

You owe it to yourself to look your best always; this isn't difficult if you prepare for the physical changes that come with time (see Chapter 4). Coping well with the stresses of major life changes also takes preparation (see Chapter 5).

To maintain your health and to detect medical problems early, you need to follow a regular schedule of medical screening tests (see Chapter 6). If you do experience a serious or chronic illness, however, there are ways to make it easier to live with (see Chapter 7). Finally, if you can minimize the environmental risks in your everyday life, you can prevent a number of health problems (see Chapter 8).

■ The information, recommendations, and visual material in LIVE LONGER, LIVE BETTER are for reference and guidance only; they are not intended as a substitute for a physician's diagnosis and care. The editors urge anyone with continuing medical problems or symptoms to consult a qualified physician.

–The Editors

"Nobody grows old by merely living a number of years. People grow old only by deserting their ideals. Years may wrinkle the skin, but to give up interest wrinkles the soul.**"**

— *Gen. Douglas MacArthur*
(1880–1964)

CONTENTS

· · · · · · · · · · · · · · · · · ·

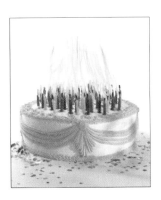

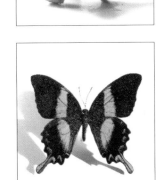

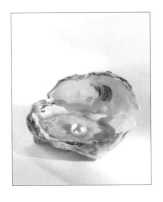

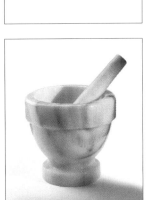

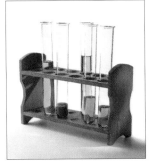

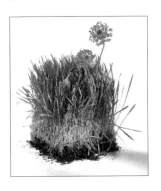

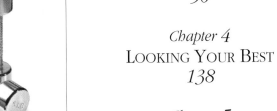

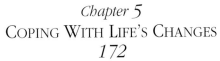

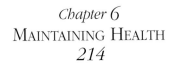

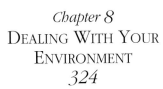

Chapter 1
PROLONGING LIFE
8

Chapter 2
EATING WELL
34

Chapter 3
SHAPING UP
90

Chapter 4
LOOKING YOUR BEST
138

Chapter 5
COPING WITH LIFE'S CHANGES
172

Chapter 6
MAINTAINING HEALTH
214

Chapter 7
LIVING WITH CHRONIC
CONDITIONS AND SERIOUS ILLNESS
262

Chapter 8
DEALING WITH YOUR
ENVIRONMENT
324

CREDITS AND ACKNOWLEDGMENTS *352*
INDEX *354*

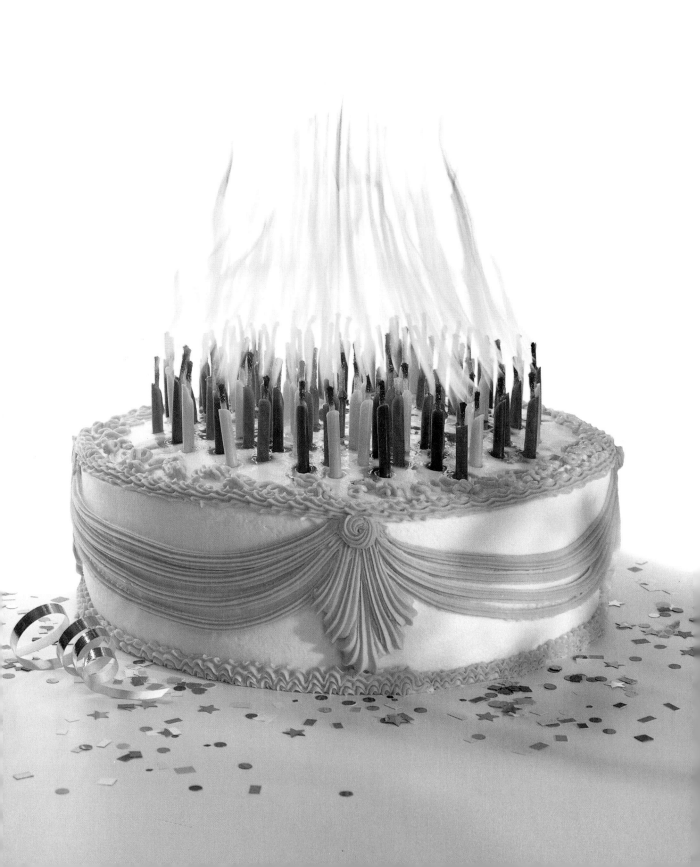

Chapter *1*

PROLONGING LIFE

. . . .

■ A Long, Healthy Life:
  An Increasingly Common Phenomenon *10*

■ How You Get Older—And Wiser *14*

■ The Aging Process Under a Microscope *22*

■ Studying the Possibility of Life Extension *26*

■ What You Can Do to Live Longer—
  And Live Better *30*

A Long, Healthy Life:
An Increasingly Common
Phenomenon

· · · · · · · · · · · · · · · · · · · ·

Americans are living longer, healthier lives than ever before—those age 65 and older are now 10 times the number they were in 1900. People in their fifties and sixties today often have parents, aunts, and uncles who are still fit and energetic.

NEW DEMOGRAPHICS IN THE UNITED STATES

The proportion of people in the oldest and youngest age groups is undergoing a shift. For every person over 65, there are now only 2 under 18. Just 10 years ago the ratio was 1 elderly person to 3 youngsters. Even the number of Americans who live to be 100—currently about 36,000—has doubled since 1980 (see *The New Centenarians—A Growing and Lively Group*, p.13).

Families in which four and even five generations live to know one another are no longer the rarity they once were.

LIFE SPAN VS. LIFE EXPECTANCY

Gerontologists, scientists who study aging, distinguish between *life span* and *life expectancy*. Life span refers to the biological limit of human life, the absolutely oldest age that an individual could possibly reach in the absence of fatal diseases, predators, or accidents. Most doctors currently estimate this theoretical figure to be 120 years for humans. Some gerontologists, however, believe that this limit will, in the future, be extended (pp.26–28).

Life expectancy is a person's average length of life based on statistical probability. A baby

AVERAGE LIFE EXPECTANCY THROUGH HISTORY
The changes in human life expectancy are depicted below. Although there were increases throughout recorded history, the greatest strides came in the early 20th century and promise to continue into the 21st.

3000 B.C.
AVERAGE LIFE:
18 YEARS

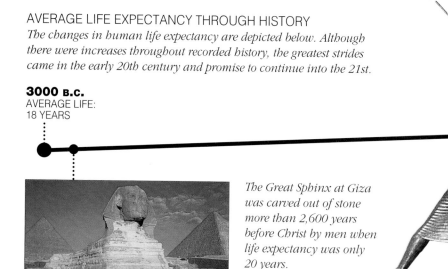

The Great Sphinx at Giza was carved out of stone more than 2,600 years before Christ by men when life expectancy was only 20 years.

King Tutankhamen of Egypt, shown harpooning from a riverboat, was born in 1370 B.C. and lived only 18 years.

born in the United States in the 1990's, for example, can be expected to live 75.4 years, an increase of 1.7 years since 1980 and 26.4 years since 1900 (see chart below).

The increase in life expectancy in industrialized countries during the 20th century is due mainly to improved hygiene and sanitation, better nutrition, and ways to prevent or treat such deadly infectious diseases as smallpox, measles, polio, and tuberculosis (now, unfortunately, making a comeback). Today the practice of preventive medicine—immunizations as well as proper diet and

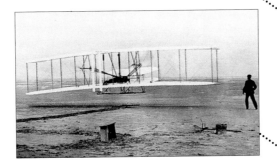

A seven-year-old boy in 1995 was quite likely to have an active grandfather in his life as well as a father.

A.D. 2010
PROJECTED
AVERAGE LIFE:
115 YEARS

A.D. 2000
PROJECTED
AVERAGE LIFE:
85 YEARS

A.D. 1990
AVERAGE LIFE:
76 YEARS

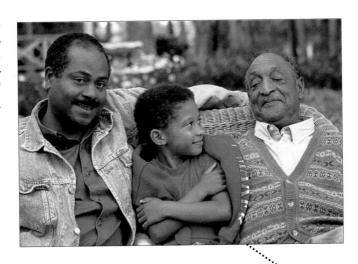

In 1903 when Orville and Wilbur Wright ushered in the age of aviation at Kitty Hawk, North Carolina, they were both in their thirties. Wilbur died at 45, a little early for the era, but Orville lived to be 77.

A.D. 1900
AVERAGE LIFE:
49 YEARS

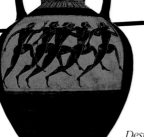

275 B.C.
AVERAGE LIFE:
26 YEARS

Despite their physical fitness, the young athletes shown racing across this Greek vase, which dates from the 6th century B.C., could not have expected to live beyond their early twenties.

regular exercise—coupled with advances in controlling such major illnesses as cancer, heart disease, and stroke promise to continue the trend, but at a somewhat slower rate.

CURRENT LIFE EXPECTANCY STATISTICS

The life expectancy for women in the United States, 78.3 years, is greater than that for men, 71.5 years. For Americans who reach the later years of life, however, life expectancy is extended. Someone born in 1925, for example, had a life expectancy of only 59 years at birth. If that person beat the odds and survived to age 65, then his life expectancy is cal-

culated in a new way and an additional 20 years of life is predicted. In Sweden, where long-term data on births and deaths go back to 1750, the number of people over 85 has increased steadily since the 1950's. Although the records are less reliable elsewhere (birth certificates were not required in the United States until 1933), the same appears to be true in other developed countries.

The United States ranks 11th among the industrial nations in life expectancy. Japan is first, with a projected life span of 78.9 years for a baby born in 1990. In contrast, life expectancy in many underdeveloped countries is in the low fifties for male babies and high fifties for female babies.

It is unclear just how high the

average life expectancy at birth can go. Many scientists believe that it is unlikely to increase beyond age 85. They say that even big drops in the current diseases of the elderly won't raise life expectancy significantly because other diseases will take their place. They claim, for example, that if a disease such as cancer were completely eliminated, the average life expectancy would increase only a few months.

More optimistic scientists believe that research will allow doctors to help their patients live significantly longer active lives. They feel confident that medical advances will prevent or cure many acute and chronic diseases associated with aging or at least delay their onset for many years.

HEALTH SPAN VS. LIFE EXPECTANCY

The work of gerontologists may or may not extend average life expectancy. But insights into how and why people age allow doctors to better understand the relationship between diseases and health habits. It is already clear that people even at middle age have the opportunity to alter their lifestyles and quite possibly postpone the onset of chronic or debilitating diseases. By so doing, they can increase their active, vital years—what doctors call their health span or active life expectancy—and possibly add to the outside number of years they will live.

A number of Americans have responded to the warnings of the medical profession. The surgeon general's report on the hazards of smoking was first published in 1964. Per capita cigarette smoking since then has decreased

LIFE SPANS OF ANIMALS

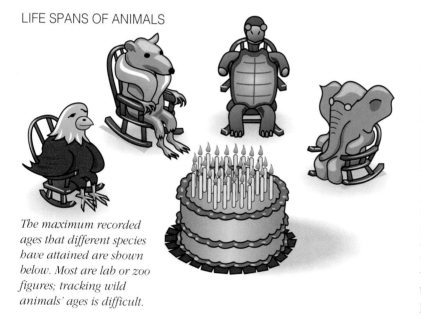

The maximum recorded ages that different species have attained are shown below. Most are lab or zoo figures; tracking wild animals' ages is difficult.

Species	Years
Shrew	2
Mouse	3
Rat	5
Skunk	13
Dog	20
Dolphin	23
Cat	30
Toad	36

Species	Years
Horse	46
Gorilla	55
Snapping turtle	58
Eagle owl	68
Elephant	70
Human	120
Galapagos turtle	150

THE NEW CENTENARIANS—A GROWING AND LIVELY GROUP

The fastest-growing group of Americans today is not the baby boomers or even the children of the baby boomers; it is the men and women who have reached their 100th birthday and beyond. The odds against living to be 100 years old in the United States have dropped from 400 to 1 in the late 19th century to 87 to 1 for children born in 1980.

The United States Census Bureau estimated there were 50,000 people 100 years old or older in 1994—more than twice the number in 1980 —and it projects there could be 1 million by 2040 if population growth and life expectancy rates continue in a predicted pattern.

According to the National Institute of Aging, women over 100 years of age outnumber men 2 to 1. About half live alone or with family members, more than half have an elementary school education or less, and three quarters were born in the United States.

Studies of centenarians are just beginning in earnest. So far, interviews suggest that most have an upbeat attitude and have had a close relationship with a spouse, a child, or a care-giver. Many have spent their lives helping others.

Centenarians themselves give various reasons for their longevity. A 100-year-old man who believes that you begin to lose your health when you get too lazy works out on a rowing machine, a stationary bicycle, and a stair machine every day. At 109, the matriarch of seven generations says that cigarettes and liquor never touched her lips and believes in hard work (she hurt her leg while chopping wood when she was 99). Another centenarian, however, broke a pledge made near the turn of the century to give up smoking (he was age 10 at the time) and now enjoys an occasional pipe.

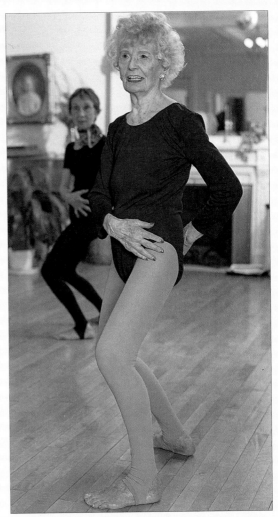

At age 100, Claire Willi donned a leotard and tights for a daily dance class. In an interview at the time, she claimed that regular exercise kept her energetic and able to look her best in the fashionable clothes she still enjoyed wearing.

more than 40 percent. In the late 1960's, the connection between a high-fat diet, a sedentary lifestyle, and heart disease was firmly established, and an association between a high-fat diet and certain types of cancer was convincingly made by medical researchers. Since then, butter consumption in the United States has dropped more than a third, the use of animal fats and oils has fallen by 40 percent, and more than 30 million health-minded citizens claim to practice regular aerobic exercise.

The changes in living habits that these statistics suggest may explain why so many Americans are living longer, healthier, more active lives. How they do it is the subject of this book.

How You Get Older— And Wiser

*R*ecent research shows that aging can no longer be regarded as an inevitable decline—and that how well you age and how long you live can depend not only on your genes and gender but also on your attitude and lifestyle.

THE DIFFERENT TYPES OF AGING

Because gerontologists regard the aging process as highly variable, they distinguish between three types of aging: chronological, biological, and psychosocial. Chronological aging is estimated in calendar years, with the arrival at old age usually set arbitrarily at 65. Measured by other criteria, however, you may literally be "as old as you feel."

Whether or not your chronological age matches your biological age depends on how well your body continues to function as the years go by. Some healthy individuals are frail in their fifties, while others are still chopping wood in their eighties. Although biological aging is genetically determined, studies show that you can slow it down by adopting a healthy lifestyle that includes a balanced diet, regular exercise, and stress reduction.

Psychosocial aging relates to mental alertness and sociability. A 70-year-old widow who belongs to a book discussion group, participates in community activities, has a part-time job, mall-walks with a group for exercise, and regularly visits with family members and friends is considered psychosocially young. The same widow would be labeled psychosocially old if, even though in good health, she had no interests and seldom left her house or saw family or friends. Because attitude can directly affect health, sometimes being psychosocially old can make a person physiologically old.

Exercising your brain is just as important to your well-being as exercising your body.

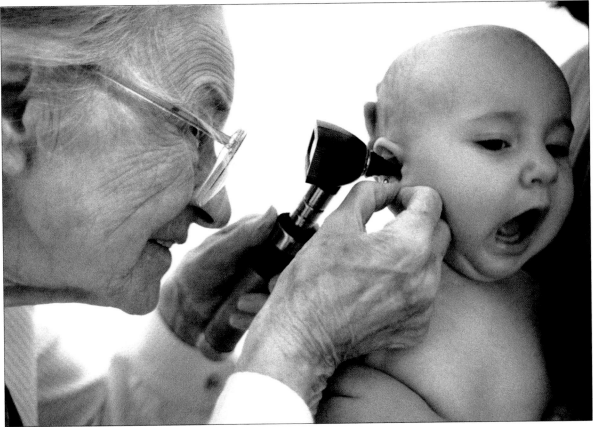

Ninety-one-year-old Dr. Leila Denmark treats a much younger patient in her Alpharetta, Georgia, office. According to Denmark, "If you love what you're doing, it's not work." She intends to continue practicing medicine "as long as I'm able."

NORMAL BODY CHANGES

As a result of studying the normal processes of aging, researchers are now able to differentiate between age-related changes that are preventable or reversible and those that are generally inevitable. No matter which category they fall into, however, it is helpful to know what to expect.

The cardiovascular system

The heart can support the regular activity of a healthy person all through life. While maximum heart rate slows with age, the heart of a healthy 80-year-old performs as well at rest as that of a 20-year-old. During exercise, the heart compensates for its slower rate by increasing the volume of blood pumped out with each beat.

Over time, the lining of the heart and its valves thicken, and the blood vessels both thicken and lose elasticity. In the absence of cardiovascular disease, however, this condition has virtually no consequences.

The digestive system

Compared with other body systems, the digestive system undergoes fewer changes over the years. Digestion generally takes longer because slight losses in muscle tone result in fewer of the contractions that move food through your alimentary canal.

The decrease in your digestive enzymes is usually minimal, although certain nutrients may not be fully absorbed. In addition, the functioning of some digestive organs slows down. The gallbladder, for example, stores less bile for the small intestine to use during the digestive process, and the liver takes longer to metabolize drugs and alcohol, thereby making these substances affect you more strongly than when you were younger.

The endocrine system

The body's precious hormone-producing glands, which regulate so many essential body functions, remain relatively intact throughout life. The output of the thyroid, adrenal gland, pituitary gland, and pancreas stays basically the same, but the production of sex hormones, especially estrogen in women, declines.

The immune system

The thymus, the coordinator of the immune system's fighter T-cells, gradually shrinks, causing a reduction in the number and functioning of T-cells, a vital component of the immune system. But while the result is an increase in autoantibodies, there is no age-related increase in autoimmune disease.

The musculoskeletal system

Although older people have less bone mass, they can counteract the harmful effects of this by developing as much of it as possible before the time loss usually begins and by maintaining and increasing current bone mass.

Because calcium helps to build bone mass, experts suggest a daily intake of 1,000 milligrams for adults and 1,500 milligrams for postmenopausal women. Hormone replacement therapy to prevent bone loss in women after menopause is also often recommended (see p.239).

Walking, running, and other weight-bearing exercises can make your bones denser as well as help improve the body's absorption of calcium. Similarly, although the body's gradual loss of muscle and nerve fibers leads to a decline in muscle mass and

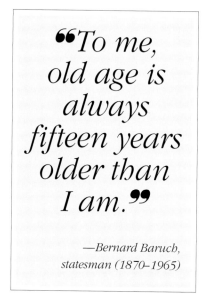

"To me, old age is always fifteen years older than I am."

—*Bernard Baruch, statesman (1870–1965)*

strength, you can build muscle mass and strength with exercise. Some experts suggest that doing so may be the best single strategy for a longer, healthier life.

The nervous system

The brain starts to lose neurons after about the age of 30. By age 80, the brain weighs roughly 7 percent less than it did at age 25. But because of the huge reserve capacity you are born with, this loss seldom makes any difference in your brain power (see *The Aging Brain*, p.18). Your reaction time, however, slows down because of the loss of neurons and the decrease in the connections between them.

The reproductive system

Changes in sexual function begin in middle age and tend to be very gradual. None of them necessarily lessen the ability to have a satisfying sex life.

As long as they remain sexually active, healthy older men continue to produce sex hormones and sperm at levels similar to

those of younger men. The prostate, however, usually enlarges, and as a result, it may press against the urethra, making urination difficult.

For the majority of older women, aging appears to have little or no effect on their sexual pleasure. The two most common symptoms of menopause, hot flashes and vaginal atrophy, vary in severity, with many women experiencing neither.

The respiratory system

The lungs, like the heart, are fully capable of supporting the normal activity of a healthy individual well into old age. Because the lungs, chest wall, and diaphragm of an older person are less elastic, however, the lungs may not be able to inflate or deflate completely or take in as much oxygen as the lungs of a younger person. Coughing, which clears mucus from the lungs, may also become less efficient.

The senses

All five senses lose some of their acuity over the years. The lens of the eye, for example, grows more rigid and is less able to shift its focus from distant to near viewing, requiring most older people to use reading glasses. Cataracts —the clouding of the eye lens that obscures vision—may be preventable. Recent research links some cataracts to smoking and sun exposure.

Your high-frequency hearing may begin to deteriorate in your twenties, but the change is not usually noticeable until your sixties, when low-frequency hearing may also begin to decline. Some hearing loss can also be caused by exposure to ear-splitting sounds such as very loud music, sirens, and jackhammers.

THE BALTIMORE LONGITUDINAL STUDY OF AGING

America's longest-running investigation into the causes and effects of human aging, the Baltimore Longitudinal Study of Aging, began in 1958 with more than 1,000 healthy volunteers.

Every 1 or 2 years, these men and women—currently ranging in age from 20 to over 90—undergo a series of tests in which researchers attempt to determine the effect of basic biological, mental, emotional, behavioral, and environmental factors on aging.

Because longitudinal studies look at the same group of people over a span of many years, they can provide a great deal more valuable information than other kinds of studies. This has certainly been the case with the Baltimore study, which has shattered many myths about aging.

One such myth is that all of a person's mind and body functions deteriorate automatically as the years go by. The actual changes caused by aging, it turns out, are slight and almost negligible as long as a person is not suffering from a major stress or disease. The reason for this is that you are born with a tremendous reserve capacity for withstanding stress or illness. Starting at age 30, you lose only about 10 percent of this reserve per decade.

Moreover, also contrary to earlier thinking, aging is not a disease. Older people are susceptible to certain illnesses, but none of these develop simply because the person has lived longer. Nor is there one inevitable pattern of aging. People age in different and highly individual ways. As a result, doctors now realize that unusual changes in an older person's physical or mental state are more apt to be caused by disease than by getting older.

The Baltimore study has also altered age norms for certain laboratory tests. For instance, the standard formerly used to measure blood sugar levels in diagnosing diabetes has been shown to be too low for anyone past middle age. Another significant finding is that most older people need lower drug doses than younger people do.

To date, the results of the Baltimore study have demonstrated that growing older is a natural and partly predictable process. This has led to a more positive attitude—and even optimism—about the aging process.

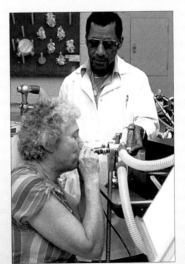

A participant in the Baltimore Longitudinal Study of Aging undergoes a pulmonary function test to measure the volume of air she is able to inhale and exhale.

THE AGING BRAIN

"Use it or lose it" applies as much to the brain as it does to the rest of the body. Just as exercise can maintain your physical strength and flexibility well into old age, so too can challenging your brain keep your memory and intelligence at high levels.

Although the brain shrinks over time and loses neurons, for the most part such changes have little effect on mental functioning. New studies show that the brain adapts to the loss of neurons by developing new dendrites, or con-nections between neurons, which are the most important factors in your ability to think and re-member. And although most people get some-what forgetful, especially when it comes to remembering new names, phone numbers, or recent events, this "benign senescent forgetful-ness" is a minor annoyance that neither pro-gresses nor interferes with normal functioning.

Changes do occur, however, in your two types of intelligence, fluid and crystallized. Fluid intelligence involves problem solving that re-quires abstract, nonverbal mental agility and a facility for swiftly assessing new situations and refiguring old ones. After peaking in early adult-hood, fluid intelligence begins to decline. An air traffic controller and a tennis player will both find that their ability to make split-second deci-sions diminishes as they get older.

Crystallized intelligence, which comprises verbal and mathematical skills and the use of accumulated knowledge, improves throughout life. For example, although a 25-year-old lawyer can usually reason more quickly than his 65-year-old colleague, it's a good bet that the vet-eran will win more cases. The younger lawyer may think faster; the older one has learned to think better.

Researchers now believe that exercising the brain stimulates it to function at its peak. In-creasing input to the brain has been shown to spur development of new dendrites. The best mental workouts provide variety, problem solv-ing, and social interaction. Get your infor-mation from several sources. If you usually read fiction, try a biography. Lis-ten to a different type of music—jazz instead of classical, for instance. Learn new skills such as ballroom dancing or a language. Examine other viewpoints—a stimulating debate may en-able you see your own views in a new light.

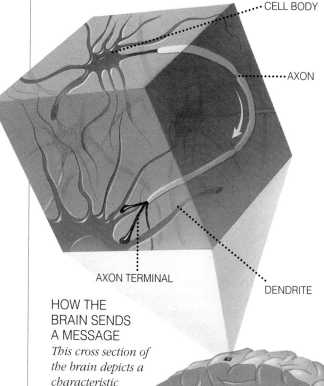

CELL BODY

AXON

AXON TERMINAL

DENDRITE

HOW THE BRAIN SENDS A MESSAGE

This cross section of the brain depicts a characteristic neuron, or nerve cell, firing a sig-nal through its axon. The signal is received by the other neuron's dendrites and sent to its cell body.

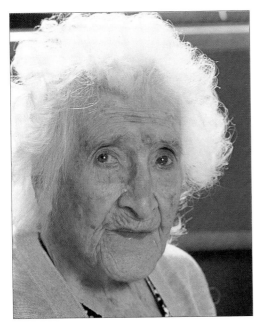
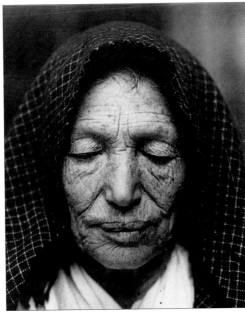

Differences in the aging of the skin: Far left, 117-year-old Jeanne Calment, in Arles, France, in 1992. Near left, a 40-year-old woman in a Chicago settlement house, about 1910.

The skin

Many wrinkles and dark spots on older skin are produced by photo-aging (sun exposure), not by the normal aging process. But normal aging does take a toll: the epidermis, the skin's top layer, becomes drier, thinner, and looser; the dermis, the second layer, grows thinner and less elastic; and the third, the subcutaneous layer, loses much of its fat. The result is that the skin begins to sag and wrinkle.

The urinary system

Although the kidneys can effectively regulate fluid volume and eliminate waste all through life, they lose some of their efficiency over the years. Blood flow to the kidneys lessens, and the number of nephrons, the kidneys' filtering units, diminishes. As a result, the kidneys need more water to excrete the same amount of urinary waste. Concurrently, the bladder's capacity is also reduced, necessitating more frequent trips to the bathroom.

DIFFERENCES IN HOW MEN AND WOMEN AGE

Men and women age similarly in most ways, but some significant differences exist. Older men are more likely to develop short-term fatal illnesses; older women, to suffer from chronic conditions. Heart disease strikes women an average of 10 to 15 years later than it does men, and men have a somewhat higher incidence of cancer. But bone fractures are more of a problem for older women; they have four times as many broken bones as men do.

The major difference between men and women, however, is in life expectancy. On average, women live about 7 years longer than men—a gap that in recent years appears to be narrowing. Experts have come up with several theories to explain why women enjoy such superior longevity:

■ *Behavior.* Men are socialized to be more active and aggressive than women, perhaps the reason they have much higher accident, murder, and suicide rates.

■ *Hormones.* At puberty, testosterone lowers the level of high-density lipoproteins (HDL's), the "good" cholesterol that helps protect against heart disease. Estrogen, on the other hand, safeguards most women from heart disease until menopause.

■ *Sex chromosomes.* Males have nonmatching X and Y chromosomes; females, two matching X chromosomes. If there is an abnormality on one X chromosome, the female has a second one that may have no abnormality; the male does not. Nor does he have a backup in case of an abnormality on his Y chromosome.

■ *Work-related stress,* possibly leading to heart disease and other disorders. Heretofore, stress has been blamed for early heart disease in men, but recent studies indicate that chronic feelings of hostility and anger may be more harmful than simple stress.

Alas, all these plausible theories have been debunked. No one

LATE-LIFE ACHIEVERS

It's never too late to embark on a new project or to develop an old interest. Many people continue to learn, to work, and to make substantial achievements even when they are no longer in what is generally considered to be the "prime of life." Indeed, when it comes to accomplishments, many people actually grow better as they grow older.

GEORGE BURNS

(1896–). Burns and his wife, Gracie Allen, were one of America's most popular comedy teams. After Allen's death in 1964, Burns carried on alone.

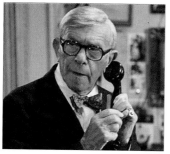

In 1976, he won an Academy Award for his first dramatic film role in *The Sunshine Boys*. Since then, he has appeared in other movies and on television specials and has written several books of humor and reminiscence, as well as a memoir of his wife.

GEORGE WASHINGTON CARVER

(c. 1861–1943). An internationally renowned agricultural chemist, Carver was born a slave. As director of the department of agriculture at Tuskegee Institute, a position he held until his death, Carver taught farmers crop diversification so that they could restore their cotton-exhausted soil. His research on peanuts, sweet potatoes, and soybeans resulted in hundreds of new by-products.

BENJAMIN FRANKLIN

(1706–1790). One of America's founding fathers, Franklin was the author and publisher of *Poor Richard's Almanac*, helped to draft the Declaration of Independence, proved that lightning was made of electricity, and invented bifocals. During the Revolutionary War, Franklin, then in his seventies, served as ambassador to France. At the age of 81, he helped to draft the Constitution.

MARTHA GRAHAM

(1894–1991). A major American choreographer and dancer, Graham was a pioneer of modern

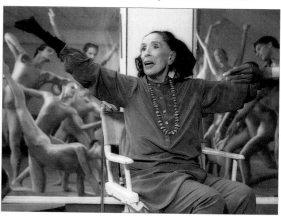

knows why women live longer than men. What is known, however, is that both men and women who refrain from smoking, drink moderately, exercise to stay in good physical condition, and maintain a desirable weight (see pp.60–61) are more likely to be fully functional and living better as they grow older.

WOMEN'S HEALTH IN THE LATER YEARS

Today women can expect to live about one-third of their lives after menopause. With its onset, however, the natural reduction in the female hormones estrogen and progesterone can cause such problems as accelerated bone loss; increased risk of heart disease and breast cancer; and discomforts that include urinary incontinence, hot flashes, and vaginal atrophy (see pp.238–239).

Scientists have only recently begun studying the unique health problems of women. The Baltimore Longitudinal Study of Aging

dance. Although her introduction of emotionally expressive, often abrupt movements at first shocked audiences, Graham's work gradually won acclaim. She continued to dance into her mid-seventies and to choreograph until shortly before her death.

OLIVER WENDELL HOLMES, JR.

(1841–1935). Appointed to the Supreme Court in 1902, Holmes greatly influenced the administration of law in the United States. Called the Great Dissenter because he disagreed with so many court edicts, Holmes persuaded his fellow judges to set aside personal opinions when making decisions, a doctrine known as judicial restraint, which now dominates American judicial policy. At the age of 91, Holmes retired from the court.

GRANDMA (ANNA MARY) MOSES

(1860–1961). During her seventies, when arthritis made embroidery too difficult for her, Moses took up painting. Although she never had a lesson, her colorful scenes of rural life brought her enormous popularity and success. When she was 79, Moses participated in a show at New York's Museum of Modern Art; the next year she had her first solo show. In the last year of her life, she painted 25 pictures.

BARBARA MCCLINTOCK

(1902–1992). A geneticist whose pioneering work was originally dismissed by her colleagues, McClintock won the 1983 Nobel Prize for that work at the age of 81. The first scientist to recognize that genes could affect heredity by shifting their positions on chromosomes, McClintock presented her then-radical discovery in 1951, but her achievement was not recognized for more than 30 years. McClintock continued her research into her late eighties, working 6 days a week.

PABLO PICASSO

(1881–1973). The Spanish painter, sculptor, and graphic artist Picasso is widely considered to be the foremost figure in 20th-century art. He continued to change and experiment throughout his life. Picasso's originality and the volume of his output were so extensive that experts generally divide his work into different periods—as though he had been not one but several major artists. A few days before his death at the age of 91, Picasso was still at work, making a selection of his recent paintings for an upcoming exhibition.

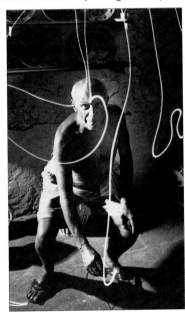

(p.17), for example, did not include women until 1978; and until recently, major research studies on heart disease have generally excluded women. Although women react differently than men to many medications because of variations in their metabolism, drugs have been tested mainly on men.

In the early 1990's, the National Institutes of Health (NIH) embarked on an ambitious 15-year study, the Women's Health Initiative, the single largest research project ever launched by the NIH. Involving more than 160,000 postmenopausal women, the study is investigating the effectiveness of hormone-replacement therapy, dietary changes, and vitamin supplements in combating depression, heart disease, stroke, cancer, and osteoporosis. Such studies are sorely needed. Older women are less likely than older men to enjoy good mental and physical health, and three times more likely to live in nursing homes.

THE AGING PROCESS UNDER A MICROSCOPE

· ·

*I*n the lab as well as in the doctor's office, research has generated many theories about how and why humans age. All have a sound scientific basis, but none are definitive. Most experts agree that no single theory will ever explain all the complexities of aging. *The answers will almost certainly combine current insights with still-undiscovered dynamics.*

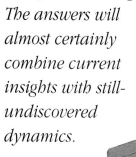

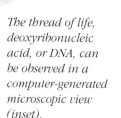

The thread of life, deoxyribonucleic acid, or DNA, can be observed in a computer-generated microscopic view (inset).

THE GOALS OF GERONTOLOGIC STUDY

Research into aging is not just an effort to extend the limits of the human life span; it also helps doctors to better understand and fight the diseases and disabilities associated with old age. Doctors often talk about the human "health span" rather than life span. Their interest is to make the later years as vital, rich, active, productive, and independent as possible, not just longer. Whatever the ultimate interplay of the various lines of research, study of the aging process is helping doctors treat patients now.

· ·

CURRENT THEORIES ABOUT AGING

Ideas about why and how people age generally fit into two broad categories: the clock theories and the damage theories. The clock theories suggest that humans carry preset timers within their genetic makeup, or DNA (deoxyribonucleic acid), and that their aging follows this biological timetable. The damage theories propose that the human body, like an old automobile, simply wears out, bit by bit, after decades of use and exposure to the elements. Each theory represents one tiny piece in a very large puzzle that no one yet sees as a whole.

MITOSIS: THE REGENERATION OF CELLS

Your body continually replaces dead or damaged cells with new ones that are created by the process of mitosis, or cell division, shown below. Some gerontologists think that each cell is capable of only a limited number of divisions, which may partly explain how people age. Others believe that aging cells begin to make mistakes in mitosis.

__1.__ Before cell division begins, the strands of the DNA double helix, which make up the chromosomes, duplicate themselves; the strands then condense into a more compact form to avoid getting tangled.

__6.__ The cell separates into two new cells, which will each mature and undergo its own mitosis.

__5.__ A nuclear envelope forms around each set of 46 chromosomes; the DNA strands begin to uncoil.

__2.__ Coiled into rods and joined at the middle, the chromosomes appear as X's.

__4.__ The chromosomes divide and are drawn to opposite sides of the cell by protein threads called the mitotic spindle.

__3.__ The chromosomes line up in the center of the cell.

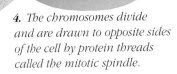

Cellular limits

Most of the body's cells are able to divide, or reproduce, only a limited number of times. After that, they either stop dividing or, when they do divide, start making defective copies of themselves that can lead to cancer-causing mutations. In addition, the older the cell, the greater the chance that it will make irreparable mistakes in reproduction.

This cellular phenomenon, called the Hayflick limit after the researcher who first described it, has been seen in human fibroblasts (the cells of connective tissue), which stop dividing after about 50 times. Fibroblasts taken from a 75-year-old person show fewer cell divisions remaining than do fibroblasts taken from a child. The longer a species' life span, the higher its Hayflick limit. Human fibroblasts, for example, have much higher Hayflick limits than do similar cells in mice. Gerontologists are now investigating the links between this cell slowdown and human aging.

Other clues to aging have been found in the tips of chromosomes, which are long genetic chains called telomeres. These structures are now known to be important in every stage of a cell's life, protecting the chromosome against damage, helping to maintain its proper position, and perhaps in some undiscovered way setting an internal clock to determine the cell's life span.

Some scientists speculate that you have a built-in genetic program that activates cells according to a predetermined schedule. The body's internal clock automatically senses when it is time to grow (during childhood and adolescence), when it is time for cells to be replaced at a normal pace (young adulthood through middle age), and when it is time to slow down (old age).

This theory may partly explain why the overall physical changes related to aging occur at different rates in different people. At the same time, people within the

THE POSSIBILITY OF A LONGEVITY GENE

Experiments with fruit flies have pointed to what may be longevity genes. Dr. Robert Arking of Wayne State University in Detroit recently completed a comparative study of two types of fruit flies, one significantly longer-lived than the other. By meticulously deleting various chromosomes from the type that lived longer, Arking was able to zero in on the location of the genes responsible for longevity—genes that were not present in the shorter-lived fruit flies.

In related research, other investigators have identified a gene that produces a powerful antioxidant called superoxide dismutase, or SOD. (Antioxidants disarm the destructive free radicals your body creates when your cells metabolize, or burn, oxygen.) Longer-lived fruit flies were found to have a more active gene than shorter-lived flies, raising the possibility that antioxidants such as SOD are a key to longevity.

Other fruit fly research has identified seven proteins that are present in much higher concentrations in the long-lived flies. These proteins may lead researchers to the specific genes that cause these flies to live longer.

Human beings are far more complex than fruit flies, but scientists believe that the insects' aging dynamics may have human counterparts.

OTHER LAB DISCOVERIES

Yeast cells have also been the subject of research into the genes linked to aging. So far, a total of 14 aging-related genes have been found. Each acts in a different way and changes its function over the course of the yeast's life span. Scientists have been able to extend a yeast cell's life by regulating one of the genes, called LAG-1. Activation of this particular gene stimulated yeast cells to reproduce many times beyond their normal limit.

In a similar way, other types of genes may limit life span. One such "death gene" has been found in roundworms; left alone, it somehow signals the worm to die at 3 weeks of age. When scientists tamper with the gene, creating a mutant version of it, the worm's life span is doubled. There is some evidence that the mutant gene created by the scientists extends life by stimulating the production of the antioxidants superoxide dismutase and catalase.

Acknowledging the difficulties, scientists are probing for principles of cell life that may also apply to human cells.

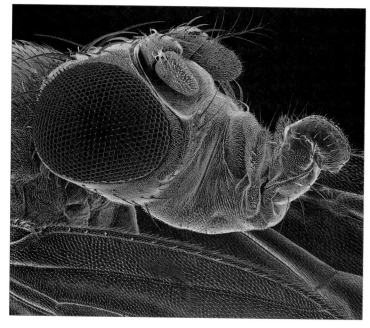

A Mediterranean fruit fly, shown 100 times its actual size, may unlock the secrets of the genes that control aging in flies and perhaps even in humans.

same family are much more likely to develop similar overall patterns of aging and susceptibility to certain diseases.

Hormonal clocks

The influence of hormones on your body's actions, development, and growth, as well as your emotions, thought processes, and appearance, is well documented if not entirely understood. There is now speculation that hormones may influence aging as well.

In women, for example, the hormone estrogen seems to help protect against atherosclerosis and osteoporosis before menopause. After the menstrual cycle stops, however, there is a marked reduction in estrogen levels. A low estrogen count is associated with an increased risk of both conditions.

Dr. Daniel Rudman's experiments that use human growth hormone to reverse some signs of aging (pp.26–27) are based on the fact that the body begins to reduce its production of this important hormone after age 30.

Immune system slowdown

A person's immunity is strongest during the early thirties. After young adulthood, marshaling your defenses against infections takes longer. In the later years, the immune system becomes impaired as a result of aging, less active T-cells. As a result, older people become more susceptible to common infections that earlier would not have threatened them. The immune system also appears to fight cancers in a younger person more successfully than in an older person. Thus, researchers theorize that cancers become more common with advancing age because the immune system may become less responsive.

Profile

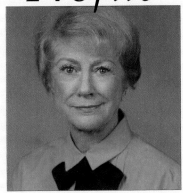

HELEN BOLEY:
A CASE OF GOOD GENES

In 1989, Helen Boley accompanied her husband to a free cholesterol screening at the University of Kansas Medical Center. While there, she decided to have the test too. Her cholesterol readings so astonished the lab technicians that they took another blood sample. The second test showed the same results: Mrs. Boley's level of high-density lipoproteins, or HDL's (the "good" cholesterol), was five times the normal reading and the highest level ever recorded. Her low-density lipoprotein, or LDL ("bad" cholesterol), level was ideal.

A sample of Mrs. Boley's blood was sent to the National Heart, Lung and Blood Institute, which studies the link between genetics and cholesterol. Researchers found that she not only had inherited a copy of a gene that leads to excessive production of HDL's from her mother but also had received another copy from her father. Called the Methuselah gene, it may be a key to increasing HDL levels in people at risk for heart disease.

Mrs. Boley's relatives routinely live into their nineties, and some, 100 years or more. She hopes that study of the gene that gives her "squeaky clean arteries" can help others live longer, healthier lives.

STUDYING THE POSSIBILITY OF LIFE EXTENSION

· ·

The dream of youth restored is slowly moving from science fiction to science fact. While there is still more that is unknown than known, many scientists no longer dismiss out of hand the possibility that there may be ways to turn the clock back—or at least off—for extended periods.

HUMAN GROWTH HORMONE

Some of the most interesting scientific research involves human growth hormone, a potent product of the pituitary gland that helps heal wounds and build bones and muscles. After about the age of 60, the pituitary gland in some people drastically slows its production of this vitality-sustaining hormone, and the body begins to age more noticeably.

In 1990, Dr. Daniel Rudman, a Wisconsin endocrinologist, speculated that it might be possible to reverse some of the signs of aging in such people by restoring their youthful levels of human growth hormone. In a 6-month experiment, 21 men in their sixties and

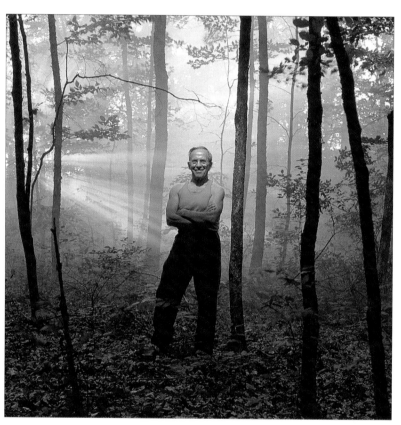

In a test to reverse symptoms of aging, Jere Gottschalk (above) injected himself with hormones three times a week for 6 months. During the experiment, he gained muscle mass, lost fat, and his skin thickened.

seventies who had low levels of growth hormone were divided into two groups. One group injected themselves three times a week with a synthetic version of the hormone in an amount equal to that produced by the pituitary gland of a healthy young man. (The dose was carefully set to natural limits because high doses can actually hasten the aging process by enlarging the heart and causing hypertension and arthritis.) Members of the control group were not given the hormone and just came in for monthly checkups.

The results were dramatic. Although all the men in the control group had lost muscle, bone, and organ mass, the opposite was true for those treated with human growth hormone. These men had regained substantial amounts of muscle mass and lost significant amounts of body fat. Their skin had become thicker and firmer, and their livers and spleens had regained mass.

The treatment essentially reversed body changes that had occurred over 10 to 20 years of aging. When the experiment ended, however, the men who had received the hormone reverted to their former condition. Researchers are now studying whether the effects of the treatment can be sustained over longer periods without serious side effects.

Because low levels of growth hormone in the elderly may not be as common as Dr. Rudman thought, some doctors feel that this therapy will have limited applicability among older people.

. . . .

CALORIC RESTRICTION

Another approach to life extension involves extreme calorie cutting. In a number of studies, researchers have found that animals fed diets containing 40 percent fewer calories but maintaining healthful levels of vitamins, minerals, and other nutrients live up to 50 percent longer than animals on typical laboratory diets. The animals on restricted diets develop such age-related illnesses as heart disease, cancer, cataracts, and kidney failure much less frequently and much later in their lives than the animals in the control group.

Early calorie-cutting research involved rodents, fish, flies, fleas, and protozoa. Following up on the encouraging results, the federal government is now supporting similar experiments with primates. One hundred fifty mon-

keys, half being fed a normal diet and half getting 30 percent fewer calories, will be monitored for age-related behavioral, physiological, and biochemical changes. Although it is still too soon to see any differences in aging between the two groups, those on the restricted diets have already shown delays in the onset of puberty similar to the delays observed in earlier experiments with mice.

Moreover, the leaner monkeys appear to be in excellent health.

Dr. Roy L. Walford, one of the pioneers in calorie-restricting research, says that he has been on such a diet himself since 1987. His life-extension theories center on gradual weight loss until you reach a target weight that is 10 to 25 percent below your individual "set point," the amount that you weigh when you eat a normal

DIET FOR LONGEVITY

In a 1978 study of the Japanese diet and the extraordinary incidence of centenarians on the island of Okinawa, a comparison was made between an average adult Okinawan's diet and the diet of other Japanese adults. The results, shown in part below, may help to explain the longevity of the tiny, physically active Okinawans. The study also revealed that Okinawan school-age youngsters ate a healthy but even more meager 62 percent of what other Japanese children ate—about 1,300 calories a day.

Diet Component	Percent of the Average Japanese Diet That an Okinawan Consumes
Cereals	76.2
Sugars	26.5
Green and yellow vegetables	309.6
Meats	203.3
Calories	83.4
Protein	91.3

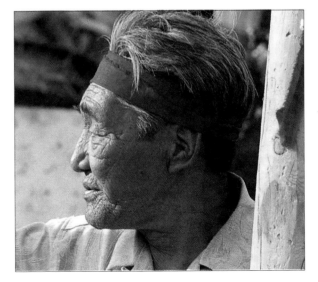

The elderly Okinawan at left is a better candidate for living to age 100 than most Japanese men.

FAST FACTS

■ Older adults can learn some types of new skills as easily as younger adults. Trouble arises when they are asked to perform two tasks at once or to process visual information too fast. If one task is learned fully before the second is added or if visual cues such as diagrams are used as a guide to learning, the difficulties are overcome.

■ Housework—along with cycling and running—was listed by men in the Baltimore Longitudinal Study (see p.17) as one of the physical activities they had significantly increased since 1970.

■ Orchestra conductors tend to lead long lives. Arturo Toscanini died at age 90, for example, and Leopold Stokowski at age 95. Researchers link the maestros' longevity to their sense of being in control of their lives and the enjoyment of their work.

■ Left-handed people, despite several well-publicized but flawed studies to the contrary, do not die younger than right-handed people. The prestigious and long-running Framingham Heart Study as well as several government surveys found no differences in mortality.

diet. The restricted diet should be fortified with vitamins and minerals, generally at officially recommended levels, he says.

If consistent calorie cutting to recommended levels were started by early adulthood, Walford estimates that the human life span could be extended to about 140 years; he thinks that less restricted diets might be able to add several years to the normal life span.

As evidence of the theory at work, Walford cites a study of the people of Okinawa, Japan. Beginning in childhood, Okinawans were found to eat as little as 38 percent fewer calories than other Japanese (see p.27). Reliable statistics show that more than 5 times as many people in

Okinawa live to the age of 100 as in the area with the next-highest rate of centenarians in Japan. Okinawa has 40 times as many centenarians as some areas of Japan.

No one understands how the connection between calorie-restricted diets and life extension might work. Possible explanations are that dietary restriction in some way protects DNA from damage, facilitates the repair of previously damaged DNA, or reduces the activity of genes that can cause cancer. Another possibility is that calorie restriction may enhance the performance of certain protective genes that, like antioxidants, help inactivate free radicals, the destructive molecules that can damage cells.

A NEW EMPHASIS ON ANTIOXIDANTS

Many scientists believe that antioxidant vitamins scavenge for free radicals before they can cause cell damage. This potential for blocking free radicals makes some experts also believe that antioxidants can slow the aging process and help protect against disease (see *Diet and Disease,* pp.38–39).

The antioxidants include vitamins C and E and beta carotene, which is partially converted into vitamin A in the body. Although there is no conclusive evidence that antioxidants are beneficial, studies suggest that they may protect against the diseases of aging. Diets that provide ample antioxidants have been associated with lower rates of these diseases. Moreover, in epidemiological studies of large populations, the higher the antioxidant level in the diet, the lower the risk of disease.

Studies of diet and cancer, for example, suggest that people

with the lowest intake of beta carotene have a risk of lung cancer up to seven times greater than those with the highest intake.

How much of these antioxidant vitamins you should consume is uncertain. Doctors usually advocate that you stick to the Recommended Dietary Allowances (RDA's) of vitamins set by the National Academy of Sciences and get your vitamins from a varied diet. However, some experts contend that older people may need higher doses to get the potential benefits of disease prevention. But at lease one long-term study found that men who took vitamin A supplements actually had a somewhat higher incidence of lung cancer than those who did not. In any event, check with your doctor before taking any supplement that provides more than 100 percent of the RDA's (see *Why You Need Vitamins and Minerals,* pp. 52–55).

TALES OF LONGEVITY: FACT OR FALLACY?

History abounds with people alleged to have lived to extraordinary ages. Genesis says that the biblical patriarchs born before the flood lived as long as 969 years (Methuselah) and 950 years (Noah). After the flood, patriarchal life spans shortened considerably. Shem lived 600 years, but Isaac lived only 180 years.

In Greek mythology, the gods kept immortality for themselves; aging and death were human problems. The search for eternal youth is depicted in Roman mythology in the story of Jupiter transforming the nymph Juventas into a fountain of youth. Whoever bathed in her sweet-smelling waters became young and healthy. In the 16th century, Juan Ponce de León discovered Florida while looking for such a fountain in the New World.

Alchemists in the Middle Ages sought an elixir to ensure eternal youth. Quacks and charlatans later sold unproven youth potions made from fetal animal tissue or animal sexual organs. In more recent times, respected scientists have touted sour milk and yogurt as the keys to longevity after studying the diet of Bulgarian mountain people who claimed an uncommon number of supercentenarians—individuals well over 100 years of age—among their population.

VERIFYING EXTRAORDINARY AGES

Carbon-14 can date an artifact, but it can't determine the birth year of an elderly individual. Researchers who try to verify the ages of self-proclaimed supercentenarians depend on official birth and marriage certificates, church records, and diaries, but many claimants come from parts of the world where such records are relatively new. In the former Soviet Union, for example, 90 percent of the churches (and their records) were destroyed between 1922 and 1940, and internal passports, first issued in 1932, recorded whatever age a person stated at the time. One man reputed to be 130 in 1959 turned out to have deserted from the army during World War I and taken over his grandfather's identity papers. He was, in fact, only 78.

In such remote mountain Shangri-Las as the Hunza province in Pakistan and Vilcabamba, Ecuador, researchers found that ages above 70 were universally—and greatly—exaggerated. Despite low-fat diets, well-maintained physical fitness, and respect given to the opinions of the elderly in village affairs—all factors that contribute to active longevity—none of these fabled old people were actually centenarians.

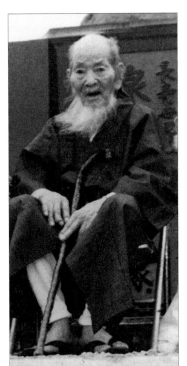

The confirmed longest-lived person in modern times was Shigechiyo Izumi, a Japanese man who died in 1986 at the age of 120 years 237 days.

WHAT YOU CAN DO TO LIVE LONGER—AND LIVE BETTER

*S*taying healthy not only helps to improve your longevity but also helps to ensure a better quality of life as you grow older. Good health, however, is no accident; there is a great deal that you can—and should—do to keep your body and mind functioning well.

MAINTAINING A HEALTHY BODY

The "secrets" of healthy living are neither mysterious nor difficult to understand—they're just a matter of common sense.

■ *Eat a well-balanced, varied diet.* One that contains more vegetables, fruits, and grains than meat and dairy products is best. Keep your intake of fat low, to protect against heart disease and cancer, and your intake of fiber high, to guard against colon cancer. To avoid hypertension, go easy on salt. In addition, women should take care to get enough daily calcium, either through diet or supplements, to help prevent osteoporosis. (See also *Dieting for Life*, pp.34–89.)

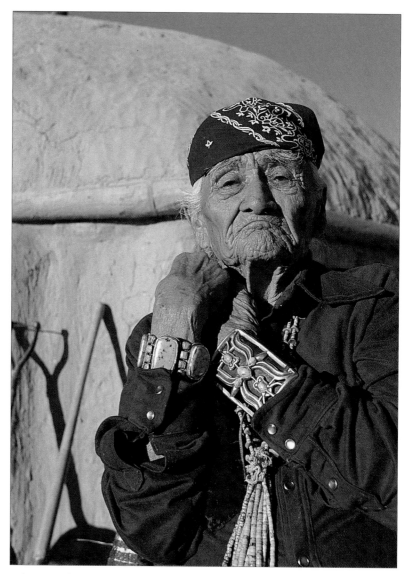

John Parrish, a 104-year-old medicine man in Monument Valley, Arizona, attributes his longevity to having run 3 miles a day until he was 84. "In the winter," says Parrish, "I would run through the snow with only my underwear on."

Exercise regularly. Experts recommend adopting a regimen of at least 20 minutes at a time three or more times a week. The easiest exercise, brisk walking, develops and maintains muscle tone, aids digestion, deepens respiration, enhances sleep, relieves depression, reduces stress, refreshes you mentally, and helps keep off excess weight. Other beneficial forms of exercise include swimming, bicycling, yoga, aerobics, and dancing. Before beginning a fitness program, however, make sure that you check with your doctor, and regardless of the exercise you choose, build up the intensity gradually to avoid injury. (See also *Shaping Up*, pp.90–137.)

Don't smoke. No matter how many years you've been smoking and how much you smoke, it's never too late to get the life-prolonging benefits of quitting. (See also *Smoking: How to Break a Bad Habit*, pp.242–245.)

Drink alcohol in moderation —if at all. Over time, drinking too much alcohol damages your nervous system, heart, and liver. If you do drink, even in moderation, hand over your car keys to someone else for the evening. (See also *The Role of Alcohol in a Healthy Diet*, pp.68–69; *Alcohol and Middle Age*, pp.196–199.)

Watch your weight. Extra pounds can compound many health problems and increase your chances of developing heart disease, diabetes, hernias, hemorrhoids, gallbladder disease, and varicose veins. The most effective way to lose weight is to eat a low-fat diet and combine it with a regular exercise program. (See also *Your Weight and Your Diet*, pp.60–65.)

Get enough sleep and rest. Although your sleeping patterns may change as you grow older— you may not sleep as long or as deeply as you did when you were younger, and you may wake up several times during the night— sufficient rest is still essential. Rest is important because it helps to relax your mind as well as your body. Stay away from sleeping pills or over-the-counter relaxants unless your doctor has specifically advised them for a particular— and usually temporary—reason. (See also *Getting a Good Night's Sleep*, pp.250–251.)

Be sure to have regular medical checkups. By doing so, you will ensure that any potential problems can be identified and treated as early as possible. You should also fill out *Your Family Medical History Tree* (see p.33) as completely as you can and then go over it with your physician to determine what your risk factors for various conditions are. Your doctor will decide what tests you should have regularly based on the current state of your health and your medical history. She may also advise you to make certain lifestyle changes. In addition, you should consider getting an annual influenza vaccination, especially if you are over the age of 65, as well as the one-time vaccination against pneumonia. (See also *Making the Most of Medical Tests*, pp.226–229.)

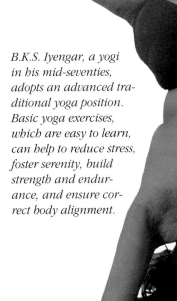

B.K.S. Iyengar, a yogi in his mid-seventies, adopts an advanced traditional yoga position. Basic yoga exercises, which are easy to learn, can help to reduce stress, foster serenity, build strength and endurance, and ensure correct body alignment.

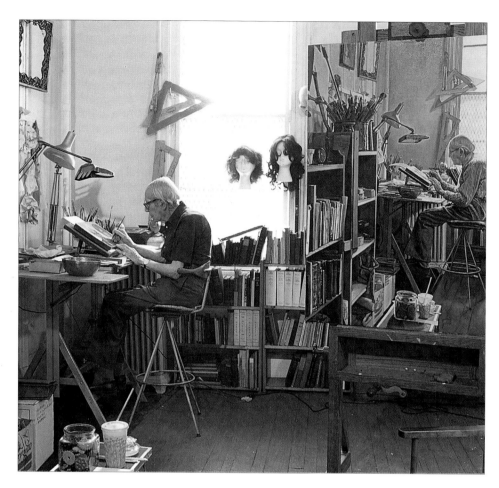

At the age of 89, John de Rosen, a Washington, D.C., artist, was still hard at work at his desk easel. Keeping him company was a mirror-image portrait of him painted by a fellow artist.

Some experts believe that many medical problems in older people are intensified or even initiated by an inactive lifestyle—and that exercising creativity and maintaining mental vitality help you to live longer. Research shows that older adults can learn new skills (such as painting) as readily as younger people can.

MAINTAINING A HEALTHY STATE OF MIND

Studies show that people who enjoy close personal relationships, have many interests, and stay in control of their lives tend to be healthier and to live longer.

■ *Nurture your ties with family and friends.* In addition, try to establish new relationships. It's a good idea to get involved with the younger generation too—arrange for special outings with your grandchildren, for example, or volunteer to help with community youth programs. Both generations will derive benefits.

■ *Become more active.* Take up a hobby, attend sporting events, go to concerts or to the movies. Investigate local organizations—for instance, amateur theatrical troupes, hiking clubs, bird-watching associations, or book discussion groups. If you have the time, consider returning to school, volunteering at a hospital, or participating in community programs.

■ *Preserve your independence.* Making your own decisions, even if you need to rely on others' expertise or physical assistance to carry them out, builds your confidence and self-esteem. Take responsibility for your financial affairs, but seek professional advice for questions about taxes, insurance, mortgages, retirement planning, charitable giving, managing assets, and making a will.

■ *Reduce stress.* Talk over a problem with friends or family members and then take action to resolve it. Keep in mind that there may be more than one solution to any dilemma and try to find ways to adjust to new situations. Maintaining your sense of humor helps put things in perspective. A regular exercise program, adequate rest, and using relaxation techniques may also be beneficial. (See also *Stress in the Middle Years,* pp.174–183.)

YOUR FAMILY MEDICAL HISTORY TREE

Fill out a family medical history tree form such as the one below; if possible, include the date at which any conditions were diagnosed as well as the date of any major surgery performed. Then discuss the information with your doctor to see what steps you should take—for example, periodic screenings or lifestyle changes—to reduce your risk.

BLOOD RELATIVES

	Parents	Grandparents	Brothers and Sisters	Uncles and Aunts	Self
Current Age or Date of Death and Age at Death					
Cause of Death					
Medical Problems					
Alcoholism					
Allergies					
Bone and Joint Problems					
Cancer					
Diabetes					
Eye Disorders					
Heart Disease					
Hypertension					
Mental Disorder					
Respiratory Problems					
Stroke					
Ulcers					
Other					

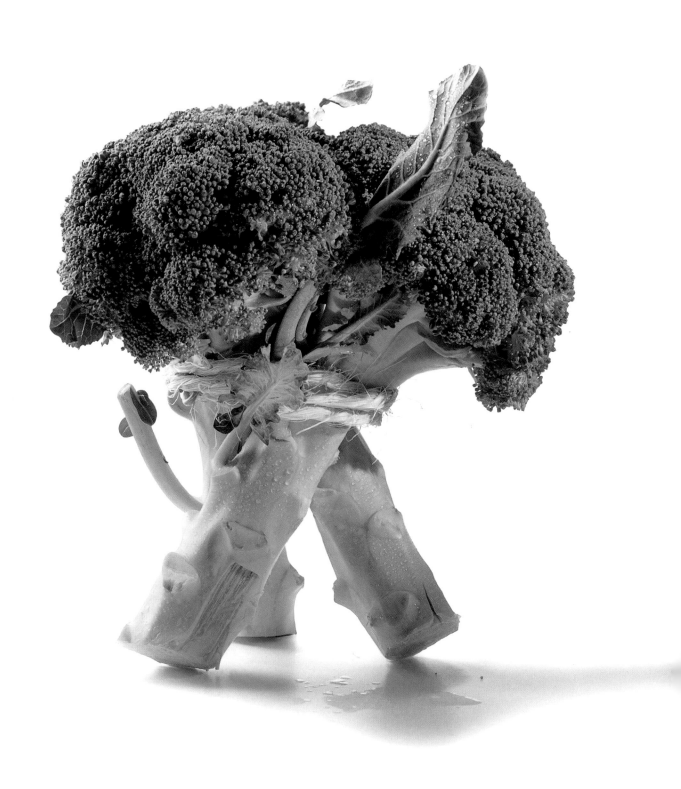

Chapter 2

EATING WELL

· ·

THE COMPONENTS OF A HEALTHY DIET *36*

DIET AND DISEASE *38*

KEEPING UP GOOD EATING HABITS *40*

PROTEIN: THE BODY'S BASIC BUILDING MATERIAL *42*

CARBOHYDRATES: THE ENERGY NUTRIENTS *44*

FAT: A LITTLE GOES A LONG WAY *48*

WHY YOU NEED VITAMINS AND MINERALS *52*

SODIUM: STRIKING A HEALTHY BALANCE *56*

CALCIUM: A KEY MINERAL *58*

YOUR WEIGHT AND YOUR DIET *60*

CAFFEINE: THE INVIGORATING TONIC *66*

THE ROLE OF ALCOHOL IN A HEALTHY DIET *68*

FOOD ADDITIVES: BOON OR MENACE? *70*

HOW FOOD CAN MAKE YOU SICK *74*

DECODING FOOD LABELS *76*

HOW TO BUY GOOD FOOD AND HANDLE IT WELL *78*

RECIPES FOR HEALTHY MEALS *80*

LEAN AND LUSCIOUS POULTRY *82*

HEARTY BASICS: RICE AND BEANS *84*

SAUCY LOW-FAT PASTAS *86*

MAIN COURSE VEGETABLE DISHES *88*

The Components
of a Healthy Diet

· ·

Food is a daily source of pleasure as well as nourishment. Picking a wholesome and savory diet from the extraordinary array of foods available at the typical American supermarket is challenging only because the choices are so broad.

EATING OUT THE HEALTHY WAY

▪ Select dishes that are steamed, baked, grilled, poached, or broiled rather than those that are pan-fried or sautéed.

▪ Request sauces or salad dressings "on the side" so that you can use them more sparingly.

▪ Order an appetizer rather than an entree to ensure a smaller serving. If a portion is too big, eat part of it and take the rest home.

▪ At a salad bar, choose leafy greens, raw vegetables, beans, and fruits. Avoid cheese, bacon bits, and creamy salads. Select a reduced-calorie dressing or oil and vinegar.

▪ In a fast food restaurant, choose a salad without dressing, a hamburger without sauce, a roast beef or grilled skinless unbreaded chicken sandwich, or a baked potato with a low-fat topping like yogurt.

THE FOOD GROUPS

Nutritionists have defined five food groups to help the public choose a healthy diet: grains, vegetables, fruits, dairy products, and meat, fish, poultry, legumes, and nuts. The pyramid shown on the facing page is the United States Department of Agriculture's visual aid to good nutrition.

Experts agree that you should eat a variety from each of the food groups every day rather than rely on a few fortified foods. Your body requires more than 40 different nutrients; only a variety of foods can meet all those needs.

· ·

LIMITING CHOLESTEROL

Most nutritionists agree that you should consume fewer than 300 milligrams a day of cholesterol (p.50). Since dietary cholesterol is found only in animal products, you can achieve this by cutting down on meat, egg yolks, and high-fat dairy products. These foods are also high in saturated fat, which is an even greater contributor to high blood cholesterol levels than dietary cholesterol.

You don't have to give up meat altogether, but you should select lean cuts without extra fat, use a low-fat method of cooking, and reduce the size of your portions (see the photos on pages 42–43). A little lean meat provides plenty of protein, as well as vital vitamins and minerals.

Design your meals around meat substitutes such as legumes (dried beans and peas) and low-fat or nonfat dairy products (milk, yogurt, and cheeses).

· ·

CUTTING DOWN ON FATS

Key to the government's dietary recommendations is a limit on fats. High fat consumption is associated with many disorders (p.38). The government guidelines suggest that fats should comprise no more than 30 percent of your total daily calories. Of these, saturated fats (animal fats and fats that harden at room temperature) should amount to less than 10 percent, and polyunsaturated fats (such as margarine and corn oil) should also amount to about 10 percent, leaving monounsaturated fats (olive, peanut, and canola oils) for the rest.

Some nutrition experts now believe that your fat intake should be even lower—25 percent or less of your daily total calories, with saturated fats cut to 8 percent. To stay healthy, most people need no more than a single tablespoon of fat a day.

FOOD AS MEDICINE

Herbs and plants—the basis of traditional medicine in many cultures—are currently being studied in the United States for their usefulness in preventing cancer, heart disease, and other serious illnesses. While the clinical significance of the research is still uncertain—animal tests may prove of no value for humans—the findings below suggest the potential value of some common foods.

■ ***Carrots, celery, coriander, and parsley*** contain an ingredient called phthalide, which substantially reduced blood pressure and cholesterol levels in animal studies.

■ ***Citrus peel*** and membrane contain pectin, which has lowered animals' cholesterol levels. (Apples are also high in pectin.)

■ ***Cruciferous vegetables,*** which include broccoli, Brussels sprouts, cabbage, cauliflower, and kale, may reduce the risk of cancer. These vegetables are rich in beta carotene and vitamins A, C, and E. They also contain a chemical called sulforaphane, which can trigger the production of cancer-fighting enzymes. Cruciferous vegetables are also a good source of indole carbinol, a chemical that breaks down the hormone estrogen, associated with the development of some breast tumors.

■ ***Flaxseed,*** a cereal grain, contains linolenic acid, which may hinder the body's production of prostaglandins, reducing inflammation.

■ ***Garlic*** may block the formation of nitrosamines, carcinogens found in cured meats and barbecued foods. Animal studies have shown that garlic may help check the substances that cause cancer of the colon, breast, esophagus, skin, and rectum. It also appears to lower cholesterol levels. As few as one or two cloves a day may offer a protective health effect.

■ ***Green tea*** (the kind served in Asian restaurants) is rich in fluoride and contains polyphenols, which may act like antioxidants. In animal studies, green tea decreased the incidence of skin, stomach, and lung cancer and lowered blood cholesterol.

■ ***Soybeans*** are a good source of lecithin, which may help prevent cirrhosis of the liver. Soybeans also contain isoflavones, which show promise in preventing liver cancer.

Scientists believe that many ordinary foods may contain ingredients that help you fight disease, as well as nutrients that maintain your health.

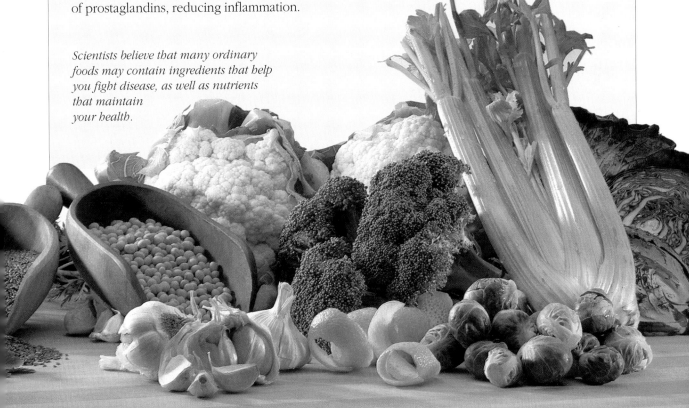

Keeping Up
Good Eating Habits

As you grow older, you may become more sedentary and consume fewer calories. The problem is that the less you eat, the harder it is to get all the nutrients you need from your diet. Staying active helps you keep a healthy appetite for good food.

POTENTIAL VITAMIN AND MINERAL DEFICIENCIES

New research suggests that age-related changes in human chemistry and the medications for chronic conditions that many older people must take affect how the body metabolizes some nutrients. A study at Tufts University shows, for example, that stomach acid production decreases with age in some people, thus hindering the absorption of certain vitamins. Vitamin deficiencies can affect alertness and memory, so as you approach your sixties, you may want to start eating slightly more than the government's Recommended Dietary Allowances (RDA's) of vitamins to ensure that your body absorbs what it needs.

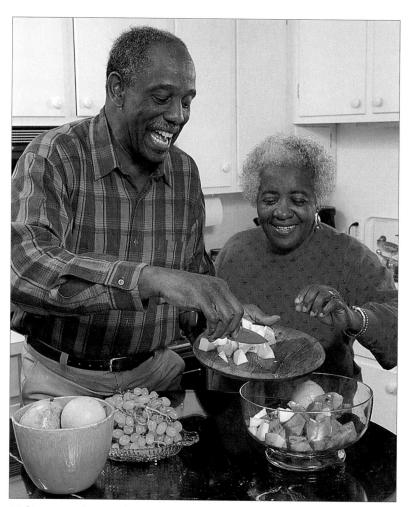

Making a meal a social occasion will probably enhance your appetite, as well as give you the opportunity to cook or taste a variety of healthy foods.

You may also have trouble getting enough minerals in your diet without supplements. Too little iron, for example, can lead to anemia (p.306). Consuming inadequate amounts of calcium contributes to osteoporosis (p.269).

ALTERED TASTE AND SMELL

What you enjoy eating may also change with age because your ability to taste deteriorates. Your taste buds for sweet and salt diminish first, which is why some older people salt their food heavily, seeking to recapture the flavor. This is an unwise practice for people with high blood pressure or those at risk for the disease. Perk up the flavor of foods with herbs, spices, and lemon juice.

Your sense of smell is as important as your taste buds in whetting your appetite for food. Age may diminish your olfactory abilities, making even your favorite dishes less appealing.

The loss of smell can also be dangerous, making you less alert to the odors of food burning or gone bad. As a precaution, use a bell-ringing timer whenever you cook and always check the expiration dates stamped on perishable foods before using them (a few days after the "sell by" date is okay). When you store leftovers in the refrigerator, date the package with a marking pen; discard outdated food.

FOOD AND MEDICATIONS

Many older people regularly take one or more medications that affect their nutrition. Diuretics, for example, can increase the body's need for potassium. Some cholesterol-lowering drugs may increase the need for the fat-soluble vitamins A and E.

Also, what you eat can reduce or enhance the effectiveness of a medication. Large amounts of vitamin K (found in broccoli, turnip greens, and cabbage), for example, may make anticoagulant drugs less effective; omega-3 fatty acids (found in salmon and other fatty fish) can increase their effectiveness. Before you start taking any new medication, ask your doctor about its possible effect on your diet and what you can do to avoid problems.

FINDING A NUTRITION EXPERT

If you have, or are at risk of developing, a health problem that requires nutritional counseling, if you want a sensible weight-loss diet that you can stick to, or if you simply want help in designing a diet for optimum good health for yourself or your family, consider consulting a professional. A good nutritionist not only will help you determine the best diet for your needs but will also advise you on how to shop for food and prepare it, how to adapt menus to the different dietary needs of family members, and how to choose a healthful meal in a restaurant.

Only 36 states have licensing procedures and standards for nutritionists, so you may have to do a little investigating to find one with valid credentials who is right for you.

Registered dietitians (RD's) are trained in clinical nutrition and are certified by the American Dietetic Association. When interviewing an RD, ask where she trained, how long she has been in practice, and what her specialty is. Some nutritionists concentrate on working with diabetics, for example, or with overweight people.

Some doctors, nurses, osteopaths, and biologists in nutrition-related fields have passed an examination given by the American College of Nutrition that qualifies them to give nutrition advice. The American Society for Clinical Nutrition is an organization of PhD's and MD's with training in nutrition.

Steer clear of practitioners with questionable credentials, those who do hair analysis and other unproven diagnostic tests (your doctor should diagnose any medical problems you have), or those who push unnecessary vitamin and mineral supplements, which they may sell themselves.

MAINTAINING YOUR APPETITE

Physical exercise, with all its other benefits, also increases your appetite. Even a walk around the block can help.

Try to make meals an anticipated break in your day. Plan a regular schedule of eating times and treat each as an event. Set an attractive table with good china and silverware rather than allowing yourself to just spoon yogurt out of the container. If you're dining alone, play music to set the mood or fix up a tray and eat while you watch a favorite television show.

As often as you can, organize meal exchanges or potluck dinners with friends and neighbors. Company and conversation can make a meal more appetizing.

An occasional problem among the elderly who live alone and have never learned to cook is the tea and toast syndrome—eating the same easy-to-fix menu day in and day out. Try to avoid this trap. Not only is a narrow diet boring, thus diminishing your appetite, but it also seriously limits the nutrients you take in.

PROTEIN: THE BODY'S BASIC BUILDING MATERIAL

Essential to all body processes, protein maintains and restores organs, muscles, connective tissues, and the blood. Enzymes, the immune system's antibodies, and many hormones are made of protein. Of its 22 amino acids, 13 are manufactured in the body; the other 9 must come from your diet.

SOURCES OF DIETARY PROTEIN

No one should worry about getting enough protein. A varied diet and an adequate caloric intake can give you all the protein your body requires.

Complete proteins, those containing the necessary amounts of the nine essential amino acids, are present in animal foods—meat, poultry, fish, eggs, and dairy products—and one plant food—soybeans. Incomplete proteins, those with an insufficient quantity of one or more of the nine amino acids, are derived from plant foods such as grains, legumes (other than soybeans), nuts, seeds, and vegetables.

Incomplete proteins can't be utilized by the body until all nine amino acids are present in the required amounts—a situation that is easily dealt with by combining two or more complementary plant foods. Any grain, nut, or seed complements any legume (dried beans and peas and peanuts). Two examples are rice and beans and a peanut butter sandwich. These proteins don't have to be eaten at the same meal or even on the same day. Another way to ensure that your body utilizes plant proteins is to add a little animal protein to them—as in pizza, for example, or macaroni and cheese, chicken soup with rice, or cereal with milk.

HOW MUCH DO YOU NEED?

The basic guideline for protein consumption for the general population is the Recommended Dietary Allowance (RDA) established by the Food and Nutrition Board of the National Academy of Sciences. For a healthy adult, the RDA is .36 grams for each pound of actual or, if you are overweight, ideal body weight (see p.61). This comes to about 55 grams for a 150-pound adult, and about 66 grams for someone weighing 180 pounds. As a general rule of thumb, if 10 to 12 percent of your total daily calories comes from protein foods, you will meet the RDA. Check the photograph below to see the correct portion sizes, and refer to the charts on pages 46 and 49 to calculate your daily intake.

EATING TOO MUCH PROTEIN

Most Americans consume more than twice as much protein as the RDA. Many people have the mistaken belief that they should eat as much protein as possible in order to be strong and healthy. But the body cannot store excess protein and converts it into fat.

Some studies show that diets high in animal protein may increase calcium loss from bones and produce high blood levels of uric acid, factors implicated in, respectively, osteoporosis and gout.

Rice and beans.
A cup each of brown rice and black beans constitutes a complete protein serving.

Another drawback to a high-protein diet is that the protein foods Americans eat most—meat, poultry, fish, eggs, and dairy products—are full of saturated fat and cholesterol, which can help cause atherosclerosis and obesity.

· · · · · · · · · · · · · · · · · · · ·

VEGETARIANISM

Many people become vegetarians because they believe that such a diet is healthier. Vegetarianism involves eating a varied and balanced diet of plant foods and greatly reducing or totally eliminating the intake of animal foods. Partial vegetarians give up red meat but include chicken, fish, eggs, and dairy products in their diet. Pescovegetarians eat fish, eggs, and dairy products; ovolactovegetarians, eggs and dairy products; and lactovegetarians, dairy products. Vegans consume only food from plant sources.

A vegetarian diet can provide all the nutrients you need, often with considerable benefits to your health. Vegetarians typically have lower blood pressure and blood cholesterol levels than non-vegetarians. Because their diet is high in fiber, vegetarians are also less likely to suffer from constipation or other digestive disorders.

Vegans, however, must make sure to get sufficient vitamin B12 (since animal foods are the main source of this nutrient) and to eat a variety of plant foods. As with any restricted diet, a vegan diet limited to one or only a few foods can be dangerous.

RECOMMENDED PROTEIN SERVINGS

Individual servings of four complete protein foods are shown here reduced to about two-thirds of their actual size. Two such servings a day should be adequate for the average adult, especially since you also get protein from grains, legumes, and vegetables.

Chicken. *A 3-ounce portion of grilled chicken breast, with the fatty skin removed.*

Fish. *A 3-ounce portion of broiled fillet of sole.*

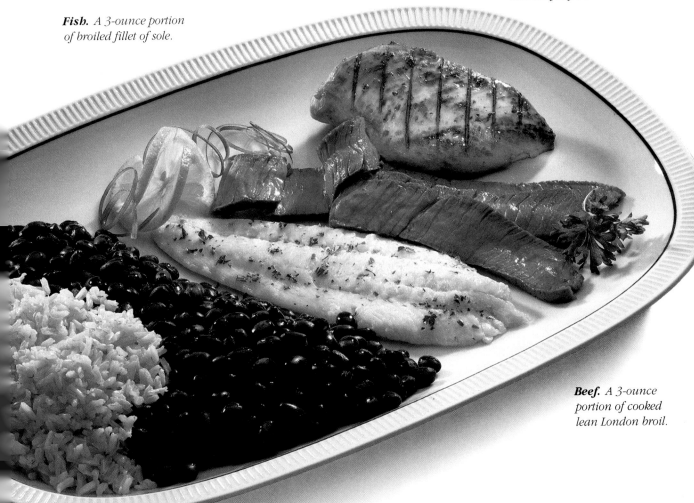

Beef. *A 3-ounce portion of cooked lean London broil.*

CARBOHYDRATES: THE ENERGY NUTRIENTS

*Y*our body gets the energy it needs from carbo-hydrates, vital nutrients present in a wide variety of foods ranging from grains, legumes, fruits, and vegetables to table sugar and pastry. Many carbohydrates also provide fiber, which, though indigestible, is crucial to your health and well-being.

TYPES OF CARBOHYDRATES

Quickly metabolized by the body, simple carbohydrates, or sugars, are available mainly in fruits, milk, and processed foods such as candy and cake.

Complex carbohydrates consist of starches, which are made up of many simple carbohydrates, and fiber, which humans cannot digest. Your digestive system breaks down carbohydrates into glucose, which is the body's major source of energy. Your body can store a half day's supply of glucose by changing it into glycogen and storing it in the liver and muscles. Any other excess glucose is stored as fat, which is used for energy only after glycogen stores have been depleted.

Because complex carbohydrates take a bit longer to be digested than simple ones, your energy level will pick up faster when you eat a candy bar than when you eat a slice of bread. But the bread contains more nutrients and supplies a steady and sustained increase in energy. This difference is crucial for diabetics; the sudden surge of glucose from simple carbohydrates requires extra insulin and dietary planning to avoid problems (see also *Living With Diabetes*, pp.281-282).

The conventional wisdom used to be that if you wanted to lose weight, you should avoid starchy foods such as grains, legumes, and potatoes. Today these complex carbohydrates are highly recommended for weight-loss diets. Per unit weight, starchy

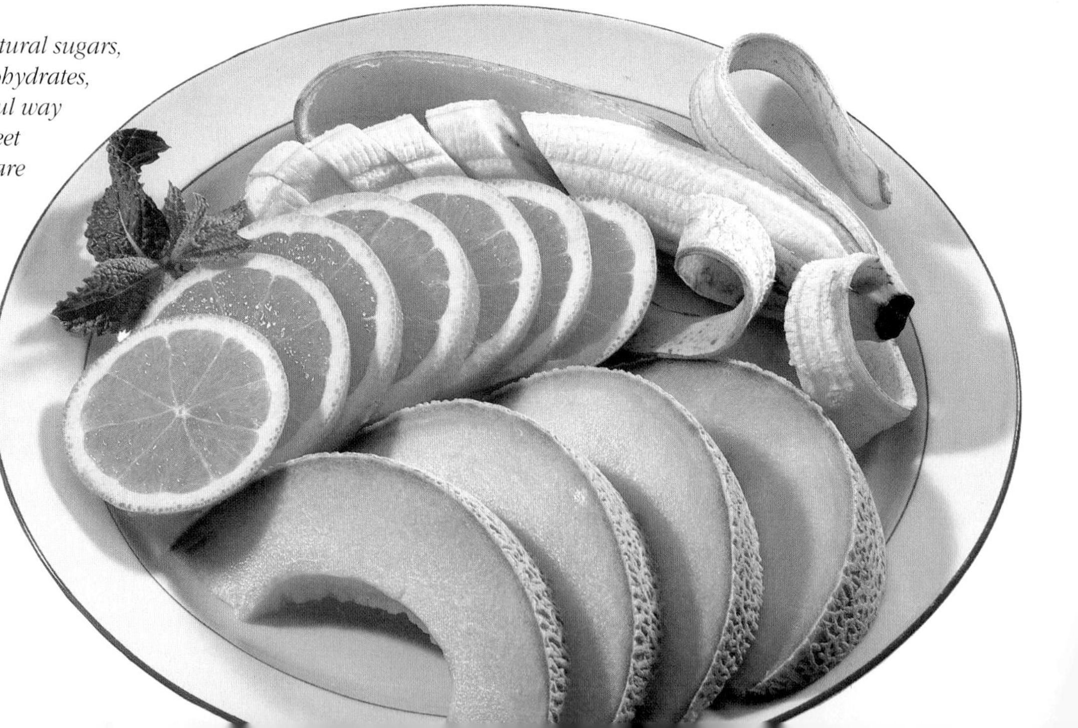

FRUITS
Providing fiber, natural sugars, and complex carbohydrates, fruits are a healthful way to indulge your sweet tooth. Shown here are recommended individual servings— one medium banana, one medium orange, and four portions (equivalent to ¹/₂ cup each) of cantaloupe.

foods have the same number of calories as protein foods and less than half the calories of fat.

Nutrition experts recommend that you get between 55 to 60 percent of your calories from carbohydrates. About 90 percent of those should be from complex carbohydrates and the natural sugars in fruits and vegetables. Consult the chart on page 46 to estimate your daily consumption.

SUGAR AND HEALTH

While sugar has been a suspected precipitating factor in conditions ranging from diabetes to hyperactivity to obesity, scientists at the Food and Drug Administration have concluded that for most people, dental cavities are the only major medical problem caused by consuming sugar. Foods that are high in sugar, however, are usually high in fat as well—and fat can lead to obesity.

Since sugar provides none of the vitamins, minerals, and other nutrients your body needs to maintain health, nutrition experts

recommend that it provide no more than about 10 to 12 percent of your daily calories. In order to limit its intake, however, you have to recognize it, something that isn't always easy. The names of sugars and sugar derivatives found in processed foods include corn syrup, dextrose, fructose, glucose, high-fructose corn syrup, honey, lactose, levulose, maltose, maltodextrin, mannitol, sorbitol, sorghum syrup, sucrose, and xylitol (see also *Decoding Food Labels,* pp.76–77).

Many people avoid sugar by indulging their sweet tooth with no- or low-calorie artificial sweeteners such as saccharin and aspartame. The Food and Drug Administration planned to ban saccharin in 1977 because animal studies showed a link to cancer, but a massive public outcry prevented this. Today most experts associate little risk of cancer with its use. Aspartame has engendered complaints that it causes headaches, nausea, mood swings, anxiety, and increased appetite, but scientific studies have not verified such correlations.

THE BENEFITS OF FIBER

The indigestible part of carbohydrates, fiber passes through your digestive system more or less intact. There are two types: water insoluble and water soluble. Most carbohydrate foods contain both types, with insoluble fiber predominating in whole grains, nuts, wheat bran, and fruit and vegetable skins; and soluble fiber in seeds, brown rice, barley, oats, legumes, fruits, and vegetables.

Because insoluble fiber absorbs many times its weight in water, it helps to prevent or relieve constipation by creating a soft, bulky stool that is more easily eliminated. Foods high in insoluble fiber can also ease the symptoms and arrest the progression of digestive disorders such as hemorrhoids (see p.258), diverticulosis (see p.310), and irritable bowel syndrome (see pp.311-312).

Although results are still inconclusive, some studies indicate that foods high in soluble fiber may help prevent colon cancer, as well as the formation of gallstones. Soluble fiber may also

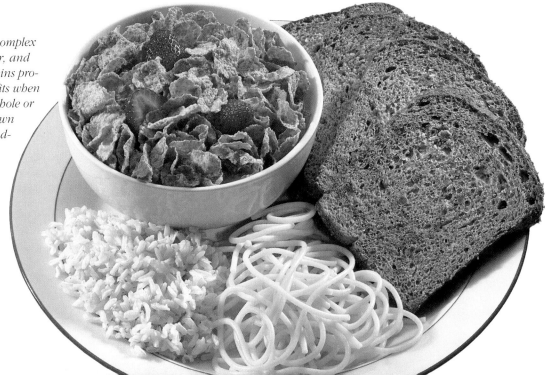

GRAINS
A major source of complex carbohydrates, fiber, and other nutrients, grains provide the most benefits when they are eaten in whole or enriched form. Shown here are recommended individual servings of four grains: a 3-ounce bowl of cold cereal, four slices, or servings, of multi-grain bread, and $^1/_2$ cup each of spaghetti and brown rice.

protect against heart disease by helping to lower blood cholesterol levels. Because soluble fiber helps to stabilize blood sugar levels, it may play a role in controlling diabetes as well.

. . . .

INCREASING THE FIBER IN YOUR DIET

The National Cancer Institute recommends that you consume between 20 and 35 grams of dietary fiber a day (see chart, right); most Americans eat only about 12 grams.

If you're not eating enough fiber-containing foods, add them to your diet gradually so that you don't suddenly overload your digestive system. Make sure to drink plenty of water to ensure that the food moves easily through your intestinal tract.

It's best to get your fiber from a variety of fruits, vegetables, legumes, and grains that are as unprocessed as possible (such as an apple instead of applesauce) and not from supplements. This way you will get the vitamins and minerals in the foods as well.

CARBOHYDRATE AND FIBER CONTENT OF COMMON FOODS

Foods	Calories	Carbohydrates (g)	Fiber (g)	Protein (g)
Apple, medium	80	20.0	2.8	0.3
Apricots, dried, 10 medium halves	91	23.3	1.0	1.8
Beans, green snap, cooked, 1 cup	31	6.8	4.2	2.0
Bread, whole wheat, 1 slice	61	11.9	1.4	2.6
Broccoli, cooked, 1 cup	40	7.0	4.0	4.8
Cake, chocolate, 2"x2"x2" (no icing)	143	20.3	1.0	1.9
Cantaloupe, cubed, 1 cup	48	12.0	1.5	1.1
Carrot, raw, 1 medium	30	7.0	2.0	0.8
Chickpeas, cooked, ¾ cup	164	27.0	3.0	9.0
Corn flakes, 1 cup (dry)	97	21.3	0.08	2.0
Grapefruit, ½	40	10.3	1.7	0.5
Kidney beans, red, cooked, 1 cup	218	39.6	11.6	14.4
Lentils, cooked, 1 cup	212	38.6	4.0	15.6
Lettuce, romaine, chopped, 1 cup	10	1.9	2.4	0.7
Oatmeal, cooked, 1 cup	132	23.3	3.7	4.8
Orange, 1 medium	71	18.1	1.6	1.1
Orange juice, 1 cup	112	25.8	0.2	1.7
Peanut butter, 1 oz.	166	5.3	1.0	7.4
Potato, baked, with skin (4¾")	145	32.8	4.0	4.0
Rice, brown, cooked, 1 cup	232	49.7	2.4	4.9
Spaghetti, cooked (firm), 1 cup	192	39.1	1.6	6.5
Spinach, cooked, 1 cup	41	6.5	4.2	5.4
Strawberries, 1 cup	55	12.5	0.8	1.0
Sugar, granulated, 1 tsp.	15	4.0	0	0
Tomato, 1 medium	20	4.3	1.0	1.0

VEGETABLES
Excellent sources of fiber, vegetables also provide some complex carbohydrates as well as many essential vitamins and minerals. Shown here are recommended individual servings of red leaf lettuce (1 cup), broccoli (½ cup), carrots (½ cup), and a baked potato sprinkled with chives (an amount equivalent to ½ cup, diced, makes 1 serving).

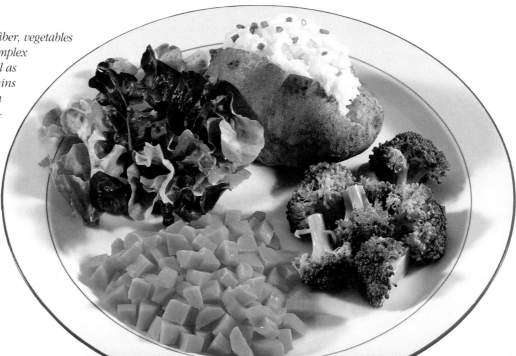

WATER: THE FORGOTTEN NUTRIENT

You can survive for several months without food, but you will die within a few days without water. Comprising between 55 and 65 percent of an adult's body, water is required for virtually every one of its functions, from digestion and elimination to the distribution of nutrients and the building of tissue. Water regulates your body temperature through perspiration, lubricates your joints, and cushions your brain and other internal organs.

The amount of water your body loses each day through perspiration, exhalation of water vapor from the lungs, and elimination in urine and feces should equal the amount you consume—about $2\frac{1}{2}$ to 3 quarts for the average adult. If you engage in strenuous exercise or heavy physical work, especially in hot weather, you will need to replace more water (see also *Outdoor Exercising in the Heat and Cold*, pp.112–113). Other factors that may increase your water requirements are eating highly salted foods and going on a weight-loss diet.

GETTING ENOUGH WATER

While thirst is a signal that your body requires water, sometimes people drink only enough to quench their immediate thirst but not enough to satisfy their body's needs. Most nutrition experts recommend drinking between six and eight 8-ounce glasses of water or other nonalcoholic fluids daily. Caffeinated beverages such as coffee, tea, and cola are acceptable sources of water, but because they also have a diuretic effect that increases urine output, you should not rely solely on them.

The rest of the water your body needs is contributed by many of the foods you eat: bread is about 30 percent water; fruits and vegetables, between 80 and 95 percent.

FAT: A LITTLE GOES A LONG WAY

*T*he body's most concentrated source of energy, fat supplies the essential fatty acids necessary for many internal processes, cushions vital organs, and facilitates the body's absorption of the fat-soluble vitamins A, D, E, and K. A modest amount of fat in your diet is necessary to maintain health. Too much of it can cause disease.

FAT AND HEART DISEASE

Saturated fat is present in meat and dairy products and to a lesser extent in all vegetable oils, especially coconut, palm, and palm kernel oils. This type of fat has been proven to raise cholesterol levels and increase your risk of heart disease if consumed in large quantities.

Monounsaturated fat and polyunsaturated fat, while also found in all fats of animal and vegetable origin, predominate in vegetable oils. Each of these fats has been shown to lower blood cholesterol levels. Both mono-unsaturated and polyunsaturated fats are generally referred to as unsaturated fat.

Most saturated fats are solid at room temperature, while unsaturated fats are liquid. The unsaturated fats in shortening and margarine, however, are

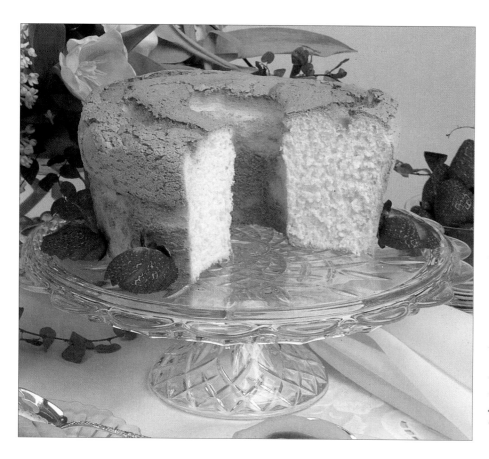

Angel food cake is both delicious and low in fat since its major ingredients consist of flour, sugar, and egg whites. A slice of a typical cake has just 0.1 gram of fat and contains only 161 calories.

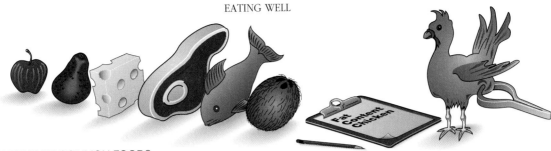

FAT CONTENT OF COMMON FOODS

Food and Portion	Calories	Fat (total, in g)	Monoun-saturated Fat (in g)	Polyun-saturated Fat (in g)	Saturated Fat (in g)	Choles-terol (in mg)	Protein (in g)
Avocado, ½	188	18.5	8.3	2.4	3.7	0	2.4
Beef, lean chuck, cooked, 3½ oz.	248	12.8	2.8	0.35	3.15	91	31.5
Butter, 1 tbsp.	102	11.5	3.8	0.3	6.3	31	0.1
Canola oil, 1 tbsp.	119	13.5	8.4	4.3	0.8	0	0.0
Cheese, Swiss, 3½ oz.	376	28.0	9.6	0.9	16.2	92	28.8
Chicken, broiled (no skin), 3½ oz.							
Light meat	165	4.0	1.4	0.7	1.0	85	31.0
Dark meat	205	7.1	2.7	1.4	2.3	93	27.0
Coconut oil, 1 tbsp.	120	13.6	0.9	0.3	11.8	0	0.0
Cod, cooked, 3½ oz.	105	1.0	<1	<1	<1	55	23.0
Corn oil, 1 tbsp.	120	13.6	3.8	7.2	1.4	0	0.0
Cottage cheese, creamed, 3½ oz.	103	4.2	1.4	0.1	2.5	15	13.6
Egg, 1 large, hard-boiled	82	5.8	2.5	0.4	1.8	213	6.5
Lamb, leg, roasted, 3½ oz.	191	16.1	5.8	0.5	9.0	89	28.0
Milk, 8 oz.: Whole (3.5% milkfat)	159	8.6	2.8	0.25	4.7	32	8.6
Skim (0.0% milkfat)	88	0.25	<1	<1	<1	4.6	8.8
Olive oil, 1 tbsp.	119	13.5	10.3	0.9	1.5	0	0.0
Pork, top loin, cooked, 3½ oz.	194	26.0	10.9	2.4	9.3	78	30.0
Safflower oil, 1 tbsp.	120	13.6	2.0	9.8	1.1	0	0.0
Salmon, pink, canned, 3¾ oz.	160	8.0	1.92	0.12	2.04	37	20.0
Shrimp, cooked, 3½ oz.	99	1.0	<1	<1	<1	195	21.0
Tuna, canned, in water, 3½ oz.	131	<1	<1	<1	<1	18	30.0
Turkey, roasted (no skin), 3½ oz.							
Light meat	135	4.4	1.9	0.9	1.3	83	30.0
Dark meat	162	9.4	4.0	2.0	2.7	112	29.0

HOW TO CUT BACK ON SATURATED FAT

▪ Eat more fruits, vegetables, and grains. Substitute fish or poultry for some or all red meat, and remove the skin from poultry before cooking. Light chicken or turkey meat is preferable to dark meat since it contains about half the fat.

▪ Select lean cuts of red meat, trim the visible fat, and roast, bake, or broil the meat on a rack so that the invisible fat drips off.

▪ Chill your soups and stews, then skim the fat off the top.

▪ Cook with unsaturated vegetable oils instead of butter, lard, or shortening.

▪ Drink low-fat or skim milk instead of whole; replace sour cream in recipes with low-fat yogurt, buttermilk, or cottage cheese.

▪ Buy margarine that has at least twice as much polyunsaturated fat as saturated fat. Make sure that a liquid oil is the first ingredient listed. The softer the margarine, the less saturated it is.

▪ Avoid prepared foods made with palm or coconut oil.

▪ Replace high-fat snacks such as potato chips and candy bars with low-fat ones such as unbuttered popcorn and fruits and vegetables.

Profile

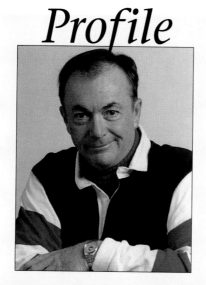

DR. ROBERT C. NORTHCUTT COUNSELS PATIENTS TO FOLLOW HIS EXAMPLE

In 1987, after doing heavy yard work, Dr. Robert C. Northcutt, an associate professor at the Mayo Medical School in Rochester, Minnesota, suffered a serious heart attack. He was 6 feet 1 inch tall, weighed 260 pounds, had a cholesterol level of 260, and smoked. Although he was an active outdoorsman, he exercised only in short, intense bursts. "The heart attack was quite a jolt," he says. "I never believed that stuff about diet and exercise applied to me."

Northcutt's road to recovery began with quitting smoking, a closely monitored exercise program, and meetings with a dietitian who changed his high-fat diet to one that was 10 to 20 percent fat and nearly vegetarian. "I called it the cardboard diet," says Northcutt. "If I liked a food, I probably shouldn't eat it." In 8 months, he lost 50 pounds and lowered his cholesterol to 210.

Today Northcutt has adjusted to his new way of eating so well that high-fat foods feel waxy on his teeth. A self-described crusader for a healthy diet and regular exercise, Northcutt always counsels his patients to follow his example.

often hardened by hydrogenation, a process that makes them chemically more similar to saturated fats.

The best way to protect yourself against heart disease is to reduce your intake of foods high in saturated fat (see chart, p.49). Besides raising your total cholesterol level, this fat increases your low-density lipoproteins, or LDL's, a component known as "bad" cholesterol because it allows plaque to accumulate on the artery walls.

DIETARY CHOLESTEROL AND HEART DISEASE

While saturated fat in the diet is a major cause of high blood cholesterol levels, dietary cholesterol, a type of fat found only in animal foods, is a significant contributor as well—especially for the 20 percent of Americans whose genetic makeup causes them to be particularly susceptible to its effects.

The American Heart Association recommends consuming no more than 300 milligrams of dietary cholesterol daily. Those foods that are high in cholesterol include egg yolks, organ meats, red meat, and dairy products (see chart, p.49).

FAT AND CANCER

Although the connection between dietary fat and cancer is less well established than the relationship between fat and heart disease, countries with the highest fat consumption usually also have the highest rates of cancer. Colon cancer is far more common in the United States, for example, than in Japan, where the population consumes much less fat.

REDUCING THE FAT IN YOUR DIET

Both the American Heart Association and the American Cancer Society recommend that you get no more than 30 percent of your daily calories from fat, as opposed to the 37 percent that most Americans currently consume. Of this 30 percent, saturated fats should make up less than a third, polyunsaturates a third, and monounsaturates the rest. Researchers estimate that if all Americans followed these guidelines, deaths from coronary artery disease and cancer of the breast, colon, and prostate would drop by 42,000 a year.

Getting 30 percent of your calories from fat is not the same as eating a diet that is 30 percent fat. Fats contain more than twice as many calories as carbohydrates and proteins (9 per gram versus 4 per gram), which is why fatty foods are more likely to cause weight gain. To determine the maximum number of fat calories you should consume daily, multiply your total calories by .30. For example, if you eat 1,800 calories a day, you should limit fat calories to 540. If you measure your fat consumption in grams, divide the 540 calories by 9 (the number of calories in a gram), which gives you 60 grams of fat.

FOODS THAT MAY HELP REDUCE YOUR CHOLESTEROL LEVEL

While a well-balanced low-fat diet is the best way to lower your cholesterol level, two foods may be particularly helpful in doing so—oat bran and fish that contains omega-3 acid.

Studies have shown that as little as 2 ounces a day of oats or oat bran can lower blood cholesterol levels—but only when the oat products are part of an overall healthy diet. Because the water-soluble fiber in oats is what makes them heart-healthy, other soluble fiber foods—fruits, vegetables, and legumes, for example—may produce the same effect (see pp.44-46).

Omega-3, a unique polyunsaturated fatty acid found in fish oil, may reduce clotting in the blood and may also lower blood cholesterol levels more significantly than other polyunsaturated oils. To make sure that you get a beneficial amount of omega-3 in your diet, eat two or more servings a week of fatty fish such as bluefish, cod, halibut, herring, mackerel, salmon, trout, and tuna, or shellfish such as crab, lobster, scallops, and shrimp. Fish oil supplements are not a good source of omega-3; in some cases, they may even be harmful.

THE FRENCH PARADOX

Considering the established link between fat consumption and heart disease, how can the French eat a rich diet—including foie gras, one of the fattiest foods imaginable—as well as drink wine regularly, exercise very little, smoke quite a lot, and still have one of the lowest rates of heart disease in the industrialized world?

One nutritionist attributes this phenomenon to the fact that high-fat diets are relatively new in France. Fat consumption only began to increase after World War II and reached 39 percent of dietary calories in 1988—a level that Americans had attained in 1923. Because it takes several decades for high-fat diets to cause heart disease, the French may begin to reap the consequences of their new way of eating in the near future.

Some experts, however, speculate that other factors may play a role in the low rate of heart disease in France—in particular, wine consumption and lifestyle. But while studies show that a moderate amount of alcohol may be heart protective (see p.68), alcohol consumption has been declining in France for the last 35 years. Today half of all French adults don't drink at all.

The effects of the French lifestyle are more difficult to assess. The French consume considerably more fresh fruits and vegetables than Americans do; they get most of their saturated fat from cheese, not from meat; and they use olive oil and goose fat for cooking instead of butter or lard. They also snack less and take care to eat their meals at a more leisurely pace.

WHY YOU NEED
VITAMINS AND MINERALS

Although required in very small amounts, vitamins and minerals—which you get from the foods you eat—are essential to your body's functioning and for maintaining good health.

TYPES OF VITAMINS AND MINERALS

Fat-soluble vitamins are stored in your body fat until they are needed, which may be weeks or even years, depending on the vitamin. Water-soluble vitamins, on the other hand, pass out of the body in the urine. As a result, they must be replenished more often (see chart, facing page).

Your body requires macrominerals, such as calcium and potassium, in relatively large amounts; trace minerals, such as iron and zinc, in minuscule amounts. Both types of minerals, however, are equally important (see chart, p.54).

GETTING THE VITAMINS AND MINERALS YOU NEED

The best way to get the vitamins and minerals your body needs is by eating a well-balanced diet. Taking pills can't make up for an unhealthy diet. Nor can vitamin and mineral supplements provide any of the energy and maintenance of body tissues and organs that you get from the proteins, carbohydrates, fats, and water in your diet.

For most healthy people, a varied low-fat diet that emphasizes whole grains, fruits and vegetables, and lean meats, fish, and poultry should provide sufficient nutrients.

As you grow older, however, your need for certain vitamins and minerals sometimes increases. New research suggests that older persons often cannot metabolize essential nutrients as efficiently as can younger people.

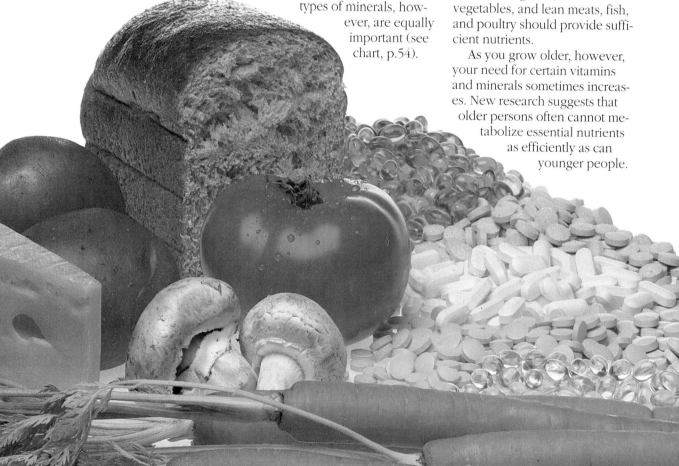

THE BENEFITS OF VITAMINS

Vitamins differ from minerals in that they are organic, that is, derived from animal or plant sources, whereas minerals are inorganic, inanimate elements originating in soil and water.

Fat-soluble vitamins

	Major Food Sources	Benefits
Vitamin A (retinol)/beta carotene	Retinol: milk and dairy products, liver, eggs. Beta carotene: dark green leafy vegetables; deep yellow and orange fruits and vegetables.	Helps keep vision sharp and skin, hair, and nails healthy; reinforces the immune system. Its precursor, the antioxidant beta carotene, which is turned into vitamin A in the body, may help protect against heart disease and some cancers.
Vitamin D (calciferol)	Fortified milk, eggs, oily fish such as canned sardines, cod-liver oil.	Maintains bones and teeth; aids in calcium absorption; may help prevent cancer.
Vitamin E (tocopherol)	Wheat germ, safflower and sunflower oils, dark green leafy vegetables, whole-grain foods.	Plays a role in the formation of red blood cells. As an antioxidant, large doses may reduce the risk of heart disease and some cancers.
Vitamin K	Dark green leafy vegetables, cereals, eggs, liver. It is also manufactured by intestinal bacteria.	Necessary for normal blood clotting; also appears to help bones retain calcium; may help to prevent some cancers.

Water-soluble vitamins

Vitamin B1 (thiamine)	Pork, organ meats, seafood, whole-grain cereals, brewer's yeast, nuts, legumes, fruits, vegetables.	Helps metabolize carbohydrates; aids digestion and nerve functions.
Vitamin B2 (riboflavin)	Organ meats, beef, lamb, chicken and turkey dark meat, fish, enriched cereals and grains, dark green leafy vegetables, fruits.	Helps metabolize all foods and releases energy to cells.
Vitamin B3 (niacin or nicotinic acid)	Poultry, fish, beef and beef liver, seeds, nuts, peanuts, enriched breads and cereals, fruits, vegetables.	Helps digestion and nerve function. Very high doses can increase blood levels of "good" HDL cholesterol while lowering "bad" LDL cholesterol (see p.298).
Vitamin B5 (pantothenic acid)	Organ meats, cereals and legumes, dark green leafy vegetables, eggs, milk, fruits.	Essential in metabolizing food and regulating nerve function.
Vitamin B6 (pyridoxine)	Meat, fish, poultry, grains and cereals, sweet and white potatoes, spinach, peanuts, bananas, walnuts, prunes, watermelon.	Plays a major role in protein and carbohydrate metabolism, red blood cell formation, and nerve function regulation. Appears to heighten the immune response in the elderly.
Vitamin B12 (cobalamin)	Meats and organ meats, poultry, seafood, eggs, milk and dairy products, fruits, vegetables.	Essential to red blood cell formation and maintenance and DNA metabolism; aids in nervous system functioning.
Biotin	Meat and liver, poultry, fish, eggs, nuts, seeds, cereals, fruits, vegetables, yeast.	Helps metabolize glucose and form fatty acids, among many other body processes.
Folic acid (folate or folacin)	Dark green leafy vegetables, chicken, liver, legumes, enriched cereals and breads, orange and grapefruit juice.	Necessary for the formation of red blood cells and DNA metabolism.
Vitamin C (ascorbic acid)	Citrus fruits and juices, strawberries, cantaloupe, watermelon, dark green leafy vegetables, potatoes, cabbage, peppers, cauliflower.	Maintains bones, teeth, and gums; helps to heal cuts and wounds; promotes resistance to infection. It may help prevent or alleviate cold symptoms. As an antioxidant, vitamin C may help to lessen the tissue damage associated with aging and may reduce the risk of cancer and heart disease.

THE BENEFITS OF MINERALS

Listed below are 16 of the 22 minerals known to be crucial to your well-being. As yet there is insufficient information on the roles of the other 6, all of them trace minerals—arsenic, boron, lithium, nickel, silicon, and vanadium.

Macrominerals

	Major Food Sources	Benefits
Calcium	Yogurt, milk, cheese, tofu, canned salmon and sardines (with bones), dark green leafy vegetables (especially collard greens and broccoli).	Essential for building and maintaining strong bones and teeth, especially in postmenopausal women at risk of osteoporosis (see p.269); facilitates blood clotting as well as muscle and nerve functioning.
Chloride	Table salt, processed foods, milk.	Helps maintain the body's fluid and acid-base balances; is an ingredient in gastric juices.
Magnesium	Dark green leafy vegetables, legumes, nuts, whole grains, milk.	Plays a vital role in the body's metabolic activities; promotes bone growth; aids nerve and muscle functioning.
Phosphorus	Fish, meat, poultry, legumes, dairy products, eggs, nuts.	Helps convert food to energy; with calcium, helps build and maintain bones and teeth; aids nerve and muscle function.
Potassium	Many fruits and vegetables—especially citrus fruits, bananas, and potatoes (with skin)—milk, yogurt, bran cereals, legumes, meat.	Essential for muscle contraction, nerve impulses, and kidney and heart functioning, as well as for blood pressure and fluid balance regulation. May help to lessen the risk of hypertension and stroke.
Sodium	Table salt, processed foods, milk.	Helps to maintain acid-base and body fluid balances.
Sulfur	Wheat germ, legumes, meat, fish.	Helps make cartilage, hair, and nails; also an essential ingredient of some amino acids.

Trace minerals

Chromium	Whole grains, meat, brewer's yeast, peanuts.	Helps metabolize carbohydrates and fats; helps to regulate the action of insulin and glucose.
Copper	Shellfish, organ meats, legumes, nuts, whole grains, potatoes.	Aids in the formation of red blood cells, connective tissue, and nerve fibers; also helps the body absorb iron.
Fluoride	Fluoridated water, foods cooked in it, canned fish (with bones), tea.	Strengthens teeth and bones; aids in the body's calcium absorption.
Iodine	Iodized salt, seafood, dairy products, vegetables grown in iodine-rich soil.	Necessary for cell metabolism and thyroid gland functioning.
Iron	Red meat and liver, poultry, fish, eggs, legumes, grains, blackstrap molasses, dark green leafy vegetables, foods cooked in cast-iron pots.	Plays a role in energy production as well as in the formation of hemoglobin (which transports oxygen in the blood) and myoglobin (which stores oxygen in the muscles).
Manganese	Whole grains, nuts, legumes, fruits and vegetables, tea, instant coffee, cocoa.	Helps tendon and bone growth and development as well as protein and energy metabolism.
Molybdenum	Legumes, whole grains, organ meats, dark green leafy vegetables.	Helps in metabolism and in regulating iron levels.
Selenium	Meat and organ meats, seafood, whole grains.	Interacts with vitamin E as an antioxidant and may help protect against some cancers. Helps facilitate immune response and heart muscle functioning.
Zinc	Beef, liver, seafood (especially oysters), eggs, grains, poultry.	Plays a major role in digestive and metabolic processes; helps to heal wounds and repair body tissues.

And some common medications for age-related ailments can interfere with vitamin absorption. If you take thiazide diuretics, for example, you may require extra potassium. Overuse of antacids containing magnesium or aluminum can weaken bones by robbing the body of phosphorus.

Another reason a dietary supplement may be beneficial is that over time your senses of smell and taste weaken, leading to appetite loss (see pp.40–41) and an insufficient intake of nutrients.

If you merely wish to supplement an already healthy diet, some experts advise taking a multivitamin-multimineral pill that provides no more than 100 percent of the DV or RDA of as many nutrients as possible. For special needs, however, check with your doctor about which supplements you should take.

· ·

THE ANTIOXIDANT VITAMINS

Recent studies have indicated that certain vitamins may be able to halt or even reverse many illnesses and disorders that are associated with aging, including arthritis, cancer, cataracts, heart disease, lung disease, osteoporosis, degeneration of the nervous system, and a failing immune system.

Much of this research has focused on the antioxidant role of vitamins C, E, and beta carotene (which the body converts into vitamin A). Antioxidants neutralize free radicals, which are unstable and highly reactive byproducts of normal body metabolism that damage DNA and kill cells. Some reseachers theorize that free radicals contribute to such illnesses as cancer and heart disease as well as to the deterioration associated with aging. Recent research suggests that antioxidants may protect against heart disease by helping to prevent blood cholesterol from sticking to artery walls and turning into plaque.

Antioxidants are available in most fruits, vegetables, and whole grains; increasing your consumption of these foods may be as important to your health as decreasing your intake of foods high in fat.

MEGADOSING

The practice of taking megadoses of vitamins (10 to 100 times the DV, USRDA, or RDA) in order to delay the aging process or to prevent chronic diseases remains controversial. Although recent tests with the antioxidants C, E, and beta carotene have involved moderately high to very high amounts of these vitamins, many of the promising results from this research are still considered preliminary.

Based on these results, however, some experts have begun to recommend that people take moderately high amounts of antioxidants. Others urge caution on the grounds that the long-term effects of increased vitamin consumption are unknown.

The short-term dangers of large doses of some vitamins, especially A and D, have been known for some time. In addition, megadoses of any one vitamin may inhibit the absorption of other nutrients. If, however, you believe that you might benefit from megadosing, be sure to check with your doctor or nutritionist first.

DAILY VALUES, USRDA's, AND RDA's

The Food and Drug Administration (FDA) has recently issued regulations to simplify and standardize food labeling. All the nutrients in a food are to be listed in terms of Daily Values, or DV's (see pp.76–77). The label must state the percentage of the Daily Value for each nutrient, based on a 2,000-calorie diet. For example, since the DV for fat is 65 grams, a food that contains 6.5 grams of fat per serving would be labeled as having a fat DV of 10 percent. With this information, consumers should be better able to plan their daily meals.

DV's replace the USRDA's (United States Recommended Daily Allowances), the values formerly used on food labels and on labels for vitamin and mineral supplements. The USRDA's should not be confused with the RDA's (Recommended Dietary Allowances), daily dietary guidelines established by the Food and Nutrition Board of the National Academy of Sciences–National Research Council and revised every few years. Most of the USRDA figures were based on the RDA's, however, as are most of the current DV figures.

SODIUM:
STRIKING A HEALTHY BALANCE

A mineral that is essential to life, sodium in large amounts is also linked to hypertension in more than 5 percent of the population. The most common source of sodium is table salt, a mixture of sodium and chloride.

HOW MUCH DO YOU NEED?

The importance of sodium is clear—it helps maintain the delicate balance of fluids in your body, aids in keeping a normal heart rhythm, and plays a role in transmitting nerve impulses to muscles—but there is no agreement on exactly how much you need. The National Academy of Sciences suggests a minimum daily sodium requirement for adults of about 500 milligrams, which you can get from a quarter teaspoon of salt. You can also meet this minimum just by eating unprocessed meat, eggs, fish, and dairy products, which naturally contain small amounts of sodium.

The average American diet contains two to three times the 2,400-milligram maximum daily amount of sodium recommended by the National Academy of Sciences. The major sources of this excess sodium are processed and preserved foods (see chart below) and salt put on food at the table. Sodium is also found in water and in many over-the-counter medications (antacids and cough syrups, for example) and a few prescription drugs (some antibiotics, for instance).

Too little sodium can cause serious problems. In older people, dehydration resulting from diarrhea or improper use of diuretics, if not treated promptly, can fatally deplete the body's supply of sodium and potassium.

SURPRISING SOURCES OF SODIUM

Chicken broth, canned, 8 oz.	**1,320 mg**
Chicken nuggets (6)	**512–840 mg**
Cheese, Cheddar, 1½ oz.	**300 mg**
Cheese, processed American, 1½ oz.	**600 mg**
Egg, ham, and cheese sandwich (fast food)	**885 mg**
Ham and egg biscuit (fast food)	**1,585 mg**
Hamburger (fast food)	**210–1,826 mg**
Hot ham and cheese sandwich (fast food)	**1,655 mg**
Pickle (dill) 2 oz.	**700 mg**
Soup, canned, 10 oz.	**up to 1,500 mg**
TV dinner, 11 oz.	**up to 2,000 mg**

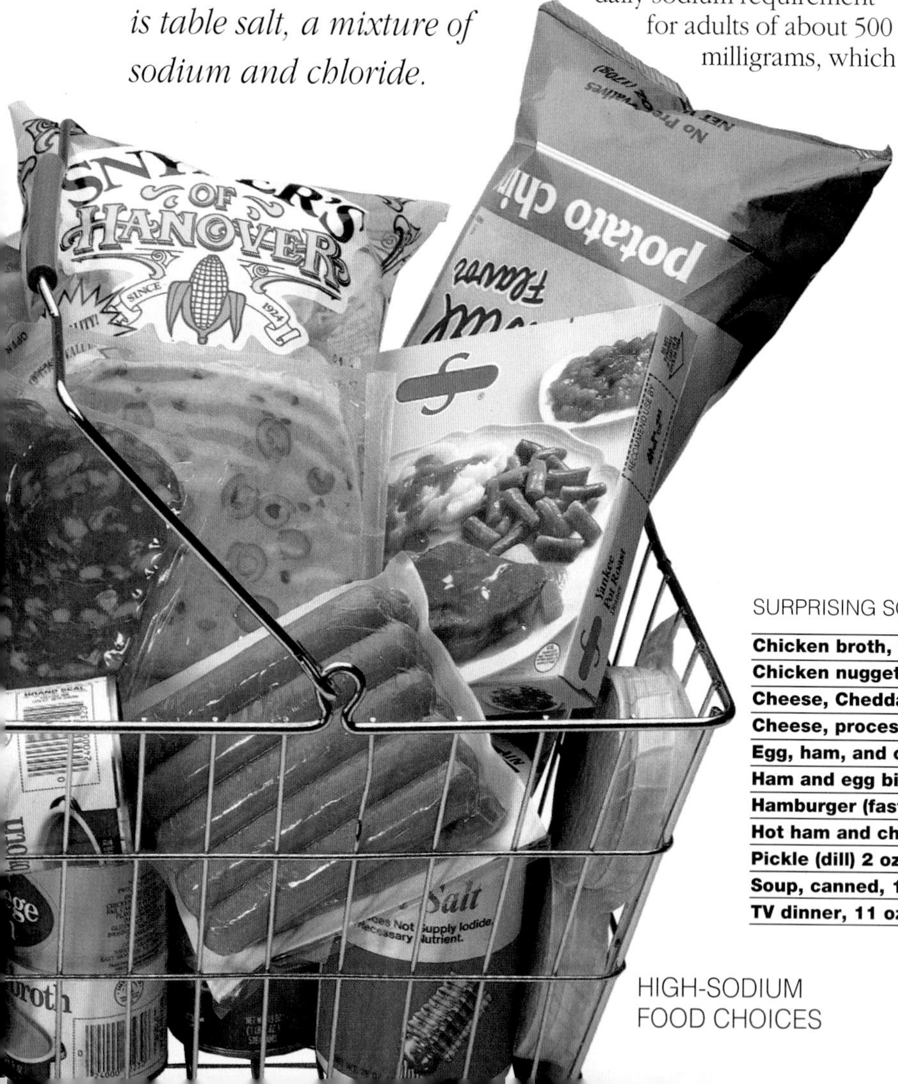

HIGH-SODIUM
FOOD CHOICES

SALT AND HYPERTENSION

Although many experts believe that Americans' heavy consumption of salt contributes to the country's high incidence of hypertension (high blood pressure) and heart disease, the link is not completely understood.

From 5 to 10 percent of Americans are sensitive to sodium; this group makes up 30 to 50 percent of those with hypertension. By restricting sodium in their diets, these people can reduce their blood pressure and sometimes even eliminate or reduce their need for hypertension drugs.

Most experts believe that people who appear not to be sodium sensitive should also limit their sodium intake. The reasoning is that it may help prevent hypertension, since it is hard to know who is sodium sensitive *before* hypertension develops. Older people have a decreased ability to excrete excess sodium, so their sodium intake may have a greater influence on their blood pressure.

SALT SUBSTITUTES

A number of commercial products are available to help people cut down on salt. These salt substitutes fall into three categories: potassium chloride; combinations of sodium chloride and potassium chloride; and mixtures of flavor-enhancing herbs and spices. Potassium chloride salt substitutes are not suitable for everyone. Some people find them objectionably bitter; others, such as people with kidney disorders, those taking diuretics that conserve potassium, or those on potassium supplements, should avoid increased potassium. Herb and spice mixtures are the safest.

REDUCING YOUR SODIUM INTAKE

■ When buying processed foods, look for "very-low-sodium" or "sodium-free" labels.

■ Gradually cut down the amount of salt you use in cooking; add herbs, spices, and lemon juice instead.

■ Taste food before you salt it and go easy on condiments like catsup, mustard, olives, pickles, and soy sauce.

■ In sandwiches, replace cured or processed meats, such as bacon, hot dogs, and luncheon meats, with fresh meats, such as turkey or chicken (use leftovers from an earlier meal).

■ Buy fresh vegetables or frozen ones without sauce.

■ Avoid salty snacks like potato or corn chips, crackers, nuts, pretzels, and prepared popcorn.

■ When eating in restaurants, avoid foods that are smoked, barbecued, or marinated.

SODIUM HIGHS AND LOWS
The grocery basket on the facing page is filled with high-sodium prepared foods. By using the fresh ingredients shown below when you prepare meals, you can drastically cut your sodium intake.

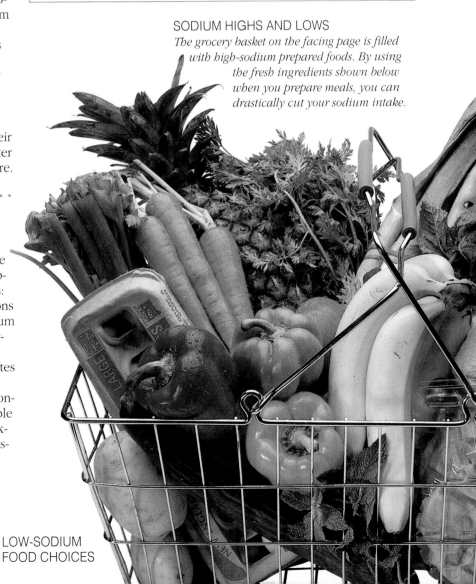

LOW-SODIUM
FOOD CHOICES

CALCIUM: A KEY MINERAL

Essential for building bones and teeth, calcium is also necessary for blood clotting and muscle contraction and may help prevent hypertension. As you grow older, it's important to consume enough calcium and to make sure your body absorbs it.

HOW MUCH CALCIUM DOES AN ADULT NEED?

The Recommended Dietary Allowance (RDA) of calcium for adults is 800 milligrams. The National Institutes of Health recommend that postmenopausal women consume 1,200 to 1,500 milligrams a day because research suggests that a high-calcium diet can slow the bone loss of osteoporosis (see p.269). Men are less prone to osteoporosis in their fifties and sixties because they usually have more bone mass than women.

Both men's and women's bodies stop increasing bone mass at around age 35; bone mass itself begins to decline slowly after the age of 50.

FACTORS THAT AFFECT CALCIUM ABSORPTION

One of the reasons that the RDA for calcium is difficult to determine is that many things can affect its absorption. One is age: children absorb up to 75 percent of the calcium they eat; adults, only about 15 to 35 percent.

Consuming the right balance of protein, vitamin D, and lactose helps your body absorb calcium. A diet too high in protein or fat reduces calcium absorption. Also, phosphorus, another mineral, is needed in about the same amount as calcium to form bone. Americans tend to consume many foods high in phosphorus (soft drinks, eggs, and meat), which may upset the phosphorus-calcium ratio and hinder calcium absorption.

Other chemicals in foods adversely affect calcium absorption—oxalic acid (found in spinach) and phytic acid (found in legumes and bran), for example. The tannins in tea and an excess of caffeine hinder absorption, as does smoking. Taking aluminum-based antacids can also affect calcium retention.

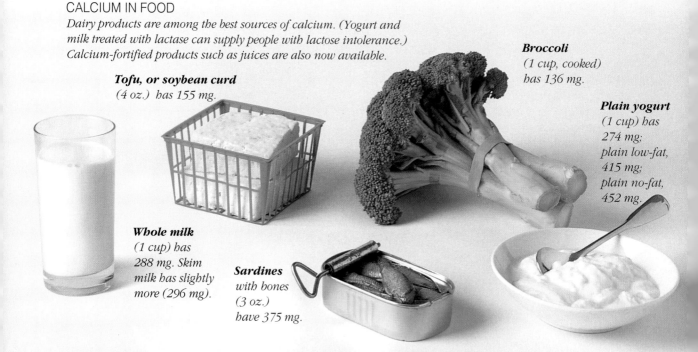

CALCIUM IN FOOD
Dairy products are among the best sources of calcium. (Yogurt and milk treated with lactase can supply people with lactose intolerance.) Calcium-fortified products such as juices are also now available.

Broccoli
(1 cup, cooked) has 136 mg.

Plain yogurt
(1 cup) has 274 mg; plain low-fat, 415 mg; plain no-fat, 452 mg.

Tofu, or soybean curd
(4 oz.) has 155 mg.

Whole milk
(1 cup) has 288 mg. Skim milk has slightly more (296 mg).

Sardines
with bones (3 oz.) have 375 mg.

In women, the hormone estrogen is important for calcium metabolism. After menopause, when the body stops producing estrogen, doctors often prescribe estrogen replacement therapy as well as calcium for those women who are at risk for osteoporosis.

A sedentary lifestyle can hinder the body's ability to absorb calcium. Regular weight-bearing exercise, such as walking and running, is essential for building and maintaining strong bones at any age (see Chapter 3).

. . . .

CALCIUM AND CHOLESTEROL

Whole-milk dairy products that are high in calcium are also high in fat. You can reduce fat by choosing lower-fat alternatives such as nonfat (skim) or 1 percent milk, nonfat or low-fat yogurt, part-skim-milk or low-fat cheeses, and frozen yogurt in place of ice cream. Low-fat dairy products have just as much calcium as the high-fat varieties, and in some cases, even more (see below).

A COMPARISON OF CALCIUM SUPPLEMENTS

Experts recommend food sources of calcium over supplements because foods often contain other nutrients that help your body to absorb the mineral. If you can't get as much calcium as you should through your diet, however, your doctor may suggest your taking a supplement.

Calcium carbonate is the least expensive supplement and contains the greatest amount of calcium. Several over-the-counter antacids are sodium-free calcium carbonate tablets (read the list of ingredients to make sure); these antacids can also serve as calcium supplements. In older people and those with decreased gastric acid, however, calcium carbonate tablets are not easily dissolved.

Calcium citrate is a good alternative. It has a lower percentage of calcium than calcium carbonate but is more easily absorbed—even with decreased stomach acid—and has fewer side effects. Calcium lactate and calcium gluconate are other alternatives,

but they contain less calcium.

Bone meal and dolomite supplements are not recommended; some have been found to be contaminated with lead and arsenic.

To test the solubility of a calcium pill (not a chewable one, however), drop it into a solution of $4\frac{1}{2}$ ounces water and $1\frac{1}{2}$ ounces vinegar, which is like stomach fluid in composition. Stir the solution periodically. After 30 minutes, the tablet should be at least 75 percent dissolved. If not, it probably won't dissolve in your stomach either and thus won't provide calcium to your body.

Supplements are best absorbed if you take them with meals that include milk or yogurt. And since only a certain amount of calcium can be absorbed at one time, spread out your dosage over your three meals

Although consuming an excessive amount of calcium is not a problem for most people, check with your doctor before taking a supplement.

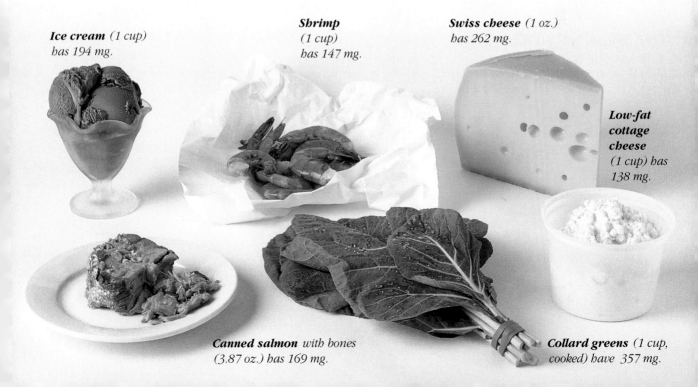

Ice cream (1 cup) *has 194 mg.*

Shrimp (1 cup) *has 147 mg.*

Swiss cheese (1 oz.) *has 262 mg.*

Low-fat cottage cheese (1 cup) has 138 mg.

Canned salmon with bones (3.87 oz.) has 169 mg.

Collard greens (1 cup, cooked) have 357 mg.

YOUR WEIGHT AND YOUR DIET

Obesity—usually defined as being more than 20 percent over your "ideal" weight—is a major risk factor in hypertension, heart disease, adult-onset diabetes, and certain cancers. It also puts extra stress on joints and bones, worsening osteoporosis and arthritis. Nevertheless, as many as a third of all Americans weigh more than they should.

WHAT SHOULD YOU WEIGH?

The weight that is healthiest for you depends on many factors, including your height, bone structure, and muscularity. Commonly used height-weight charts can sometimes be misleading. Muscle and bone are heavier than fat tissue; a football player could be considered obese according to a standard weight chart but actually have a low percentage of body fat because of his large frame and well-developed muscle mass.

On the other hand, an older and less active computer programmer might weigh what the chart suggests is ideal but have very little muscle. Falling within the normal range on the chart, she would actually be carrying too much body fat.

CHANGES THAT CREEP UP

Your basal metabolic rate (BMR)—the rate at which your body burns calories when it is completely at rest—drops about 2 percent per decade starting at age 20, particularly if you cut back on exercise. This means that every 10 years, you need to eat about 100 fewer calories a day just to maintain the same weight.

As middle age approaches, people often decrease their physical activity but keep their old eating habits. This generally results in more body fat in relation to muscle tissue. And because fat requires fewer calories to maintain than muscle does, when this happens, your calorie needs decrease even more. If you don't curb your eating, you gain weight.

THE PROS AND CONS OF GAINING WEIGHT AS YOU GROW OLDER

There is a continuing controversy among health professionals over whether putting on a few pounds as the years pass is unhealthy. According to the U.S. government's 1990 *Dietary Guidelines for Americans* (see chart), you need not worry about a few extra pounds.

Some studies have indicated that people who gain a pound a year have a lower death rate, while people who stay thin or lose weight as they age have a relatively high death rate. Other research suggests that women who gain a modest amount of weight with age seem to have a lower risk of osteoporosis.

Scientists who believe that staying thin is healthier argue that the studies cited above are flawed because they excluded heavier people who were sick as a result of their weight and included thin people who had lost weight because of illness.

A number of researchers who believe in maintaining a low weight for life say that there should be a return to the Metro-

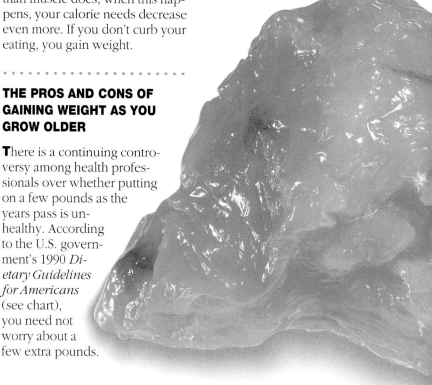

politan Life Insurance height-weight tables of 1959, which recommended lower "ideal" weights for everyone. They cite a study that indicated that thin men in general died at a lower rate of all causes than did heavier men.

Most experts on both sides of the controversy agree that your goal should be to avoid extremes at either end of the weight spectrum. Don't allow yourself to become obese, but don't diet excessively in an effort to stay very thin. Either extreme invites health problems.

A 3¾-pound blob of fat (shown in a life-size replica) dramatizes what carrying around just a few extra pounds really means to your body in heft and bulk.

HEALTHY WEIGHTS FOR ADULTS

The government recommendations for a healthy weight allow you to safely put on a few pounds after you pass age 34. The higher weights generally apply to men. (Heights are without shoes, and weights are without clothes.)

Height	Weight (in pounds)	
	Ages 19–34	Over age 34
5'0"	97–128	108–138
5'1"	101–132	111–143
5'2"	104–137	115–148
5'3"	107–141	119–152
5'4"	111–146	122–157
5'5"	114–150	126–162
5'6"	118–155	130–167
5'7"	121–160	134–172
5'8"	125–164	138–178
5'9"	129–169	142–183
5'10"	132–174	146–188
5'11"	136–179	151–194
6'0"	140–184	155–199
6'1"	144–189	159–205
6'2"	148–195	164–210
6'3"	152–200	168–216
6'4"	156–205	173–222
6'5"	160–211	177–228
6'6"	164–216	182–234

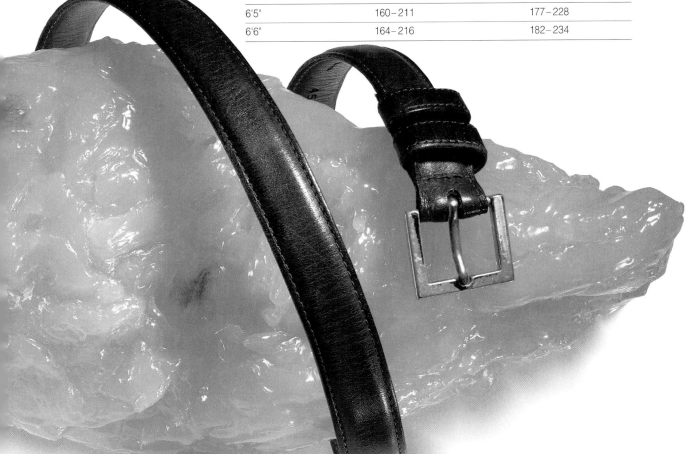

EASY WAYS TO CUT THE FAT

Basic strategies for lowering the amount of fat in the daily diet are listed on page 49. If you are trying to lose weight, however, you may want a few other low-fat tricks.

▩ Experiment with commercial no-fat versions of cottage cheese, sour cream, yogurt, and mayonnaise. With a few herbs, you can mix up a delicious dressing for baked potatoes and pasta or a dip for raw vegetables.
▩ Use nonstick pots and pans to minimize—and sometimes eliminate—your use of fat in cooking.
▩ Try balsamic or herbed vinegar alone on salads instead of an oil-based salad dressing.
▩ Avoid putting butter or mayonnaise on breads and rolls. Buy fresh loaves of bread from the bakery, such as whole grains and other flavorful varieties like pumpernickel and rye, which are tasty by themselves. Restrict spreads on sandwiches to various types of mustard.
▩ Choose low-fat bagels or pita bread over rich pastries like croissants and oversize muffins.
▩ Substitute broth for oil in homemade tomato sauce.
▩ Cook vegetables in broth instead of butter when you are making soups. Make a cool summer gazpacho by substituting tomato juice for the oil.

WHO NEEDS TO LOSE WEIGHT?

Experts offer a simple three-step method for determining whether or not you need to lose weight. First, ask yourself if you have, or are at risk for, a medical condition such as diabetes or high blood pressure that is aggravated by your being overweight.

Second, calculate how much of your body fat is located around your middle. To do this, measure around your waist at navel level, then measure your hips at their widest point. Divide the waist measure by the hip measure to get your "waist-to-hip ratio." A ratio of .95 or higher for a man or .80 or higher for a woman means you may need to lose weight.

Third, check your weight on the height-weight table on page 61. If you pass steps 1 and 2, you probably will fit within the range of healthy weights for your height and age.

FAT PATTERNS: MEN VS. WOMEN

Where your body stores fat helps to determine your healthy weight (see figure at right). It's generally believed that a broad-hipped woman can more safely gain a few extra pounds than a pot-bellied man.

In all adults, as the years go by, fat tends to shift from the arms, legs, face, and neck to the middle. Subcutaneous fat (just under the skin) relocates around the internal organs.

For men, gaining only 5 to 10 pounds can tip the balance toward poor health in those at risk for diabetes, with borderline high blood pressure, with high levels of triglycerides, or with low levels of high-density lipoproteins.

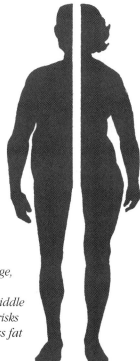

MEN
In most men, fat collects around the stomach, where it is associated with an increased risk of heart disease.

THE FAT TRAP
In both sexes, with age, extra fat starts to be stored around the middle of the body, but the risks in carrying the excess fat are greater for men.

WOMEN
In most women, fat collects on the hips and thighs, which seem to be safer areas for storing a few extra pounds.

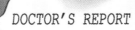

HEALTHY EATING
FOR A HEALTHY WEIGHT

The key to weight control is a low-fat diet, not calories per se. Fats provide 9 calories per gram, compared to 4 per gram for proteins and carbohydrates. And recent studies indicate that your body may more easily convert the fat in your diet to fat on your stomach, hips, and thighs than it does carbohydrates or proteins. A study at Harvard Medical School, involving 141 women, found virtually no link between calorie intake and body weight. Rather, excess weight was linked to the amount of fat in the women's diets.

Although the American Heart Association recommends that you derive no more than 30 percent of your daily calories from fat, a growing number of experts believe that figure should be closer to 10 or 20 percent—an effective but difficult way to lose weight.

CHANGING EATING BEHAVIOR

Experts agree that for weight to stay off, you must permanently change your eating habits. In other words, stop thinking "diet" and start thinking "healthy eating" for the rest of your life. To accomplish this, consider the following suggestions:

Set realistic goals for yourself. You don't have to become model thin. According to researchers at Harvard Medical School, losing as little as 10 percent of your body weight can improve blood pressure, cholesterol, and blood sugar levels.

Don't expect to lose a lot of weight fast. Experts typically recommend that you lose no more than a pound or two a week. If you lose weight too quickly, your metabolism may slow down. This is the body's way of conserving energy and maintaining fat stores. Researchers have also found that quick weight loss may cause gallstones to form.

Don't skip breakfast and lunch, then eat all your day's food in the evening. Skipping meals triggers a drop in the body's blood sugar and glycogen levels, which causes the brain to send out hunger signals.

Be aware of why you eat. Stress and anger are common eating triggers and can be addressed by exercise, relaxation techniques, or counseling.

Keep a diary of everything you eat (it's easy to underestimate).

Join a support group of people who are struggling with the same problems. They can provide emotional support and share practical tips on how to cope with the urge to eat.

THE ROLE OF EXERCISE

Exercise is an essential part of weight loss—and weight maintenance. Exercise not only burns calories but also builds muscle. And muscle requires more calories to maintain than fat. Muscle tissue is also more compact and, pound for pound, takes up less space, making you appear slimmer, even if the number on the scales stays the same.

Walking is an excellent exercise for burning calories. It's cheap, it's easy, and it's readily accessible (see pp.116–123).

"To lengthen thy life, lessen thy meals."

—*Benjamin Franklin*
in Poor Richard, *1733*

THEORIES OF OBESITY

Obesity results from a complex mix of factors ranging from a genetic predisposition for storing body fat to psychological problems. Recent animal studies identified a "fat" gene that promotes excessive weight gain. Experts don't know which factors are most important because each patient is different. But they do recognize that the condition is not, as many people believe, caused by simple lack of will power.

Researchers have proved that some people who are obese have a genetic tendency to use the food they eat more efficiently than most; as a result, they store more body fat. And their bodies are more likely to keep that fat.

Other people have a faulty mechanism for regulating their appetites, a function of the hypothalamus. They don't get their body's signal that they have had enough food.

In many obese people, the tendency toward overweight begins in childhood. A youngster who overeats may develop an excessive number of fat cells that he carries with him into adulthood. Even if he loses weight and the fat cells shrink, the same number of cells lie waiting to be filled with fat again.

DISTORTED PERCEPTIONS OF FOOD CONSUMPTION

Dieters who fail to lose weight are often accused of cheating. But new research at St. Luke's-Roosevelt Hospital in New York City shows that while some severely overweight people actually eat up to twice as much as they report, the deception is innocent. Underreporting often reflects a badly warped perception of serving size. A person may truly think he is eating a 1-ounce slice of cake, for example, when in fact, the serving is triple that. Such discrepancies, added up over time, translate into extra and, in the dieter's mind, completely unaccounted for pounds.

Doctors agree that having dieters weigh and measure their portions on a well-calibrated scale is the only way to correct their distorted perceptions of serving sizes.

A TALE OF TWO SHIPS

During a 6-month tour at sea, the 380-member crew of the destroyer U.S.S. *Scott* were a captive test group for the American Cancer Society's nutritional guidelines.

The sailors got 30 percent or less of their calories from fat and were encouraged to fill up on fruits, vegetables, and other high-fiber foods. Cold cereal with low-fat milk and fruit replaced fried eggs and home-fried potatoes for breakfast. At lunch and dinner, barbecued ribs gave way to leaner roast beef, vegetables were seasoned without butter, and fruits replaced richer desserts. The sailors could eat all they wanted, but fat was restricted, and alcohol was unavailable. They were encouraged to exercise during their free time. At the end of the tour, the *Scott* crew on average had lost nearly 12 pounds each and reduced their waist measurement 2 inches. The sailors' serum cholesterol rates were universally down. When questioned, more than half the *Scott* sailors said they liked the food aboard. In fact, 44 percent even said that they would follow a similar diet ashore.

Sailors on another destroyer, U.S.S. *Peterson,* acted as the control group in the experiment. They ate traditional Navy food during a similar 6-month tour of sea duty. At the end, the *Peterson* sailors had gained an average of 7 pounds, added 1½ inches to their waists, and experienced a general rise in blood cholesterol.

Doctors from the American Cancer Society felt the test proved that their eating guidelines were not difficult to implement or to follow. Some nutritionists, however, think the program is much harder for individuals to follow on their own.

COMMERCIAL WEIGHT-LOSS PROGRAMS

Americans spend more than $30 billion a year on commercial weight-loss programs. Why, then, are both dieters and obesity experts increasingly unhappy with these plans? A panel of experts convened by the National Institutes of Health in 1992 concluded that about 90 to 95 percent of dieters regain most or all of the weight they've lost within 5 years, a phenomenon called yo-yo dieting (see *The Issue of Yo-yo Dieting*, right). The dropout rate for some weight-loss programs is disturbingly high. In one study of obese people on a very-low-calorie liquid diet at a hospital, one-quarter of the dieters called it quits within the first 3 weeks.

But not everyone who signs up for a weight-loss program drops out or fails to lose weight. In a survey of its readers, *Consumer Reports* found that 25 percent of those who responded to a questionnaire had kept off most of the weight lost in a commercial program for 2 years.

There are several types of commercial diet programs available. Most include nutrition counseling, an exercise schedule, and behavior modification. Depending on the program you choose, the number of pounds you want to lose, and the amount of time you stick with it, costs range from several hundred to several thousand dollars.

Some programs offer daily individual counseling sessions, and dieters can choose between food provided by the program and specifically prescribed food they purchase themselves. Dieters are required to purchase packaged food in other programs; regular food is reintroduced gradually for

THE ISSUE OF YO-YO DIETING

Whether you choose a commercial program or go it alone, yo-yo dieting—losing weight only to regain it within a matter of months or even years—is a common occurrence. A long-term study of residents of Framingham, Massachusetts, found an increased incidence of heart disease and early death among people who repeatedly lost and regained weight compared to those whose weight remained stable. A more recent report of another long-term study, however, concluded that even a short-lived weight loss is preferable to uninterrupted obesity. Still, maintaining a stable ideal weight is the best course.

Researchers have found that significant weight loss may slow metabolism permanently. That may explain, in part, why people who repeatedly lose weight often regain it more quickly after each diet.

Another consequence of yo-yo dieting is that people who lose weight rapidly lose significant amounts of muscle tissue as well as fat. If they regain the weight, it is primarily fat, not muscle, so even if they ultimately return to their original weight, they are, in fact, "fatter" than before. What's more, this rebound weight tends to accumulate around the abdomen, which is associated with higher risks of heart disease and diabetes (see p.62).

weight maintenance only after the target number of pounds has been lost.

Other programs offer regular support-group meetings and emphasize long-term healthy eating habits. Doctors often refer patients to these programs.

Very-low-calorie diets are designed for people who are more than 20 to 30 percent above their ideal weight. The diets typically consist of liquids or powders available only through doctors or hospitals. Frequent medical ex-

ams are required. At some point, food is gradually reintroduced.

If you feel that a certain style of program is appropriate for you, try it. Statistics suggest, however, that the odds are not in your favor in the long run. That's why more and more experts are recommending that you learn to lose weight yourself by changing your basic eating habits. The plan most often recommended? A reduced-fat diet combined with regular exercise (see *Healthy Eating for a Healthy Weight*, p.63).

CAFFEINE:
THE INVIGORATING TONIC

America's most popular drug, caffeine wakes many people up, improves their mood, and increases their ability to concentrate. Only in excessive amounts does caffeine pose problems for most of the adults who depend on it.

HOW CAFFEINE WORKS

One of a group of compounds called methylxanthines, which stimulate the central nervous system, caffeine works by preventing the calming chemical adenosine from binding to nerve cell receptors in the brain. The result is increased mental alertness. The drug heightens the senses and quickens physical reaction time. It may also help to set the body's biological clock and, in susceptible people, prevent depression.

Caffeine, by constricting blood vessels in the brain, helps relieve migraine headaches and is included in some analgesics. In cold and allergy drugs, it offsets the drowsiness caused by antihistamines. It is also the active ingredient in over-the-counter pills to counteract sleepiness.

CAFFEINE AND HEALTH

Because caffeine is so widely consumed, it has been a target of intense medical scrutiny. So far, however, researchers have found little evidence that caffeine in moderate amounts causes any serious health problems.

Studies linking heavy coffee consumption with heart disease have been criticized for failing to also consider the effects of diet, exercise, and stress on the test subjects. And reports of elevated blood cholesterol among coffee drinkers have included

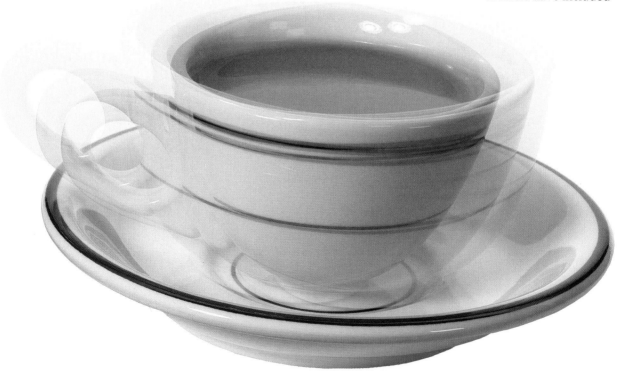

people who drank boiled, unfiltered coffee, which skewed the results. Research on filtered-coffee drinkers has found no significant increase in cholesterol. The only heart problem that has been definitely linked to caffeine intake is arrhythmia, or an irregular heartbeat. Doctors generally advise people with this condition to avoid caffeine.

Researchers have also found that if some hypertensive people exercise immediately after consuming caffeine, it can result in a temporary but dangerous rise in blood pressure. Hypertensive people may be wise to cut out caffeine altogether.

Caffeine was long thought to aggravate ulcers by increasing the production of gastric juices in the stomach and intestines, but it has been discovered that decaffeinated coffee has the same effect. Ulcer sufferers should avoid both kinds of coffee.

Doctors often advise the 10 to 20 percent of women who have painful lumpy fibrocystic breasts to limit or abstain from caffeine. Several studies, however, have failed to confirm a statistical link between caffeine intake and fibrocystic breasts.

Over the years, reports have occasionally linked caffeine with bladder, pancreatic, colon, and ovarian cancers. These studies have been criticized for not being properly designed or controlled. To date, no definitive link has been found between caffeine and cancer of any kind.

SIDE EFFECTS

Because caffeine keeps people awake, doctors often advise patients with insomnia to avoid it, especially within 2 to 3 hours of

SOURCES OF CAFFEINE

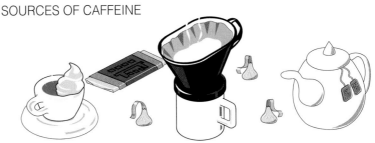

Coffee (5-oz. cup)	Caffeine (mg)
Regular, drip	60–180
Regular, percolated	40–170
Regular, instant	30–120
Decaffeinated, brewed	2–5
Decaffeinated, instant	1–5

Tea (5-oz. cup)	Caffeine (mg)
Brewed	20–50
Iced (12-oz. glass)	67–76
Instant	20–36

Chocolate	Caffeine (mg)
Baking chocolate (1 oz.)	26
Chocolate-flavored syrup (1 oz.)	4
Cocoa (5-oz. cup)	2–20
Milk chocolate (1 oz.)	1–15
Semisweet chocolate (1 oz.)	5–35

Soft drinks	Caffeine (mg)
Cola (12-oz. glass)	36–48
Cherry cola (12-oz. glass)	30–58

bedtime. Some people must stop drinking coffee as early as noon.

Too much caffeine can cause irritability, nervousness, frequent urination, and diarrhea in people who are especially sensitive to it. If you are on a medication, ask your doctor how much caffeine you can drink; it sometimes magnifies the effect of compounds that are similar to it, such as theophylline, an asthma drug.

CUTTING DOWN

Despite the scare stories and conflicting research, most doctors agree that moderate amounts of caffeine—the equivalent of two to three 6-ounce cups of coffee a day—pose no health risk for the average person. Tolerance for caffeine declines with age, however. If you are sensitive to caffeine, you may want to reduce your intake or eliminate it entirely to avoid unpleasant side effects as you grow older.

Cutting back on caffeine can trigger its own disagreeable side

effects. At Johns Hopkins Medical School, researchers recently proved that even those who drink only one to three cups of coffee a day can experience serious withdrawal symptoms, such as migraine-type headaches, fatigue, nausea, and muscle pain or stiffness, when they quit drinking coffee cold turkey.

The key to painless caffeine withdrawal is to taper off gradually. To cut back on coffee, try reducing your consumption by a half cup a day over the course of a week or two. If you usually drink from a large mug, switch to a coffee cup, which is smaller. You can also substitute decaffeinated beans for a part of your regular coffee in the coffee maker or try a cup of decaffeinated coffee for one of your morning breaks. Or try a cup of instant coffee—it contains less caffeine than freshly brewed.

Some people find it easier to switch to a less potent source of caffeine like tea. Remember to take into account other sources of caffeine as well (see chart above).

THE ROLE OF ALCOHOL IN A HEALTHY DIET

A highball before dinner, a beer at a picnic, a glass of wine with a meal provide pleasure to many people and, it appears, protection from heart disease. More than a drink or two a day, however, can lead to serious health problems (pp.196-199).

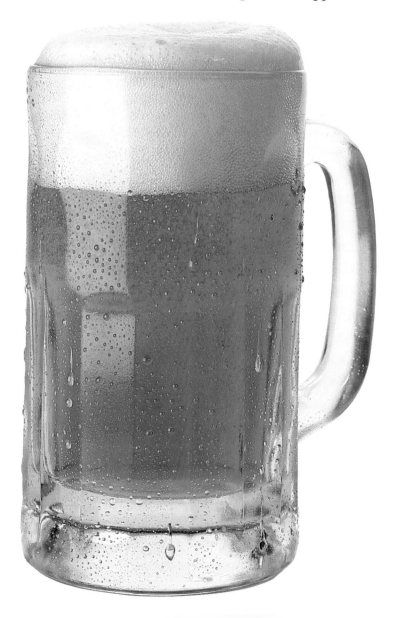

THE BENEFITS OF ALCOHOL IN MODERATION

Experts generally agree that for most adults, drinking in moderation—two drinks a day for men, one for women, and one for older people—is unlikely to cause harm. (A drink is generally defined as 12 ounces of beer, 4 to 5 ounces of wine, 3 ounces of sherry, or about 1 ounce of hard liquor.) In fact, a moderate level of drinking may actually have some benefits.

Researchers at Harvard's School of Public Health found that men who drank moderately had a 25 to 40 percent lower chance of developing heart disease than nondrinkers. The reason may be that alcohol consumed in modest amounts seems to boost levels of high-density lipoproteins, or HDL's, the "good" kind of cholesterol thought to help lower the risk of heart disease.

Other research has found a similar effect for women. One study indicated that post-menopausal women who drank moderately had higher levels of estrogen than nondrinkers. The hormone helps protect pre-menopausal women from heart disease and osteoporosis. A Harvard study, however, found that the benefits of drinking for women may be offset by statistics suggesting that even one drink a day may increase the risk for breast cancer in some women.

WHAT A PRUDENT DRINKER SHOULD KNOW BEFOREHAND

Because women have only about half as much of the enzyme that breaks down alcohol in the stomach as men, they feel the effects of alcohol more rapidly. Twice as much alcohol is absorbed directly into a woman's bloodstream.

How you react to alcohol depends on how strong your drink is. The alcohol concentration of a liquor, wine, or liqueur is described in terms of "proof." Divide the proof in half to get the percentage of alcohol in the drink. For example, whiskey that is 80 proof is actually 40 percent alcohol. Hard liquors, such as bourbon, gin, Scotch, vodka, and brandy, are 40 to 50 percent alcohol. Table wines are 10 to 14 percent alcohol. Most American beers are 4 percent alcohol; light beers are about 3 percent.

The carbon dioxide in sparkling wines and in the carbonated mixers used in some drinks speeds alcohol's absorption. Undiluted hard liquor is absorbed more quickly than wine or beer. You can slow the process somewhat, however, by eating some food high in protein or fat before you take your first drink.

. . . .

ALCOHOL AS A SOURCE OF EMPTY CALORIES

Technically, alcohol is a food because it supplies calories to the body—7 per gram. However, like sugar, alcohol has calories

BEHIND A BEER BELLY

The calories in beer or any other alcoholic drink aren't the only reason heavy drinkers develop paunches; evidently alcohol slows down the way your body disposes of the fat in your diet. Studying a group of young men, Swiss researchers discovered that imbibing alcohol actually slows the rate at which the body burns fat by about one-third. Whether the alcohol was added to their regular diets or substituted for part of their food allotment, the test subjects' bodies burned less fat when they consumed alcohol. On the other hand, the young men burned extra carbohydrates easily. The conclusion of the study director was that if you want to drink socially and not gain weight, you should substitute the calories in alcoholic drinks for fat calories.

HOW ALCOHOL AFFECTS YOU

The amount of alcohol in your blood determines your condition. In most states, a driver with a .1 concentration of blood alcohol is considered intoxicated.

Body Weight (pounds)	Percentage of Blood Alcohol Concentration Number of Drinks in 2 Hours				
	2	4	6	8	10
120	.06	.12	.19	.25	.31
140	.05	.11	.16	.21	.27
160	.05	.09	.14	.19	.23
180	.04	.08	.13	.17	.21
200	.04	.08	.11	.15	.19

Blood Alcohol Concentration	Effect
.05%	Relaxed state; judgment not as sharp.
.08%	Everyday stress lessened.
.10%	Movements and speech become clumsy.
.20%	Very drunk, loud, and difficult to understand; emotions unstable.
.40%	Difficult to wake up; incapable of voluntary action.
.50%	Coma and/or death.

that are empty, containing almost no vitamins, minerals, or other important nutrients.

Because alcohol typically provides between 75 and 120 calories per serving (mixed drinks may have even more), people who are trying to lose weight would be wise to pass up alcoholic drinks and concentrate on more nutritious foods. (Alcohol may, in fact, whet your appetite.) When you drink, try to see that the calories from the alcohol that you consume replace the fat calories in your day's diet (see *Behind a Beer Belly*, above).

FOOD ADDITIVES: BOON OR MENACE?

*S*ugar, salt, and corn sweeteners (in that order) by weight account for 93 percent of the food additives consumed by Americans. Baking soda, yeast, and flavorings make up nearly 7 percent. Controversial additives represent only a minute part of the total.

WHY ADDITIVES ARE USED

Additives are substances that don't occur naturally in foods. Food producers and manufacturers use them to improve nutritional value, preserve freshness, extend shelf life, provide consistency or texture, enhance flavor and appearance, and retain moisture and prevent caking.

Many of the foods you consume have vitamins added to replace those lost in processing. Others are fortified with extra vitamins and minerals to ensure against deficiencies; that's why vitamin D is added to milk, and iodine to salt.

Preservatives retard spoilage, prevent oils from becoming rancid, maintain color and flavor, and increase the safe edible life of perishable foods.

Emulsifiers, such as those in peanut butter, keep liquid particles mixed. Stabilizers and thickeners are used to create a particular texture in foods.

Flavors are the largest category of food additives and include vanilla, spices, seasonings, and artificial flavorings. Flavor enhancers, such as monosodium glutamate, modify the taste of food. Sweeteners include natural sugars and syrups and artificial sweeteners.

Coloring agents give foods the colors that you associate with them, such as green for mint and brown for hot dogs. Some coloring agents are natural food components, such as the carotene used to make some cheeses yellow, and others are synthetic.

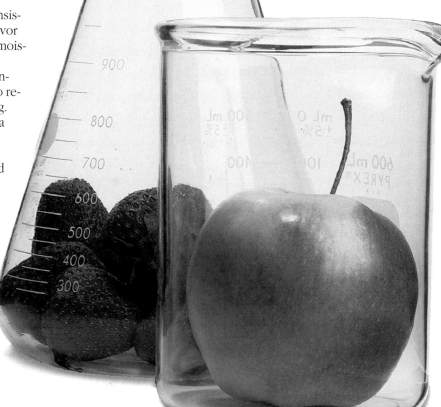

HOW ADDITIVES ARE REGULATED

In 1958, an amendment to the Food, Drug, and Cosmetic Act prohibited the use of any food additive that had been shown to cause cancer in animal or human studies. At the same time, however, about 700 "generally recognized as safe" (GRAS) additives were exempted from the amendment because they had been used for many years, presumably without any harmful effect. In recent years, the Food and Drug Administration (FDA) has been re-evaluating the GRAS list. Some GRAS additives have since been banned or their use restricted, and the review continues. The manufacturer of any new additive must prove its safety; the FDA reviews the tests and then sets guidelines for the additive's use.

. . . .

WHAT ARE THE CONCERNS?

The Food and Drug Administration maintains that most additives are safe and useful. It feels that bacterial contamination and nutrient deficiencies are of far greater concern than any potential health problems related to additives. The Committee on Diet and Health of the National Research Council concurs.

Other experts feel that certain additives are dangerous for some people and may be responsible for an array of health problems ranging from childhood hyperactivity to adult cancer (see *Suspect Additives,* right). They also argue that additives shown to be safe in animal studies may still prove to be harmful over the long term in human use. Potentially dangerous interactions among additives are another concern.

SUSPECT ADDITIVES

▪ *Artificial colorings.* Many food dyes have been banned by the FDA, including Red No. 2. Of the few certified (and numbered) artificial dyes that remain, all are suspected carcinogens, especially Red No. 3, used in maraschino cherries, pistachio nuts, and gelatins. The FDA has banned it for some purposes but is still studying other uses. Another popular dye, Yellow No. 5, can cause allergic reactions in some people.

▪ *Aspartame.* Most studies find no harmful effects from this artificial sweetener. Some scientists, however, have linked it to altered brain function and behavioral changes in people, and one study found an increased risk of brain tumors in rats given aspartame. Aspartame is dangerous for people with phenylketonuria (PKU) and for pregnant women.

▪ *BHT* (butylated hydroxytoluene) and *BHA* (butylated hydroxyanisole). These preservatives are used in vegetable oils, potato chips, and cereals. Although both are on the "generally recognized as safe," or GRAS, list, they are controversial. There is some evidence that BHT causes cancer in rats but also that it protects against disease. BHA has also produced conflicting reports. Both are under review by the FDA, but in the meantime, some companies have stopped using them.

▪ *Monosodium glutamate (MSG).* Many people are sensitive to MSG, the sodium salt of glutamic acid. It occurs naturally in many foods, such as cheese and tomato sauce, and is often used to enhance flavor, particularly in Asian cooking. In some people, too much MSG may cause headaches and tightness in the chest. Hydrolized vegetable protein (HVP) may also contain MSG.

▪ *Saccharin.* Another noncaloric sweetener, saccharin was linked to cancer in lab animals and was banned by the FDA in 1977. After a public uproar, Congress interceded and saccharin returned to the market. Today aspartame has replaced it in many foods, but saccharin, with a warning label, is still in use.

▪ *Sodium nitrite and sodium nitrate.* These chemicals inhibit the growth of the bacteria that cause botulism and are used for curing bacon and other processed meats. During frying and digestion, nitrate is converted to nitrite; nitrite combines with secondary amines to form cancer-causing nitrosamines. The U.S. Department of Agriculture, which regulates meat and poultry, has banned nitrate from most processed meats and reduced the level of nitrite permitted.

▪ *Sulfite.* The FDA has banned sulfite preservatives on fresh fruits and vegetables (except potatoes) because many people have adverse reactions to them, ranging from hives to breathing difficulties. Sulfites are still allowed in wine and beer to prevent the growth of molds and bacteria and in dried fruits to maintain moisture, but the label must indicate their presence.

A COMMONSENSE APPROACH TO FOOD ADDITIVES

Since neither the safety nor the benefits of all food additives has been clearly established, you may want to be conservative about the suspect additives (p.71) you consume. Concentrate on eating a healthy diet based on additive-free unprocessed foods, as described on pages 36–37. If you eat prepared and packaged foods, you can limit your exposure to any particular additive by eating a variety of them. Many foods that are particularly high in artificial colors and other questionable additives—cookies, potato chips, ice cream, and sodas, for example—are also high in calories, fats, sugar, and sodium. Such foods are of little nutritional value and ought to be eaten sparingly for that reason.

Read the ingredients list on food labels for the additives that you want to avoid and don't buy foods that include them. There may be safer alternatives on a nearby shelf.

FOOD CONTAMINANTS

Not all additives are put in food purposely; contaminants can enter crops through the ground, water, or air. Herbicides, insecticides, and fungicides, which are commonly used in farming, can remain on the food. Of particular concern are the organochlorine insecticides, which have caused cancer and birth defects in animal studies. These insecticides are stored in body fat and can accumulate to high levels over time. Organochlorines can remain in the soil and the water supply for 50 to 75 years. DDT, for example, was banned some years ago, but its residues are still found in food.

The Environmental Protection Agency sets tolerance levels for pesticide residue for each food type based on the safety of the pesticide and how much the average American eats of that food over the course of a lifetime. The FDA tests samples of foods for pesticide residues, but the tests can detect only about a third of the chemicals for which tolerance levels have been set. Also, some pesticides banned in the United States are still sold to other countries from which food is imported.

Some scientists believe that contaminant levels in the U.S. food supply are low enough for the body to detoxify. They point to the natural toxins in some foods. Sprouting potatoes, for example, contain solanine, which can cause digestive upset. Moldy nuts and grains may carry aflatoxins, carcinogenic mold by-products. The fiber and vitamins in these foods may protect the body against the poisons. Other scientists remain concerned about contaminants and the proven vulnerability of children to them.

· ·

PROTECTING YOURSELF AGAINST PESTICIDES

To reduce your exposure to pesticides, peel fresh fruits and vegetables or wash them in a mild solution of detergent and water.

GENETICALLY ENGINEERED FOOD

Genetic engineering involves altering an organism's characteristics by suppressing the action of a gene or by adding a gene from another plant or animal. Fruits and vegetables, from cantaloupes to cucumbers, have been genetically engineered to be more nutritious, tastier, and longer lasting, and pest-resistant genes have been introduced into some crops. More consistent yeasts have been created for fermenting beer and wine. Trout genes have been spliced into catfish to make them grow faster.

The FDA allows some bioengineered fruits and vegetables onto the market without pretesting and without a warning label. Foods in this category are those whose nutritional value hasn't been lowered, those that incorporate new substances that are already present in other foods, and those that haven't had new allergenic substances added (such as peanut oil, to which many people have severe allergies).

Only if the new genes in a food significantly change the amount of its important nutrients, form new substances, or create allergens are companies asked to consult voluntarily with the FDA before sending the new food to market. The new foods may still appear on grocery shelves, but the genetic changes must be spelled out on the label.

Look for organically grown produce, which should be free of pesticides as well as chemical fertilizers. Some states have very strict organic farming laws, but the term varies from state to state. Develop your own sources. Talk to the producers at a farmers' market about their growing methods or check around for a reputable health food store or organic farm stand. Organic produce may cost more and look less perfect than what is sold in supermarkets. Also, produce that isn't treated with wax and chemicals doesn't stay fresh as long as treated produce, so you will have to market more often and use up what you buy right away.

THE USE OF ANTIBIOTICS

For years, some scientists have encouraged a ban on the use of antibiotics in livestock feed. They are concerned that the drugs may promote the development of strains of infectious organisms that are resistant to the antibiotics now in use.

Some growers have responded and raise livestock without antibiotics. Their meat and poultry products are more expensive but can be found in most areas.

FOOD IRRADIATION

Like pasteurization, canning, or freezing, food irradiation is a method for preserving food. Food passes through a chamber containing radioactive cobalt-60 or cesium-137. The gamma rays destroy salmonella and other dangerous organisms found in meat and poultry, control insects and microorganisms in spices, fruits, and vegetables, and delay ripening of fruits and vegetables, thereby increasing their shelf life.

Advocates of irradiation contend that the process is a safe and effective way of eliminating harmful organisms in food. Critics charge, however, that irradiation may cause carcinogenic by-products, that it destroys a relatively high percentage of a food's nutrients, and that it threatens the environment. Environmentalists question the value of creating more atomic waste to protect the food supply when there are other, less hazardous methods for safeguarding what Americans eat.

The Food and Drug Administration has already approved the use of irradiation for poultry, pork, herbs and spices, wheat and wheat powder, and fresh produce such as strawberries and potatoes.

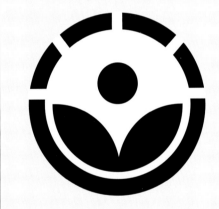

Whole foods such as fruits or meats that are irradiated must be labeled with the words "Treated With Radiation" and the logo at left. Prepared or packaged foods that contain irradiated ingredients and irradiated food sold in restaurants or schools don't have to be labeled.

FINDING SAFE MEAT, POULTRY, AND FISH

Look for meat and poultry from producers who don't use antibiotics in their feed. The label on the package will specifically say that no antibiotics were used. Find a reputable butcher who will answer your questions about the sources of his supply. If you can't be sure that meat or poultry is antibiotic-free, avoid organ meats, which contain the highest con-

centration of toxins. Remove any visible fat before cooking, since toxins accumulate in fat.

Despite pollution of rivers, lakes, and the ocean, the National Academy of Sciences says that fish and shellfish are safe to eat—if they are cooked. You should avoid all raw seafood.

To buy fish, find a reputable fish market that will tell you its

fish sources. Alternate between deep-water ocean fish, freshwater varieties, and farm-bred fish to limit contamination from a single source. Buy younger, smaller fish, which will have accumulated fewer toxins. Like other animals, fish retain pollutants in fat. Remove the skin and the fatty layer beneath it, as well as any other visible fat, before cooking a fish.

How Food Can Make You Sick

Even the most nutritious food can be dangerous to your health if it has become contaminated, was improperly handled, prepared, or stored— or if the food is one to which you have an allergy or an intolerance.

FOOD HANDLING AND PREPARATION

Never allow cooked food to touch uncooked food. If cooked fish is displayed alongside raw fish, don't buy it; bacteria may have spread from one to the other. Also, because raw eggs harbor bacteria, don't taste cake or cookie batter made with eggs or eat any foods, such as Caesar salads, that are prepared with raw eggs.

When cooking meat, use a meat thermometer to make sure that the internal temperature reaches at least 160°F, the point at which most food-borne bacteria are killed. Chicken should be cooked to a temperature of 180°F, or until all the juices run clear. Stuff poultry just before roasting to avoid bacterial contamination. Cook pork until it loses its pink color. Never reuse the liquid fat left over from frying bacon or sausage; such fat has been linked to an increased risk of cancer.

FOOD STORAGE

Refrigerate leftovers and other perishables promptly to prevent bacteria from multiplying. To ensure that your foods will cool evenly, don't overload the refrigerator or crowd items together.

When you freeze food, put it into several small containers, which can be frozen and thawed more safely and quickly than a large one. Thaw food in the refrigerator, the microwave, or in a plastic bag under cold running water, never at room temperature.

Discard meat that shows signs of mold. Hard salami is the only exception—cut away the moldy area and an inch around it. You can also cut away mold on hard cheese, but throw out moldy soft cheeses and milk products. Also dispose of moldy bread, cereal, grain products, or nuts.

Store bread, dry foods, and canned foods in a cool, dark, dry, and insect-free place. In hot weather, put the bread in the refrigerator. Throw away cans with rust, bulges, or leaks; they may be tainted with bacteria. Do the same if the cans have lumpy seams; these may have been soldered with lead, which can leach into food.

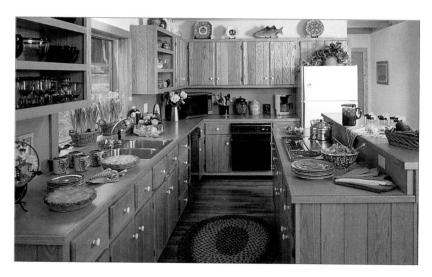

ENSURING FOOD SAFETY

Refrigerator. *Keep the temperature between 35° and 40°F; the freezer should be 0°F.*

Countertops and cutting boards. *The bacteria in meat and poultry can migrate to other foods via hands, utensils, cutting boards, and countertops; wash any of these that come in contact with food with hot, soapy water.*

Cabinets. *Clean your cabinets regularly; wait until they are completely dry to restock them.*

FOOD POISONING

More than 30 million Americans a year suffer from food poisoning. The primary cause is unrefrigerated meats and salads. Salmonella, the microorganism most often implicated in food poisoning, is found in undercooked meats, poultry, poultry stuffing, eggs, dairy products, and seafood from polluted waters. Recent outbreaks of *E. coli* infections have been traced to undercooked hamburgers and other contaminated meats. Other bacteria can be transmitted by food handlers and can also grow in foods kept on steam tables. (See *Food Poisoning Facts*, pp.256–257.)

Contaminated canned foods are the usual cause of botulism, a potentially fatal type of food poisoning. Onset is generally 12 to 48 hours after infection, but may be longer. Symptoms include impaired speech, headaches, double vision, difficulty in breathing and swallowing, and paralysis.

To prevent food poisoning, take the precautions described on these pages whenever you handle, prepare, and store food.

FOOD ALLERGIES

Any adverse reaction to perfectly good food is considered to be a food sensitivity, whether it is caused by a food allergy or by a food intolerance.

A true food allergy provokes an immune system response that produces the allergic reaction. This may vary in different people. The symptoms, which can occur at once but usually are delayed, may include diarrhea, abdominal pain, vomiting, hives, nasal congestion, asthma, and swelling of the eyes, lips, tongue, and throat.

Some people, however, may experience a more severe allergic reaction or even anaphylaxis, a life-threatening condition that causes difficulty in breathing, a rapid pulse, lowered blood pressure, heart irregularities, and shock. Anaphylaxis requires immediate emergency medical help.

Most food allergies are caused by cow's milk, legumes, wheat, eggs, and shellfish. Less common allergens include berries, chicken, corn, citrus fruits, fish, yeast, and Yellow Dye No. 5. The most practical way to treat a food allergy is to avoid the offending food.

FOOD INTOLERANCES

The symptoms of a food intolerance are similar to those of a food allergy, but the cause is entirely different: the lack of an enzyme needed to digest a specific food. As with allergies, the treatment for most intolerances is to avoid the foods that trigger the reaction.

Lactose—the sugar in milk—is the most common food that people can't digest. Symptoms of lactose intolerance include abdominal cramps, diarrhea, and flatulence. Many lactose-intolerant people can eat dairy products such as hard cheese, yogurt, and sour cream because the lactose in them has been partially predigested. They can also drink milk fortified with the enzyme lactase and use lactase drops or tablets with the dairy products they consume.

Other foods to which people may be intolerant include gluten (found in grains), tyramines (found in cheese and chocolate), broccoli, peas, and mushrooms. Some people are intolerant to food additives, such as sulfite, a preservative in wine, beer, champagne, and dried fruits.

FAST FACTS

■ A 6-ounce can of tuna has 800 milligrams of sodium. Rinsing the tuna in running water for 2 minutes can lower its sodium level by about 80 percent.

■ Honey, which has some minerals and B vitamins, is only slightly better for you than sugar. In addition, 1 tablespoon of honey has about 30 percent more calories than sugar does.

■ Wooden cutting boards get a clean bill of health from researchers at the University of Wisconsin, who contaminated both wood and plastic boards with the bacteria that can cause food poisoning. Within 3 minutes, the wooden boards became virtually germ free; the plastic boards, however, even after a thorough scrubbing with soap and water, still harbored bacteria.

■ To cool a hot pepper burn in your mouth, drink milk. The hot chemical in peppers is capsaicin, which binds to your taste buds. Casein, the principal protein in milk, washes away the fiery compound.

■ You would have to eat 32 cups of unbuttered air-popped popcorn to equal the calories in 1 cup of roasted peanuts.

DECODING FOOD LABELS

Thanks to the 1990 Nutrition Education and Labeling Act, food labels have become much more informative. The law, designed to make food labels less confusing and more reliable, addresses public concerns about healthy eating.

INGREDIENT LABELING AND HEALTH CLAIMS

The Food and Drug Administration (FDA) requires a list of all ingredients on the label of most packaged foods (the exceptions are spices and foods prepared in retail stores, such as potato salad and coleslaw). Ingredients should be listed in descending order by weight, from most to least.

Labels also must reveal if the product contains color additives or protein hydrolysates and give the percentage of juice in beverages that claim to contain fruit or vegetable juice.

Stated health benefits are now limited to well-established relationships, such as calcium's role in preventing osteoporosis or the benefit of fiber, fruits, and vegetables in preventing cancer and heart disease.

LABELING OF FRESH FOODS

Grocery stores, under a voluntary program, are asked to supply nutritional information for the 20 most common fresh fruits and the 20 most common fresh vegetables sold in the produce department, as well as for the 20 most common fresh fish offered for sale. As long as the information is near the food it describes, it can appear on shelves or in a poster or booklet.

The U.S. Department of Agriculture (USDA) is responsible for voluntary labeling on or near 45 cuts of raw meat and poultry in retail stores, as well as the mandatory labels—identical to the new FDA labels—on frozen and canned foods that contain meat or poultry in their ingredients.

GLOSSARY OF LABELING TERMS

The FDA now regulates many of the terms producers put on food labels. The following are common labeling terms and their official meanings.

■ *Calorie-free* foods have fewer than 5 calories a serving.

■ *Low-calorie* foods have 40 or fewer calories a serving.

■ *Reduced-calorie* foods have at least one-fourth fewer calories a serving than a comparison food.

■ *Light or "lite"* foods have at least one-third fewer calories in a serving than a comparison food, contain no more than half the fat in a serving of a comparison food, or have a light texture or color that is noted on the label.

■ *Cholesterol-free* foods have fewer than 2 milligrams of cholesterol in a serving and no more than 2 grams of saturated fat in a serving.

■ *Low-cholesterol* foods have no more than 20 milligrams of cholesterol or 2 grams of saturated fat in a serving.

■ *Reduced-cholesterol* foods have at least 25 percent less cholesterol and 2 grams or less saturated fat in a serving than a comparison food.

■ *Fat-free* foods have less than 0.5 gram of fat in a serving.

■ *Low-fat* foods have no more than 3 grams of fat in a serving.

■ *Low-saturated-fat* foods have 1 gram or less fat in a serving and not more than 15 percent of their calories from saturated fat.

■ *Reduced-fat* or *less-fat* foods have at least 25 percent less fat a serving than a comparison food.

■ *Reduced-saturated-fat* or *less-saturated-fat* foods have at least 25 percent less saturated fat a serving than a comparison food.

LOOKING AT A LABEL

The Nutrition Facts part of a typical food label (right) gives you all the information you need to design a healthy diet.

The FDA *has established a uniform serving size for many products based on commonly eaten portions rather than what the manufacturer specifies. Serving size is given in both household and metric measures.*

A breakdown *of the components in a healthy 2,000- and 2,500-calorie daily diet helps teach the basics of eating well. If you consume fewer calories a day, reduce the amounts of each component proportionately.*

Nutrition Facts

Serving Size ½ cup (114g)
Servings per Container 4

Amount per Serving		
Calories 90	Calories from Fat 30	
		% Daily Value*
Total Fat 3 g		**5**%
Saturated Fat 0 g		**0**%
Cholesterol 0 mg		**0**%
Sodium 300 mg		**13**%
Total Carbohydrate 13 g		**4**%
Dietary Fiber 3 g		**12**%
Sugars 3 g		
Protein 3 g		

Vitamin A	80%	Vitamin C	60%
Calcium	4%	Iron	4%

*Percent Daily Values are based on a 2,000-calorie diet. Your daily values may be higher or lower depending on your calorie needs:

		Calories	2,000	2,500
Total Fat	Less than		65 g	80 g
Sat. Fat	Less than		20 g	25 g
Cholesterol	Less than		300 mg	300 mg
Sodium	Less than		2,400 mg	2,400 mg
Total Carbohydrate			300 g	375 g
Dietary Fiber			25 g	30 g

Calories per Gram:
Fat 9   Carbohydrate 4   Protein 4

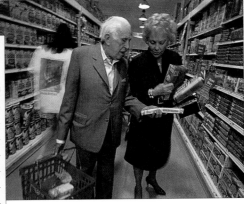

Some 70 percent of American shoppers read nutritional labels before buying a new food.

The calories from fat *figure helps you keep your fat intake to 30 percent or less of your daily calorie total.*

Daily Value *replaces the U.S. Recommended Daily Allowance for nutrients on labels. The Daily Value is the recommended daily intake of a nutrient, based on the National Research Council's Diet and Health Study (p.55). Percent Daily Value on food labels shows how a serving of a food fits into your overall daily diet. It is based on a daily diet of 2,000 or 2,500 calories.*

■ **High-fiber** food has at least 5 grams a serving.

■ **Good source of fiber** means a food has 2.5 to 4.9 grams of fiber a serving.

■ **More** or **added fiber** means a food has at least 2.5 grams more a serving than a comparison food.

■ **Sodium-free** or **salt-free** foods have fewer than 5 milligrams of sodium a serving.

■ **Very-low-sodium** foods have no more than 35 milligrams of sodium in a serving.

■ **Low-sodium** foods have no more than 140 milligrams of sodium in a serving.

■ **Reduced-sodium** or **less-sodium** foods have at least 25 percent less sodium in a serving than a comparison food.

■ **Unsalted foods** have no salt added during processing.

■ **Sugar-free** foods have less than 0.5 gram of sugar in a serving.

■ **Reduced sugar** or **less sugar** means a food has at least 25 percent less sugar in a serving than a comparison food.

■ **No added sugar** means that no sugar was added to the food during processing.

■ **Fresh** refers to raw foods that have not been cooked, preserved, or frozen.

■ **More** means that one serving provides at least 10 percent more of the recommended Daily Value of a nutrient than the comparison food.

■ **Good source** means that one serving provides 10 to 19 percent of the Daily Value of a nutrient.

■ **High** means that one serving provides at least 20 percent of the Daily Value of a nutrient.

■ **Lean** foods have fewer than 10 grams of fat, 4 grams of saturated fat, and 95 milligrams of cholesterol in a serving.

■ **Extra-lean** foods have fewer than 5 grams of fat, 2 grams of saturated fat, and 95 milligrams of cholesterol in a serving.

HOW TO BUY GOOD FOOD
AND HANDLE IT WELL

I t's not enough to pick the plumpest, freshest ear of corn or snag a bluefish just off the boat. How you store and prepare food is equally important in ensuring that you get the maximum nutrients from what you eat.

CHOOSING THE FINEST PRODUCE

Although many varieties of produce are available year round, it's still best to shop for produce in season. Fruits and vegetables that have traveled a long way have probably been picked before they were ripe—which means they will never reach their optimum flavor and nutrition—or they have been picked ripe and are past their prime by the time they reach the supermarket. The most nutri-tious and flavorful produce is frequently grown on local farms.

Choose fresh produce that appears to be at its peak, and buy only as much as you can use in a few days. If you can't shop often, buy frozen fruits and vegetables for later in the week. They generally contain more nutrients than less-than-fresh produce.

Pick small, young vegetables with good color. Choose bright orange carrots and dark-green leafy vegetables like spinach and collard greens. Select lettuce with crisp whole leaves; broken or limp leaves decay quickly.

Citrus fruits, melons, and pineapples should feel heavy for their size. Cantaloupes and strawberries should smell good. Look for peaches, nectarines, and plums that are firm but not hard, and berries that are brightly colored. Apples and pears should be firm and unbruised.

*A **wok** lets you sauté foods quickly with a minimum of oil.*

*A **fish poacher** cooks with no fat.*

*A **steamer** holds food above the water and prevents vitamin loss.*

*A **stove-top grill** allows convenient broiling.*

HANDLING PRODUCE

Scrub fruits and vegetables under cold running water with a vegetable brush just before you plan to use them. If you are concerned about pesticide residue, use a little dishwashing detergent, then rinse thoroughly.

Many of a vegetable's nutrients are concentrated in or just below the skin. Don't discard the outer leaves of cabbage, for example, which are higher in calcium, iron, and vitamin A than the pale inner leaves. In general, the leaves of vegetables are richer in nutrients than the stems. Broccoli leaves, for example, contain far more vitamin A for their weight than either the stalk or florets.

Make fruit or vegetable salads just before serving them. Exposed to air, cut-up fruits and vegetables lose some of their vitamins.

A pressure cooker speeds cooking times and preserves nutrients.

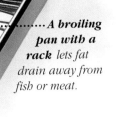

............*A broiling pan with a rack* lets fat drain away from fish or meat.

SELECTING MEAT, POULTRY, AND SEAFOOD

Look for a whitish-pink color in veal and a bright red color in beef or lamb. Legs and wings of poultry should spring back into place when pulled back. Bruised, rough, or dry skin on a chicken or turkey can indicate that the bird was improperly handled.

The smaller the cut of meat, the more perishable it is. If a chop or package of ground meat is not going to be used within a day or two after purchase, rewrap and freeze it until you're ready to cook it. Defrost it in the refrigerator overnight.

The protein content of meat or poultry remains intact even after lengthy cooking. Meat and poultry should reach a high enough internal temperature (check with a meat thermometer) to kill contaminants (see p.74, pp.256–257). Don't char, or blacken, meats, particularly over a charcoal fire; this increases the concentration of possible carcinogens.

Buy fish that is displayed unwrapped on ice. Fresh fish should not have a strong fishy or ammonia odor. Whole fish should have clear and bulging eyes, tight scales, and a light color. Gills should be bright red, and the flesh should feel firm when lightly pressed. Slimy-feeling fish is old or has been stored improperly. The edges of fillets should not be browned or curled.

Clams, oysters, and mussels should have tightly closed shells at the market, but discard any that don't open during cooking. Buy only live lobsters and crabs. Use fresh seafood within a day or two of buying it and keep it well chilled in the meanwhile.

Fish can be steamed, braised, broiled, fried, or microwaved, an especially easy and healthful method. Don't overcook it, which makes it tough and dry. For the best flavor, cook fish just until the flesh becomes opaque.

BUYING AND HANDLING EGGS AND DAIRY PRODUCTS

If you see cartons of eggs waiting to be refrigerated in the supermarket, don't buy them; unrefrigerated eggs spoil quickly. Select grade AA or A eggs that are clean and uncracked. Brown eggs are no more nutritious than white eggs; they are simply laid by a different breed of hen (and often cost more). Keep eggs in their carton in the refrigerator.

The nutritional value of eggs remains the same regardless of the way you cook them. You must, however, cook them long enough to destroy any salmonella bacteria that may be present, or until the yolk and white are no longer runny (no more 3-minute boiled and poached eggs or soft scrambled eggs).

If dairy product cartons—for milk, cottage cheese, or yogurt—are stacked up in the supermarket, select yours from the bottom. The cartons on top may not be properly cooled. Check the "sell by" date and pick the latest one.

When you buy milk, don't linger on your way home. Refrigerate it within 15 to 30 minutes. If milk in plastic containers is exposed to light for long periods of time, it can lose B vitamins; bag it in brown paper for the trip home.

RECIPES FOR HEALTHY MEALS

*L*ow-fat, high-fiber, nutritious cooking is neither difficult nor time-consuming. These meat dishes and the recipes on the following pages are as tasty as their richer versions and suggest ways you can adapt your own favorites to make them healthier.

LEAN BUT HEARTY BEEF STEW

PREPARATION TIME: 14 MIN.
COOKING TIME: 1 HR. 27 MIN.

1 pound boneless beef round, cut
 into ¾-inch cubes
3 tablespoons all-purpose flour
1 tablespoon olive or vegetable oil
1 large yellow onion, finely chopped
 (1 cup)
6 cloves garlic, slivered
1 cup water
4 all-purpose potatoes (1 pound),
 peeled and cut into ½-inch cubes
3 small carrots, peeled and sliced
 ½ inch thick (1¾ cups)

2 medium-size parsnips (6 ounces),
 peeled and sliced ½ inch thick
 (1 cup)
¾ cup canned crushed tomatoes
½ teaspoon each dried thyme,
 crumbled, and salt
2 cups cooked cannellini (white
 kidney beans) or navy beans

1. Preheat the oven to 350°F. On a sheet of wax paper or in a shallow pan, dredge the beef in the flour, shaking off the excess. In a 5-quart Dutch oven, heat the oil over moderate heat. Add the beef and cook, stirring frequently, for 5 minutes or until lightly browned all over.
2. Push the meat to one side of the pan. Add the onion and garlic and cook, stirring frequently, for 7 minutes or until the onion has softened. Add the water and bring the liquid to a boil. Transfer to the oven and bake, covered, for 30 minutes.
3. Stir in the potatoes, carrots, parsnips, tomatoes, thyme, and salt and bake, covered, 40 minutes longer or until the meat is tender. Stir in the beans and bake, uncovered, 5 minutes more or until heated through. Serves 4.

Per serving: Calories 473; Saturated Fat 2 g; Total Fat 9 g; Protein 37 g; Carbohydrate 62 g; Fiber 9 g; Sugar 7 g; Sodium 788 mg; Cholesterol 65 mg; Percent Calories From Fat 17. Percent Daily Values: Vitamin A 129; Vitamin C 48; Calcium 7; Iron 22

ONE-DISH MEAT LOAF DINNER

PREPARATION TIME: 8 MIN.
COOKING TIME: 1 HR.

1 large yellow onion
4 all-purpose potatoes (1 pound),
 peeled and cut into ½-inch cubes
1 medium-size carrot, peeled and
 sliced ½ inch thick (¾ cup)
¾ cup water
⅔ cup no-salt-added tomato sauce
1¼ pounds ground chicken
12 ounces lean ground beef
3 tablespoons plain dry bread
 crumbs
1 large egg white
½ teaspoon each mild chili powder
 and salt

1. Preheat the oven to 375°F. Cut ¾ of the onion into 1-inch chunks and finely chop the remainder.
2. In a 13" x 9" x 2" baking pan, combine the onion chunks, potatoes, carrot, and water. Bake, uncovered, for 20 minutes.
3. While the vegetables are baking, combine the chopped onion and tomato sauce in a 10-inch skillet. Cover and cook over low heat for 8 minutes or until the onion has softened.
4. In a large bowl, combine the chicken, beef, bread crumbs, egg white, chili powder, salt, and onion and tomato sauce mixture. Form into a 9- by 5-inch loaf and place on top of the baked vegetables. Bake 40 minutes longer or until cooked through. Serves 8.

Per serving: Calories 162; Saturated Fat 1 g; Total Fat 2 g; Protein 17 g; Carbohydrate 17 g; Fiber 2 g; Sugar 2 g; Sodium 227 mg; Cholesterol 50 mg; Percent Calories From Fat 13. Percent Daily Values: Vitamin A 26; Vitamin C 11; Calcium 2; Iron 6

PORK CHOP AND SWEET POTATO BAKE

PREPARATION TIME: 6 MIN.
COOKING TIME: 34 MIN.

*3 medium-size sweet potatoes
  (1 pound), peeled and thinly sliced*
2 cloves garlic, slivered
4 teaspoons olive oil
½ teaspoon salt
1 cup low-sodium chicken broth
½ teaspoon ground sage
¼ teaspoon sugar
¼ teaspoon black pepper
*4 loin pork chops, about ½ inch
  thick (5 ounces each)*
4 sprigs fresh sage (optional garnish)

1. Preheat the oven to 400°F. Arrange the sweet potatoes and garlic in a single layer in an 11- by 7-inch baking dish. Drizzle 2 tea- spoons of the oil over the pota- toes and sprinkle with ¼ tea- spoon of the salt. Add the broth and bake for 20 minutes.

2. In a small bowl, combine the sage, sugar, pepper and remain- ing salt and rub the mixture onto both sides of the pork chops. In a 12-inch nonstick skillet, heat the remaining 2 teaspoons of oil over moderately high heat. Add the chops and cook for 4 minutes or until browned on both sides.

3. Place the chops on top of the sweet potatoes and bake 10 min- utes longer or until the chops are cooked through and the sweet potatoes are tender. Garnish with fresh sage if desired. Serves 4.

Per serving: Calories 344; Sat- urated Fat 3 g; Total Fat 13 g; Protein 27 g; Carbohydrate 29 g; Fiber 3 g; Sugar 13 g; Sodium 366 mg; Cholesterol 71 mg; Percent Calories From Fat 34. Percent Daily Values: Vitamin A 248; Vitamin C 48; Calcium 4; Iron 10

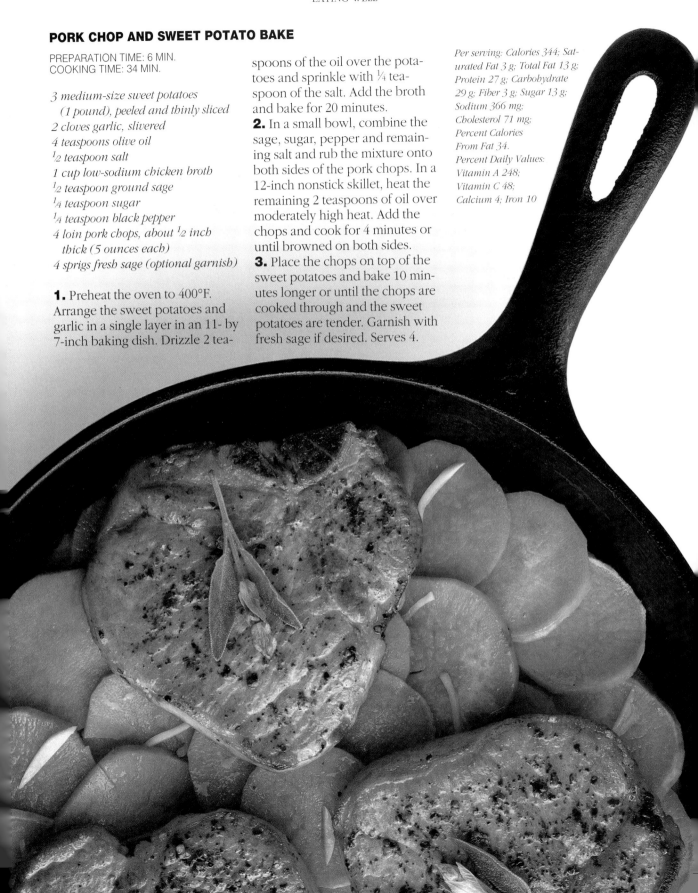

LEAN AND LUSCIOUS POULTRY

*I*f a recipe like the turkey legs (below) derives more than 30 percent of its calories from fat, compensate with lower-fat choices elsewhere in the day's menu.

OVEN-FRIED CHICKEN

PREPARATION TIME: 5 MIN.
MARINATING TIME: 1 HR.
COOKING TIME: 34 MIN.

CHICKEN

2 cups buttermilk, or 2 cups low-fat or skim milk mixed with 1 tablespoon plus 1 teaspoon lemon juice
¼ teaspoon each salt and black pepper
⅛ teaspoon each ground nutmeg and ground red pepper (cayenne)
1 whole broiler-fryer (3 pounds), cut into eight pieces and skinned
Nonstick cooking spray
½ cup all-purpose flour
1 tablespoon vegetable oil

GRAVY

2 tablespoons all-purpose flour
1 cup low-sodium chicken broth
½ cup evaporated skim milk
¼ teaspoon salt
¼ teaspoon black pepper

1. To prepare the chicken, in a large bowl, stir together the buttermilk, salt, black pepper, nutmeg, and ground red pepper. Add the chicken, turning to coat. Cover and refrigerate for 1 hour.
2. Preheat the oven to 425°F. Coat a jelly-roll pan with nonstick cooking spray. Remove the chicken from the milk mixture. In a shallow dish, dredge the chicken in the flour, shaking off the excess. Place the chicken in the prepared pan and drizzle with the oil. Bake for 25 minutes or until lightly browned, carefully turning the chicken pieces halfway through the cooking time. Transfer the chicken to a serving platter, reserving the pan drippings.
3. To prepare the gravy, pour 1 tablespoon of the pan drippings into an 8-inch skillet. Add the flour and cook over moderate heat, stirring constantly, for 4 minutes or until lightly browned. With a wire whisk, gradually stir in the chicken broth, evaporated milk, salt, and pepper. Cook, stirring frequently, for 5 minutes or until thickened. Spoon the gravy over the chicken. Serves 4.

Per serving: Calories 325; Saturated Fat 2 g; Total Fat 9 g; Protein 42 g; Carbohydrate 15 g; Fiber 0 g; Sugar 2 g; Sodium 389 mg; Cholesterol 121 mg; Percent Calories From Fat 27. Percent Daily Values: Vitamin A 4; Vitamin C 2; Calcium 13; Iron 10

TURKEY LEGS "OSSO BUCCO STYLE"

PREPARATION TIME: 8 MIN.
COOKING TIME: 1 HR. 17 MIN.

4 small or 2 large turkey legs (2½ pounds), skinned
2 tablespoons all-purpose flour
1 tablespoon olive oil
1¼ cups low-sodium chicken broth
1 large yellow onion, diced (1 cup)
1 small carrot, peeled and coarsely chopped (½ cup)
3 cloves garlic, slivered
½ cup orange juice
½ cup canned crushed tomatoes
¼ teaspoon each salt and black pepper

1. In a shallow dish, dredge the turkey legs in the flour, shaking off the excess. In a 12-inch nonstick skillet with an oven-safe or removable handle, heat 2 teaspoons of the oil over moderate heat. Add the turkey and cook, turning frequently, for 5 minutes or until browned on all sides. Remove the turkey legs from the skillet; set aside.
2. Preheat the oven to 350°F. Add the remaining 1 teaspoon of oil to the skillet and reduce the heat to low. Add ¼ cup of the broth and the onion and cook, stirring occasionally, for 7 minutes or until the onion is soft. Stir in the carrot and garlic and cook 5 minutes longer. Add the orange juice, tomatoes, remaining broth, salt, pepper, and turkey legs. Bring the liquid to a boil. Transfer to the oven and bake, covered, for 1 hour or until the turkey is tender. If using large turkey legs, remove the meat from the bone before serving. Serves 4.

Per serving: Calories 253; Saturated Fat 2 g; Total Fat 9 g; Protein 28 g; Carbohydrate 13 g; Fiber 2 g; Sugar 6 g; Sodium 384 mg; Cholesterol 88 mg; Percent Calories From Fat 34. Percent Daily Values: Vitamin A 40; Vitamin C 41; Calcium 3; Iron 18

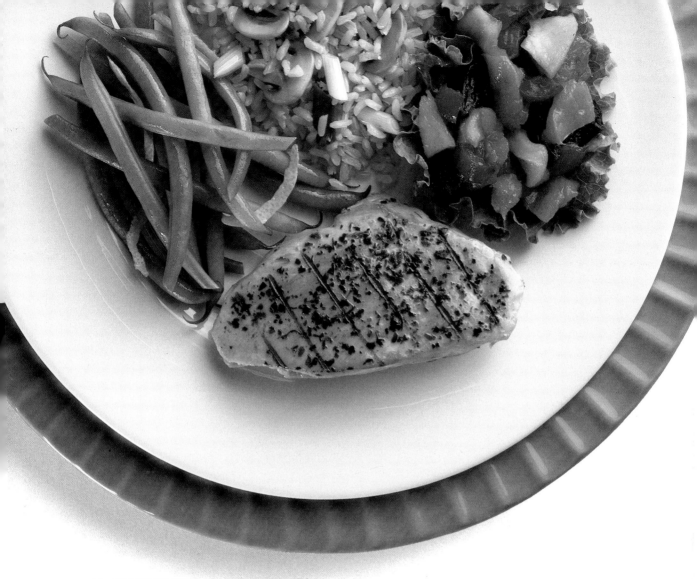

GRILLED CHICKEN WITH FRUIT CHUTNEY

PREPARATION TIME: 8 MIN.
COOKING TIME: 25 MIN.

CHUTNEY

*1 medium-size sweet red pepper,
  cored, seeded, and diced (¾ cup)*
1 small yellow onion, diced (¾ cup)
½ cup cider vinegar
*8 ounces mixed dried fruit, coarsely
  chopped (2 cups)*
¼ cup apple cider or juice
3 tablespoons sugar
½ teaspoon ground ginger
1 teaspoon prepared mustard

CHICKEN

1¼ teaspoons dried oregano, crumbled
½ teaspoon salt

½ teaspoon sugar
⅛ teaspoon black pepper
*3 whole skinned and boned chicken
  breasts (1½ pounds), halved*

1. To prepare the chutney, in a medium-size saucepan, combine the red pepper, onion, and vinegar and bring to a boil. Reduce the heat and cook for 3 minutes. Stir in the fruit, cider, sugar, and ginger. Reduce the heat to low; simmer, covered, for 15 minutes. Remove from the heat and stir in the mustard. Serve warm or transfer to a container, cover, and refrigerate until chilled.

2. To prepare the chicken, preheat the broiler, setting the rack 7 inches from the heat. Combine the oregano, salt, sugar, and pepper and rub it onto both sides of the chicken. Arrange the chicken in a broiler pan. Broil for 4 minutes. Turn and broil 3 minutes longer or until the chicken is cooked through. Serves 6.

*Per serving: Calories 264; Saturated Fat
(trace); Total Fat 2 g; Protein 28 g;
Carbohydrate 38 g; Fiber 3 g; Sugar 27 g;
Sodium 267 mg; Cholesterol 66 mg;
Percent Calories From Fat 5.
Percent Daily Values: Vitamin A 11;
Vitamin C 25; Calcium 4; Iron 10*

HEARTY BASICS: RICE AND BEANS

*L**ean meat and beans or beans alone can make satisfying, stick-to-the-ribs eating well within your daily quota of fat. A surprisingly low-fat risotto can be as creamy and rich tasting as the classic Italian version of this rice dish.*

CHUNKY PORK AND BEANS

PREPARATION TIME: 8 MIN.
COOKING TIME: 1 HR. 5 MIN.

*1 pound boneless lean pork, cut into
    ¾-inch chunks
2 tablespoons all-purpose flour
1 tablespoon vegetable oil
1 large yellow onion, chopped (1¼
    cups)
2 small carrots, peeled and thinly
    sliced (¾ cup)
4 cloves garlic, crushed
1 cup water
½ cup canned crushed tomatoes
1 tablespoon plus 1 teaspoon
    molasses
2 teaspoons cider vinegar
½ teaspoon each ground ginger,
    dried oregano, crumbled, and salt
2 cups cooked cannellini (white
    kidney beans) or pinto beans*

1. Preheat the oven to 350°F. On a sheet of wax paper or in a shallow pan, dredge the pork in the flour, shaking off the excess.
2. In a 5-quart Dutch oven, heat the oil over moderately high heat. Add the pork and cook for 5 minutes or until browned on all sides. Reduce the heat to moderate. Stir in the onion, carrots, and garlic and cook, stirring occasionally, for 5 minutes or until the vegetables have softened.
3. Stir in the water, tomatoes, molasses, vinegar, ginger, oregano, and salt. Bring the liquid to a boil and remove from the heat. Cover the Dutch oven and place it in the middle of the oven. Bake for 50 minutes or until the meat is tender. Stir in the beans and bake, uncovered, 5 minutes longer or until the beans are heated through. Serves 4.

Per serving: Calories 367; Saturated Fat 3 g; Total Fat 12 g; Protein 33 g; Carbohydrate 31 g; Fiber 5 g; Sugar 8 g; Sodium 763 mg; Cholesterol 71 mg; Percent Calories From Fat 30. Percent Daily Values: Vitamin A 78; Vitamin C 18; Calcium 4; Iron 10

BLACK BEAN CHILI

PREPARATION TIME: 6 MIN.
COOKING TIME: 28 MIN.

*1 tablespoon olive oil
1 medium-size green pepper, cored,
    seeded, and diced (¾ cup)
8 green onions, including tops,
    thinly sliced (1 cup)
3 cloves garlic, minced
¾ teaspoon minced canned jalapeño
    pepper or ½ teaspoon hot red
    pepper sauce
¾ cup bulgur
1½ cups water
½ teaspoon each salt, dried oregano,
    crumbled, and chili powder
3½ cups cooked black beans
3 tablespoons chopped parsley
2 tablespoons lime juice*

1. In a large saucepan or 5-quart Dutch oven, heat the oil over low heat. Add the green pepper and cook, stirring occasionally, for 5 minutes or until the pepper has softened. Add the green onions, garlic, and jalapeño pepper and cook 2 minutes longer. Add the bulgur, stirring to coat.
2. Stir in the water, salt, oregano, and chili powder and bring to a boil. Reduce the heat to a simmer and cook, covered, for 20 minutes or until the bulgur is tender. Stir in the black beans, parsley, and lime juice and cook, stirring frequently, until heated through. Serves 4.

Per serving: Calories 332; Saturated Fat 1 g; Total Fat 5 g; Protein 17 g; Carbohydrate 59 g; Fiber 13 g; Sugar 1 g; Sodium 285 mg; Cholesterol 0 mg; Percent Calories From Fat 12. Percent Daily Values: Vitamin A 8; Vitamin C 45; Calcium 7; Iron 22

SEAFOOD RISOTTO WITH ASPARAGUS

PREPARATION TIME: 5 MIN.
COOKING TIME: 46 MIN.

1 teaspoon olive oil
1 large yellow onion, finely chopped
   (1 cup)
1 medium-size sweet red pepper,
   cored, seeded, and diced (¾ cup)
2¼ cups water
1¼ cups long-grain rice
⅔ cup dry white wine
1 bottle (8 ounces) clam broth
8 ounces asparagus spears,
   trimmed, peeled, and cut in
   1½-inch pieces (1¼ cups), or
   thawed frozen spears
1 tablespoon unsalted butter
12 ounces raw or cooked shrimp,
   shelled and deveined, or 1 can

(14½ ounces) salmon, flaked
2 tablespoons chopped parsley
¼ teaspoon freshly ground pepper

1. Heat the oil in a large
saucepan over moderately low
heat. Add the onion, red pepper,
and ⅓ cup of the water and cook,
uncovered, stirring occasionally,
until the onion is very soft—12 to
15 minutes. Add the rice, stir to
coat, and add ⅓ cup of the wine.
Cook, stirring, until the wine has
been absorbed—about 2 minutes.
Add the remaining wine and cook
until it has been absorbed.
2. Combine the remaining water
and the clam broth and add ⅓ cup

to the rice. Stir frequently, keeping the mixture at a simmer, until
all of the liquid has been absorbed—about 3 minutes. Continue adding the liquid ⅓ cup at a
time until just 1½ cups remain.
3. Add the asparagus and, if using, the raw shrimp. Continue
adding the broth ⅓ cup at a time,
stirring frequently, until almost all
of the liquid has been absorbed
and the rice is creamy and tender—12 to 14 minutes more. Stir
in the butter, parsley, black pepper, and, if using, the cooked
shrimp or salmon. Cook until all
the ingredients are heated
through. Serves 4.

*Per serving: Calories 399; Saturated Fat 2 g;
Total Fat 6 g; Protein 24 g; Carbohydrate
54 g; Fiber 2 g; Sugar 3 g; Sodium 274 mg;
Cholesterol 139 mg; Percent Calories
From Fat 14. Percent Daily Values:
Vitamin A 8; Vitamin C 38;
Calcium 9; Iron 30*

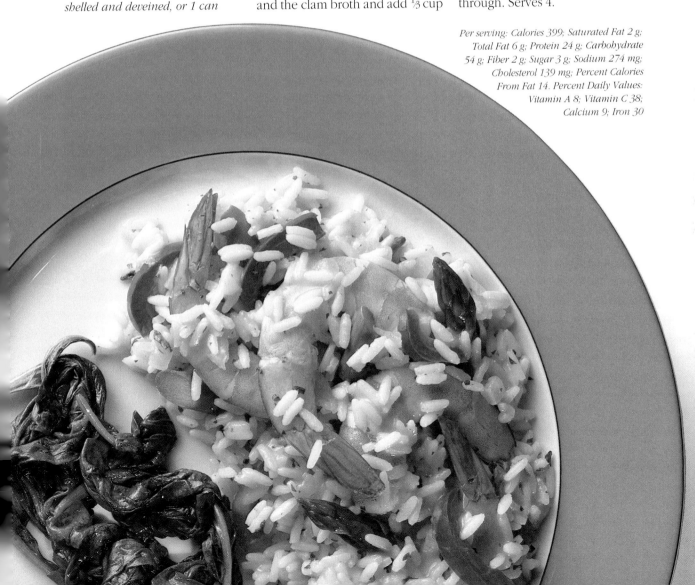

SAUCY LOW-FAT PASTAS

· ·

Macaroni and noodles, nourishing and filling by themselves, have gotten a bad reputation because of the rich sauces that often accompany them. These dishes suggest delicious low-fat ways you can serve pasta for wholesome eating.

FETTUCCINE WITH CREAMY BROCCOLI SAUCE

PREPARATION TIME: 5 MIN.
COOKING TIME: 15 MIN.

2 cups broccoli florets (1 medium-
    size head)
8 ounces fettuccine or spaghetti
2½ cups skim or low-fat milk
3 tablespoons all-purpose flour
4 cloves garlic, minced
¼ teaspoon each salt and black
    pepper
2 tablespoons reduced-calorie sour

cream, at room temperature
¼ cup grated Parmesan cheese

1. Bring a large saucepan of water to a rolling boil over high heat. Add the broccoli and cook for 2 minutes or until crisp-tender. With a slotted spoon, remove the broccoli from the saucepan, reserving the water. Set the cooked broccoli aside.

2. Cook the pasta in the reserved water for 8 minutes or until tender but still firm to the bite. Drain.
3. While the pasta is cooking, whisk together the milk, flour, garlic, salt, and pepper in a 12-inch skillet. Cook over moderate heat, stirring frequently, for 5 minutes or until the sauce is slightly thickened. Stir in the broccoli. Remove the skillet from the heat and stir in the sour cream and Parmesan cheese.
4. Add the cooked pasta to the broccoli sauce and toss well to coat. Serves 4.

Per serving: Calories 342; Saturated Fat 3 g; Total Fat 5 g; Protein 17 g; Carbohydrate 58 g; Fiber 1 g; Sugar 8 g; Sodium 353 mg; Cholesterol 7 mg; Percent Calories From Fat 12. Percent Daily Values: Vitamin A 17; Vitamin C 72; Calcium 31; Iron 18

· ·

EGGPLANT AND MUSHROOM LASAGNE

PREPARATION TIME: 12 MIN.
COOKING TIME: 35 MIN.

1 tablespoon olive oil
1 can (16 ounces) no-salt-added
    tomato sauce
½ cup water
1 large eggplant, peeled, halved
    lengthwise, then sliced ½ inch
    thick
2 cups low-fat (1% milkfat) milk
3 tablespoons all-purpose flour
¼ teaspoon each salt and black
    pepper
⅛ teaspoon ground nutmeg
8 ounces (9 sheets) lasagne noodles,
    cooked according to package
    directions
6 ounces mushrooms, sliced
    (1½ cups)
6 tablespoons grated Parmesan
    cheese

1. Preheat the oven to 450°F. Lightly grease an 11- by 7-inch baking dish. In a small bowl, whisk together the oil, ⅓ cup of the tomato sauce, and the water. Arrange the eggplant slices in a single layer in a jelly-roll pan and top with the sauce mixture. Cover the pan with aluminum foil and bake for 10 minutes or until the eggplant is tender.
2. In a medium-size saucepan, using a wire whisk, combine the milk and flour. Cook over moderate heat, stirring frequently, for 5 minutes or until the sauce is thickened and smooth. Stir in the salt, pepper, and nutmeg.
3. Spoon 2 tablespoons of the remaining tomato sauce over the bottom of the prepared dish. Lay

3 lasagne noodles over the sauce, then top with half of the baked eggplant, half of the mushrooms, ⅓ of the white sauce, and half of the remaining tomato sauce. Sprinkle with 2 tablespoons of the Parmesan cheese. Repeat layers.
4. Top the layers with the remaining 3 lasagne noodles. Spoon the remaining white sauce over the noodles and sprinkle with the remaining Parmesan cheese. Bake for 20 minutes or until the top is golden and the mixture is bubbling. Serves 6.

Per serving: Calories 195; Saturated Fat 2 g; Total Fat 5 g; Protein 10 g; Carbohydrate 26 g; Fiber 2 g; Sugar 4 g; Sodium 275 mg; Cholesterol 21 mg; Percent Calories From Fat 25. Percent Daily Values: Vitamin A 7; Vitamin C 5; Calcium 21; Iron 6

PASTA SALAD NIÇOISE

PREPARATION TIME: 8 MIN.
COOKING TIME: 13 MIN.

½ cup low-sodium chicken broth
¼ cup minced parsley
3 tablespoons red wine vinegar
1 tablespoon olive oil
1 teaspoon prepared mustard
8 ounces green beans, trimmed
*   (2 cups)*
6 ounces medium-size pasta
*   shells, rotini, penne, bow-*
*   ties, or wagon wheels*
2 cans (6½ ounces each)
*   tuna in water, drained,*
*   rinsed, drained again,*
*   and flaked*
6 ounces mushrooms,
*   trimmed and quartered*
*   (2¼ cups)*
6 ounces cherry
*   tomatoes (1 cup)*
½ cup thinly sliced red
*   onion*
¼ cup pitted black olives,
*   sliced*

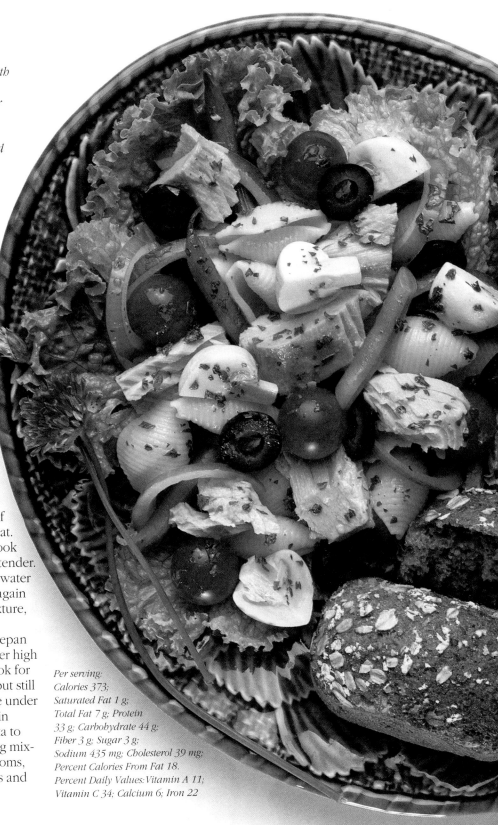

1. In a large serving dish or salad bowl, combine the chicken broth, parsley, vinegar, oil, and mustard to make a dressing; set aside.

2. Bring a large saucepan of water to a boil over high heat. Add the green beans and cook for 3 minutes or until crisp-tender. Drain and rinse under cold water to stop the cooking. Drain again and add to the dressing mixture, tossing to coat.

3. Bring another large saucepan of water to a rolling boil over high heat, add the pasta, and cook for 10 minutes or until tender but still firm to the bite. Drain, rinse under cold water to cool, and drain again. Add the cooked pasta to the green bean and dressing mixture. Add the tuna, mushrooms, tomatoes, onion, and olives and toss well. Serves 4.

Per serving:
Calories 373;
Saturated Fat 1 g;
Total Fat 7 g; Protein
33 g; Carbohydrate 44 g;
Fiber 3 g; Sugar 3 g;
Sodium 435 mg; Cholesterol 39 mg;
Percent Calories From Fat 18.
Percent Daily Values: Vitamin A 11;
Vitamin C 34; Calcium 6; Iron 22

MAIN COURSE VEGETABLE DISHES

*N*o longer relegated to the side, vegetables now join fruits and grains at center stage on many menus. These recipes—with the addition of some crisp bread, a salad, and some fresh fruit for dessert—make tasty, wholesome, and filling meals.

CABBAGE AND CARROT SOUP WITH DILL

PREPARATION TIME: 15 MIN.
COOKING TIME: 42 MIN.

2 teaspoons olive oil
1 medium-size yellow onion, chopped (1½ cups)
3 cloves garlic, minced
3 cups water
1 medium-size head green or savoy cabbage, cored and cut into 2-inch chunks (10 cups)
4 cups low-sodium chicken broth
1 smoked ham hock (12 ounces)
1 can (11½ ounces) mixed vegetable juice
2 small carrots, peeled and thinly sliced (¾ cup)
½ cup canned crushed tomatoes
½ teaspoon dried marjoram, crumbled
¼ cup snipped dill or minced parsley
½ cup plain low-fat yogurt or light sour cream (optional)

1. In a stockpot or 5-quart Dutch oven, heat the oil over moderately low heat. Add the onion and garlic and cook, stirring occasionally, for 7 minutes or until the onion has softened, gradually adding 2 tablespoons of the water while cooking to prevent sticking.
2. Stir in the cabbage and cook, covered, for 5 minutes. Stir in the broth, ham hock, vegetable juice, car-rots, tomatoes, marjoram, and remaining water and bring the liquid to a boil. Reduce the heat and simmer, covered, for 30 minutes. Remove the ham meat from the bone and return the meat to the soup, discarding the bone. Stir in the dill or parsley and serve each portion with a tablespoon of the yogurt or sour cream if desired. Makes eight 1½-cup servings.

Per serving: Calories 121; Saturated Fat 1 g; Total Fat 4 g; Protein 11 g; Carbohydrate 13 g; Fiber 3 g; Sugar 6 g; Sodium 656 mg; Cholesterol 19 mg; Percent Calories From Fat 26. Percent Daily Values: Vitamin A 46; Vitamin C 115; Calcium 7; Iron 10

VEGETABLE PIZZA

PREPARATION TIME: 8 MIN.
COOKING TIME: 20 MIN.

1 medium-size zucchini (10 ounces), thinly sliced
8 ounces mushrooms, sliced (2 cups)
1 small yellow squash (6 ounces), thinly sliced
1 small red onion, sliced
¼ cup water
2 cloves garlic, minced
½ teaspoon each salt, dried oregano, and dried basil, crumbled
1 tablespoon olive oil
1 can (16 ounces) no-salt-added tomato sauce
1 cup shredded part-skim mozzarella cheese (1 cup)

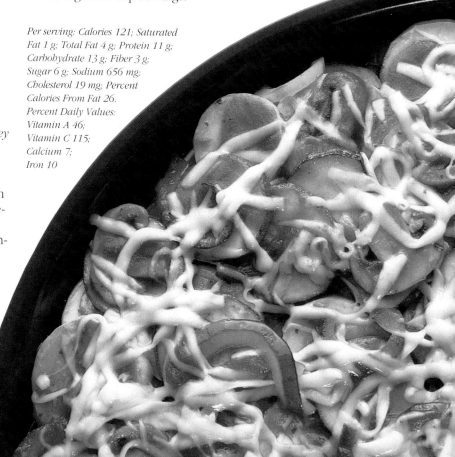

1. Preheat the oven to 450°F. In a large bowl, combine the zucchini, mushrooms, yellow squash, onion, water, garlic, salt, oregano, basil, and oil. Transfer to a 10-inch round or 9" x 9" x 2" baking pan, cover with aluminum foil, and bake for 10 minutes.

2. Spoon the tomato sauce over the vegetables and bake, uncovered, 5 minutes longer. Sprinkle with the cheese and bake 5 minutes or until the cheese is melted. Serves 4.

Per serving: Calories 189;
Saturated Fat 3 g; Total Fat 8 g;
Protein 12 g; Carbohydrate 19 g;
Fiber 4 g; Sugar 3 g; Sodium 437 mg;
Cholesterol 16 mg;
Percent Calories From Fat 38.
Percent Daily Values:
Vitamin A 9; Vitamin C 21;
Calcium 22; Iron 7

CRUSTLESS POTATO AND CHEESE PIE

PREPARATION TIME: 6 MIN.
COOKING TIME: 37 MIN.

Nonstick cooking spray
2 tablespoons plain dry bread crumbs
5 medium-size all-purpose potatoes
  (1¾ pounds), peeled and cubed
1 container (16 ounces) low-fat
  (1% milkfat) cottage cheese or
  part-skim ricotta cheese
2 large eggs
1 large egg white
2 tablespoons grated Parmesan
  cheese
2 tablespoons chopped parsley
¼ teaspoon salt
½ teaspoon black pepper
1 large sweet red pepper, cored,
  seeded, and diced (1 cup), or
  2 pimientos, diced
3 green onions, including tops,
  sliced (⅓ cup)

1. Preheat the oven to 400°F. Lightly coat a 9-inch round pan with nonstick cooking spray. Dust with bread crumbs; set aside.

2. Bring a large saucepan of water to a boil over high heat, then add the potatoes. When the water returns to a boil, cook the potatoes 6 to 7 minutes or until tender. Drain the potatoes and rice or mash them until smooth.

3. In a food processor or blender, whirl the cottage or ricotta cheese for 1 minute or until very smooth and creamy. Add the potatoes, eggs, egg white, Parmesan cheese, parsley, salt, and black pepper and whirl until well combined. Transfer to a large bowl and stir in the red pepper or pimientos and the green onions.

4. Pour into the prepared pan and bake for 30 minutes or until a toothpick inserted in the center comes out clean. Let cool for 10 minutes. With a spatula, loosen the edges of the pie, then invert onto a serving platter. Serves 4.

Per serving: Calories 331; Saturated Fat 2 g;
Total Fat 5 g; Protein 23 g; Carbohydrate 47 g;
Fiber 3 g; Sugar 7 g; Sodium 732 mg;
Cholesterol 114 mg; Percent Calories
From Fat 11. Percent Daily Values:
Vitamin A 11; Vitamin C 64;
Calcium 15; Iron 7

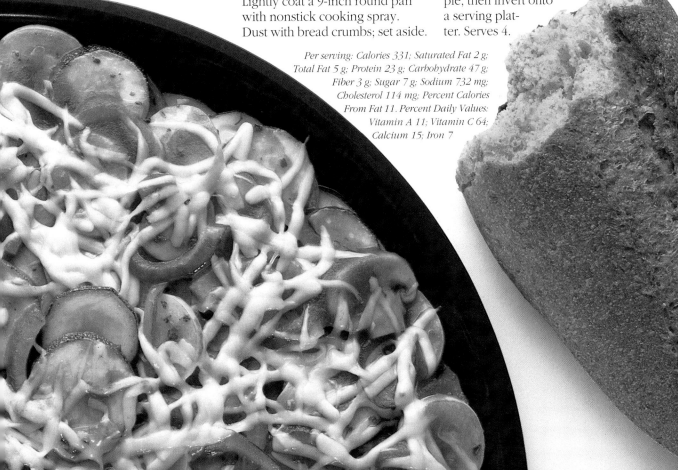

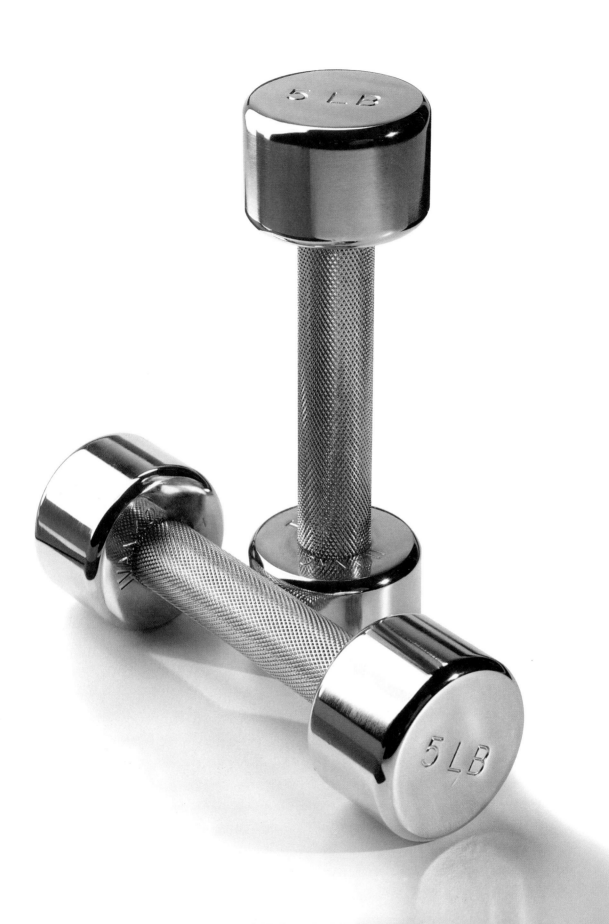

Chapter 3

SHAPING UP

· · · · · · · · · · · · · · ·

▦ THE BENEFITS OF EXERCISE *92*

▦ HOW FIT ARE YOU? *96*

▦ THE IMPORTANCE OF GOOD
  BREATHING AND POSTURE *102*

▦ GOOD AND BAD STRETCHES *104*

▦ DESIGNING YOUR OWN BALANCED
  EXERCISE PROGRAM *106*

▦ OUTDOOR EXERCISING IN THE
  HEAT AND COLD *112*

▦ AVOIDING AND OVERCOMING INJURIES *114*

▦ WALKING FOR HEALTH *116*

▦ SWIMMING: THE KINDEST SPORT *124*

▦ BICYCLING: GOING THE DISTANCE *128*

▦ JOGGING: AEROBICS IN A HURRY *130*

▦ EXERCISING AT HOME *132*

▦ WEIGHT TRAINING FOR STRENGTH *134*

▦ EXERCISING AS YOU AGE *136*

THE BENEFITS
OF EXERCISE

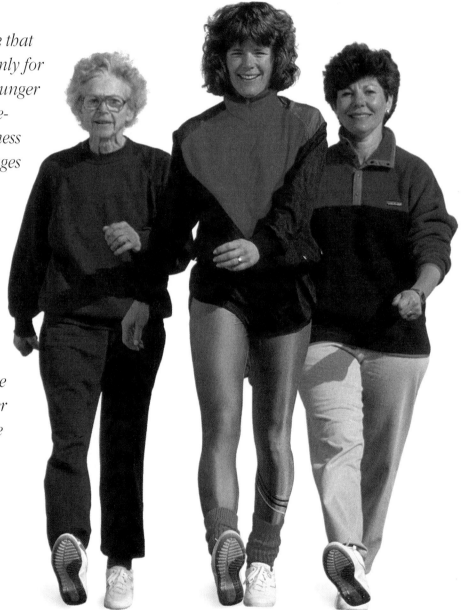

You may think that fitness is mainly for athletes or younger people. But current research shows that fitness is important at all stages of life and especially as you grow older. Exercise can help counteract what were once believed to be the inevitable effects of aging. While you can't turn back the clock, say the experts, you can lower your "functional" age by exercising.

It's never too late—or too early—to begin an exercise program. The body's need for physical activity is lifelong. You can exercise alone or make it a social event with friends and family members.

LIFE EXTENSION

Studies show that exercise cuts the risk of life-threatening illnesses, including heart disease, cancer, and stroke, which together account for 80 percent of all deaths in this country. Happily, it appears increasingly clear that exercise can mean just about any physical activity, from running in marathons to raking leaves.

In 1986 compelling evidence of exercise's life-lengthening benefits came from data on 16,936 Harvard University alumni. Those men expending at least 2,000 calories a week in exercise—mostly simple activities like yard work and stair climbing—lived on average more than 2 years longer than those exercising less. In another study, the American Cancer Society surveyed more than a million people and found that death rates from all major diseases were lower in the active population.

MORE YEARS OF HEALTH

No one can promise you a longer life if you exercise. But there is a virtual guarantee you will be healthier. The USDA Human Nutrition Research Center on Aging at Tufts University reports that active people can take care of themselves longer than inactive people. Active people are also less prone to ailments that impair quality of life, such as diabetes, arthritis, and osteoporosis. As exercise expert Dr. Kenneth Cooper says, exercise is about "improving the quantity of life a little and the quality of life a whole lot." Improvement occurs at any age; in one study, people in their nineties tripled their muscle strength after lifting weights for 8 weeks.

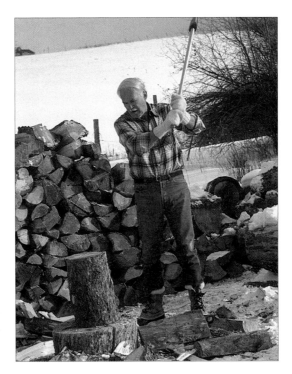

Keeping physically active is one secret to enjoying a lively and vigorous old age. Almost any kind of exertion counts, whether it's ballroom dancing, hiking, mowing the lawn, chopping wood for the fireplace, or engaging in a structured exercise program—or all of these.

IMPROVED QUALITY OF LIFE

The fact that heart-rate-raising physical activity improves the status of depressed patients has often been documented, as has the fact that, depressed or not, most people feel better after a workout. Active people report less depression and anxiety and more self-confidence than inactive people. The reasons are not totally understood, but may be related to endorphins, morphine-like chemicals secreted by the pituitary gland, brain, and some nerve tissue. Endorphins help suppress pain and elevate mood, and physical activity increases their level.

For many people, however, the most important benefits of exercise remain somewhat intangible. Quite simply, being physically active improves their quality of life. They look better, feel better, and know they have a reduced risk of illness.

MENTAL FITNESS

There is convincing evidence that being fit can help you think and react more clearly and improves your ability to solve problems and make choices. This seems to hold true at all ages. Studies conducted at California State University at Fullerton have shown that older women who exercised an average of three times a week for 15 years had physical and verbal response times equal to those of sedentary college-age women. Other studies have supported these findings.

WEIGHT CONTROL

Inactivity is associated with excess weight at all ages. As you grow older, you may find that extra pounds creep on more easily than they used to. According to current theory, this is due to the

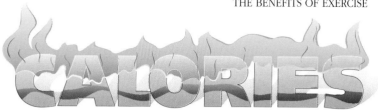

YOU CAN FIGURE OUT HOW MANY CALORIES YOU'VE BURNED
BY DOING THE CALCULATIONS BELOW.

Activity	Calories Burned per Minute per Pound	X	Your Weight	X	Minutes	=	Total Calories Burned
Chopping wood, fast	.135	x		x		=	
Swimming, backstroke	.076	x		x		=	
Snowshoeing, soft snow	.075	x		x		=	
Swimming, fast crawl	.071	x		x		=	
Basketball	.063	x		x		=	
Running, 11.5-minute mile	.061	x		x		=	
Swimming, slow crawl	.058	x		x		=	
Climbing hills	.055	x		x		=	
Skiing, cross-country	.054	x		x		=	
Lawn mowing	.051	x		x		=	
Tennis	.049	x		x		=	
Aerobic dance, moderate	.046	x		x		=	
Cycling, 9.5 mph	.045	x		x		=	
Badminton	.044	x		x		=	
Weight training, circuit training	.042	x		x		=	
Weight lifting, free weights	.039	x		x		=	
Golf	.038	x		x		=	
Walking, normal pace	.037	x		x		=	
Weeding	.033	x		x		=	
Table tennis	.031	x		x		=	
Gymnastics	.030	x		x		=	
Window cleaning	.026	x		x		=	
Raking	.025	x		x		=	
Dancing (ballroom)	.023	x		x		=	
Volleyball	.023	x		x		=	
Piano playing	.018	x		x		=	
Sitting still	.009	x		x		=	

STRESS REDUCTION

Stress is unavoidable in life, but you can control how it makes you feel. Research shows that regular exercise can generate feelings of calm and relaxation. In one study, physically active people who were asked to solve a series of unsolvable problems suffered less stress trying to do so than an inactive control group. People who exercise also report sleeping better and feeling less anger, hostility, and frustration. Chronic stress is also associated with a number of illnesses, including hypertension, digestive problems, allergies, and minor infections. By improving your ability to cope with stress, exercise can offer protection against these ailments.

INCREASED MUSCLE STRENGTH

"Use it or lose it," we are told, and the advice couldn't be more apt. From age 30 on, people lose 3 to 6 percent of their muscle mass per decade. It's not yet clear to what extent exercise can arrest this progression, but studies of people of all ages who start exercising show that physical activity builds bigger, stronger muscles.

Why should you worry about having strong muscles? The health and lifestyle reasons are compelling. Strength allows you to keep on performing tasks you might otherwise have to depend on other people to do for you. These can range from removing a jar lid to picking up a child. Strength also helps to prevent injury—for example, if you have strong back and abdominal muscles, you have a reduced risk of incurring a back injury or of developing chronic back problems.

body's gradual loss of bone and muscle mass, which causes a drop in BMR (basal metabolic rate), the rate at which the body burns calories at rest. From age 20 on, BMR drops about 2 percent every 10 years, which means that the average person needs roughly 100 fewer daily calories each decade. Once considered a "natural" part of aging, this reduced calorie need is now believed to result mainly from inactivity. Ex-

ercise can halt or reverse this decline by raising your metabolism. You burn more calories during exercise, so you can lose weight even if you don't change your diet. Regular exercise also stimulates muscle growth, and muscle tissue uses more calories to maintain itself than fat tissue does. If you can control your weight, you can reduce your risk of heart disease, hypertension, stroke, diabetes, and some forms of cancer.

EXERCISE AND YOUR HEART

When you exercise, your heart pumps blood faster and harder in order to supply the working muscles with nutrients and oxygen. The blood vessels supplying the muscles dilate to accommodate the increased flow. The vessels supplying other areas, the digestive system in particular, reduce flow so that as much blood as possible can be diverted to the working muscles. Over time, the heart grows stronger and can fuel the muscles with progressively less effort.

EXERCISE AND YOUR LUNGS

You have to breathe harder, deeper, and faster when you are working out. In order to accomplish this, your airways expand to allow as much air as possible to be inhaled. The oxygen taken in by your lungs is transported through the bloodstream to help fuel the increased activity of your muscles. Over time, your lung capacity and efficiency increase so that you expend less effort to take in and process the oxygen your body needs to have for your workouts.

BLOOD FLOW IN THE BODY

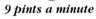

9 pints a minute

When you are at rest, your heart pumps about 9 pints of blood through your body per minute.

54 pints a minute

When you exercise, your blood flow can rise to as much as 54 pints a minute, depending on how fit you are and how hard you are exercising.

AIR FLOW IN THE LUNGS

12 pints a minute

When you are at rest, the volume of air passing in and out of your lungs is about 12 pints a minute.

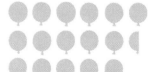

200 pints a minute

When you exercise, the air passing in and out of your lungs can increase to more than 200 pints a minute, depending on your fitness level and the intensity of your workout.

HOW FIT ARE YOU?

Experts divide fitness into five basic components: aerobic fitness, muscle strength, muscle endurance, body composition, and flexibility. A description of each of these elements is provided on the following pages, along with tests you can use to determine where you need to improve.

AEROBIC FITNESS

Aerobic fitness (also called cardiorespiratory fitness or cardiovascular fitness) concerns your body's ability to perform sustained physical activity that taxes your heart above its resting rate.

When you become fit, your heart is able to deliver increasingly larger amounts of blood and oxygen to fuel your working muscles. Aerobic fitness is considered the most important fitness component because of its beneficial effect on your health, in particular on your cardiovascular system.

While aerobic fitness has been shown to decline significantly with age, much of that decline appears to be associated with inactivity and can be reversed with a program of regular aerobic exercise. One recent study of men and women in their sixties showed that their cardiorespiratory function improved 25 to 30 percent during 12 months of regular moderate aerobic activity.

To develop and maintain aerobic fitness, the American College of Sports Medicine (ACSM) recommends sustained physical activity lasting between 20 and 60 minutes, performed 3 to 5 days a week, that raises your heart rate into your target heart-rate zone (see right). How long your exercise session should be depends on how vigorous your activity is.

For instance, 20 minutes of running is approximately comparable to between 40 and 60 minutes of brisk walking.

What activities qualify as aerobic? For most people, any exercise consisting of rhythmic, continuous movement that utilizes the large muscle groups of the body is fair game. Walking, hiking, jogging, swimming, bicycling, cross-country skiing, dancing, jumping rope, rowing, skating (ice or roller), and stair climbing are all aerobic exercises. Games that involve sustained, vigorous movement (such as soccer and competitive tennis) can also improve or maintain aerobic fitness. On the other hand, activities that either tax the heart very little (such as golf, bowling, or softball) or require exertion only in short bursts (such as weight lifting or football) are not considered aerobic and do not improve aerobic fitness.

AEROBIC FITNESS TEST

The One-Mile Walk. *Designed for healthy adults, this test involves walking a mile as fast as you can without straining. Find a flat, measured course. A track is ideal, or you can mark off a mile using a pedometer or your car's odometer. Use a stopwatch to record your time. When you finish, check the chart to determine your aerobic fitness level.*

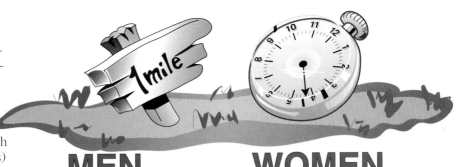

	MEN Minutes/Seconds		WOMEN Minutes/Seconds
Excellent	Less than 11:45	Excellent	Less than 13:10
Good	11:45 – 13:15	Good	13:10 – 14:40
High average	13:15 – 14:45	High average	14:40 – 16:10
Low average	14:45 – 16:15	Low average	16:10 – 17:35
Fair	16:15 – 17:55	Fair	17:35 – 19:05
Poor	More than 17:55	Poor	More than 19:05

WHAT IS YOUR TARGET HEART RATE?

To know if you are obtaining aerobic benefits, measure your heart rate during or just after exercise. Your rate should be in your target zone, figured as 70 to 85 percent of your maximum heart rate, or MHR (some experts suggest 60 to 90 percent). To figure your MHR, subtract your age from 220; then multiply by 0.70 and 0.85 to get your zone. If you are 50 years old, your MHR is 170, and your zone is between 119 and 144.5. (Don't go past your zone; it could be dangerous.) If you are new to exercise, stay in your zone's lower end. If you are on medication or have diabetes, follow your doctor's advice.

Two basic ways to measure your heart rate:

Pulse taking: You can take your pulse wherever a large artery lies near the skin—your wrist and temple are the most convenient places. Your wrist artery is ½ inch below the heel of your hand on the thumb side. Your temporal pulse is in the wide, shallow groove in front of and slightly above each ear. Press lightly with your first two fingers, count the beats for 10 seconds with your watch's second hand, and multiply by 6 to get the beats per minute.

RPE (Rate of Perceived Exertion): RPE is your estimate of how hard you are working on a scale of 6 (no effort) to 20 (all-out effort). To achieve your target heart rate, try for the "light" to "hard" range between 11 and 15 (or what your doctor advises). The rationale for RPE is that heart rate is less important than how hard you feel yourself working. With practice, exercisers can stay in their target zone without taking their pulse.

MUSCLE STRENGTH

Strength is a measure of the force of one muscle contraction, which is usually computed as an amount of weight lifted, pushed, pulled, or resisted. While some degree of strength is established by factors beyond your control, such as your gender and the types of muscle fibers you were born with, virtually anyone can increase muscle strength through exercise. Studies suggest that the average sedentary adult who begins a strength-training program will be able to see a 25 to 30 percent increase in strength over the course of 6 months.

Having muscle strength is important for several reasons: it helps you to maintain good posture and body alignment; it helps keep bones strong; and it helps prevent the risk of chronic knee and back problems, as well as other injuries. It also ensures that you will be able to continue participating in your regular everyday activities into old age, thus preserving your independence and general well-being.

As you age, muscle strength declines somewhat. But, as with other fitness components, that decline can be reversed with regular exercise, and this change can be effected at any age.

MUSCLE STRENGTH AND ENDURANCE TESTS
Since there is some overlap between muscle strength and muscle endurance, these tests measure both at once.

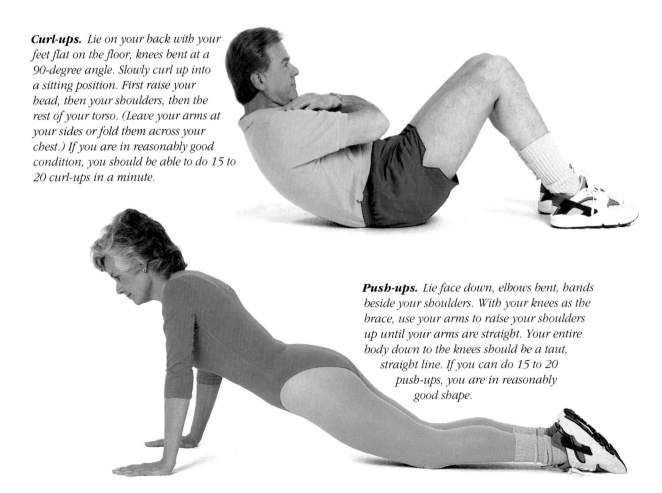

Curl-ups. *Lie on your back with your feet flat on the floor, knees bent at a 90-degree angle. Slowly curl up into a sitting position. First raise your head, then your shoulders, then the rest of your torso. (Leave your arms at your sides or fold them across your chest.) If you are in reasonably good condition, you should be able to do 15 to 20 curl-ups in a minute.*

Push-ups. *Lie face down, elbows bent, hands beside your shoulders. With your knees as the brace, use your arms to raise your shoulders up until your arms are straight. Your entire body down to the knees should be a taut, straight line. If you can do 15 to 20 push-ups, you are in reasonably good shape.*

MUSCLE ENDURANCE

The ability of a muscle to contract repeatedly over time (for example, when you do as many sit-ups as possible in 1 minute) defines its endurance. Muscle endurance activities, when done with large muscles such as the legs, can also improve cardiorespiratory function. For instance, running or walking for 20 minutes or more develops both aerobic fitness and muscle endurance. A 1-minute leg endurance exercise with weights, however, helps develop your muscle endurance but has no aerobic benefit. A basic rule of thumb you can follow is that heavy weights you work a few times are best for improving your strength, and that light weights you resist many times in a row are best for enhancing your endurance.

Step-ups. *Using a sturdy step stool or box 12 inches high, step up with one foot, then the other; bring the first foot back down, then the other. Do this 24 times a minute (2.5 seconds each) for 3 minutes. Use a stopwatch or a clock's second hand to time yourself. Take your pulse for 1 minute to determine your heart's response and speed of recovery right after undergoing this endurance exercise. Check the chart (right) to see how you rate. (Note: Skip this test if it provokes knee pain.)*

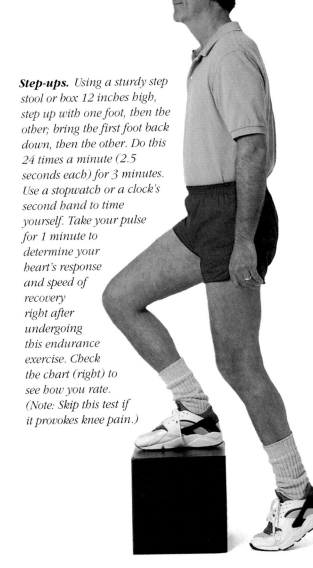

STEP TEST RESULTS

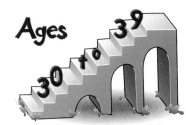

	Male	Female
Excellent	83 or less	77 or less
Good	84–105	78–99
Average	106–122	100–109
Fair to poor	123–136	110–126

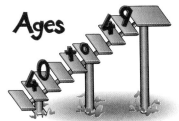

	Male	Female
Excellent	87 or less	79 or less
Good	88–108	80–100
Average	109–118	101–112
Fair to poor	119–131	113–126

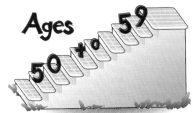

	Male	Female
Excellent	91 or less	85 or less
Good	92–113	86–105
Average	114–123	106–115
Fair to poor	124–137	116–131

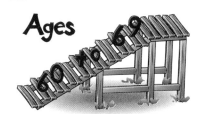

	Male	Female
Excellent	94 or less	89 or less
Good	95–117	90–108
Average	118–127	109–118
Fair to poor	128–141	119–131

BODY COMPOSITION

In general, staying in the weight ranges recommended in federal government and insurance company tables is healthful in terms of reducing your risk of major diseases. But your actual weight is less important than how much of it is fat. A football player, for instance, may be overweight according to the charts, but most of that weight is muscle and bone. The two tests here will give you a rough idea of whether you are carrying too much fat.

BODY COMPOSITION TESTS

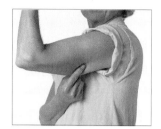

Underarm Pinch. *If you can pinch more than ½ inch of fat on the back of your arm in the area halfway between your armpit and elbow, you could stand to lose some weight.*

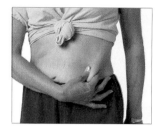

Abdominal Pinch. *With your thumb and index finger, pinch a fold of flesh in the stomach area around your navel. If you pinch more than 1 inch of fat, you are overfat.*

FLEXIBILITY

Flexibility involves the muscles' stretchability and their ability to move through their joints' full range of motion. It declines with age and lack of activity. But many people who complain of being stiffer than they used to be often find that their flexibility improves considerably when they start a regular exercise program.

Anyone can improve flexibility with the appropriate exercise. Stretching through the full range of motion and gentle movement exercise, such as swimming, appear to be the most effective.

FLEXIBILITY TESTS

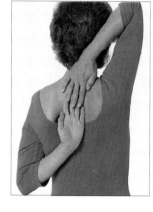

Hands Across the Back. *For this test of arm and shoulder flexibility, place one hand behind your neck. Put the other, with the palm facing outward, behind your back. Try to connect the fingers of both hands. Switch hand positions and try again. Rate yourself as follows: hands clasped, excellent; fingers touching, good; 1 to 3 inches apart, average; several inches apart, fair to poor.*

Sit and Reach. *To test the flexibility of your back muscles and hamstrings (backs of your legs), stretch your arms slowly forward; do not bounce or strain. Rate yourself as follows: if you reach up to 6 inches past your feet, excellent; touching your feet, very good; if you fall short of your feet by 1 to 6 inches, average; by more than 6 inches, below average.*

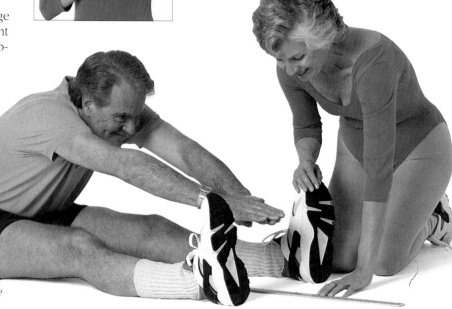

BEFORE YOU EXERCISE

Most doctors and fitness experts advise anyone over the age of 35—no matter how healthy—to seek medical approval before launching even the most modest fitness program. Their main rationale is that an undiagnosed health problem can make exercise dangerous, even life-threatening in rare cases. Some conditions may have no symptoms. For example, hypertension (high blood pressure) affects 50 million Americans, many of whom don't know they have it. Moderate aerobic exercise helps control hypertension because it can lower the resting heart rate and help reduce obesity. But high-intensity activities, such as sprinting and strenuous weight lifting, can cause blood pressure to rise, sometimes to dangerous levels.

Besides assessing your health, your doctor can help you plan a safe and balanced exercise program. See a doctor if:

▓ You are over 35

▓ You have been totally sedentary

▓ You are on any regular prescription medication, especially one that affects heart rate

▓ Your blood pressure and/or cholesterol levels are considered high

▓ A parent, grandparent, or sibling developed heart disease before the age of 55

▓ You have diabetes

▓ You are 20 percent or more over the recommended weight range for your height and age

▓ You smoke

Your doctor may recommend that you take an exercise stress test, which involves physical work, usually walking or jogging on a treadmill or riding a stationary bicycle. The test is conducted in a doctor's office or laboratory while you are hooked up to an electrocardiograph, a machine that records the heart's electrical activity. A specialist monitors the information being recorded, known as an electrocardiogram (ECG or EKG), to see if you have undiagnosed coronary artery disease (CAD). At the same time, blood pressure, heart rate, and heart rhythm are also measured. If you know you have diseased coronary arteries or have had a heart attack, this test can help determine the maximum safe level at which you can exercise.

You are so carefully monitored that the test is a low-risk procedure. Its aim is not to tire you out but to see if your heart muscle gets adequate blood and oxygen at increasing levels of physical effort. At any sign of trouble, the test is stopped immediately.

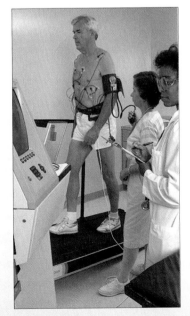

Some conditions can't be diagnosed when you are at rest. A stress test makes you exercise at a pace that raises your heart rate to a level where such problems as reduced blood flow to the heart muscle are detected.

THE IMPORTANCE
OF GOOD BREATHING
AND POSTURE

. . . .

Two fitness areas to check out before you begin exercising are breathing and posture. Both are important tools for getting the maximum benefit out of your exercise program.

BREATHING AND YOUR EXERCISE ROUTINE

The lungs bring oxygen into the body and allow carbon dioxide to leave. When you inhale, a portion of the oxygen in your breath enters the bloodstream and is carried throughout the body. At the same time, carbon dioxide is transferred from the bloodstream to the lungs and exhaled. The more air the lungs can process, the more oxygen is made available for the body's use, and the more carbon dioxide is expelled.

Making this exchange as efficient as possible not only is essential for all life processes but also enhances your body's ability to work hard during exercise. Therefore, optimum breathing is very important to your oxygen delivery system.

Most adults breathe shallowly, from the throat and upper chest, and as a result fill only the top part of their lungs. Shallow breathing may be adequate to meet the demands of sedentary living, but it isn't adequate for fitness exercises that require your heart rate to increase.

Deep breathing (also called belly breathing or diaphragmatic breathing) fills the lungs more completely. Try to practice deep breathing every day. Be careful not to breathe quickly, or else you may hyperventilate, that is, blow out more carbon dioxide than is safe. Stop at once if you feel faint or dizzy. Keep in mind that not smoking, avoiding polluted air, and improving your posture can help improve your breathing capacity too.

Many people find they get an emotional as well as a physical lift from deep breathing. It can also help you to relax and focus your thoughts and feelings.

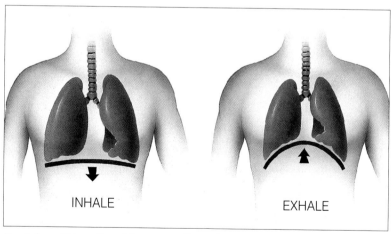

INHALE   EXHALE

Deep breathing. *Breathing more efficiently means using your diaphragm, the dome-shaped muscle below the lungs that contracts to expand them to their full capacity. With your hand just under your rib cage, fingers at the center of your chest, inhale slowly through your nose or mouth. Feel your abdomen push out as your lungs fill. Hold the breath for a second, then slowly exhale through your mouth. Breathe this way for 5 to 10 minutes.*

IMPROVING YOUR POSTURE

Because of the constant force of gravity, it is not unusual for your posture to deteriorate over time. Some signs of this gravitational compression are a head that is thrust forward, rounded shoulders, a swayed or hunched back, and a protruding stomach. Poor posture puts extra pressure on the back muscles, especially those of the lower back, and can cause pain and/or spasm. It also inhibits breathing; stresses (and can cause pain in) the head, neck, and shoulders; compresses the spine; and can be psychologically draining as well. Correcting bad postural habits makes exercise easier and more comfortable and helps you avoid injury.

Most people know bad posture when they see it; these same individuals may also think that the ramrod-straight, military-style, chest-out/shoulders-back/stomach-in stance is good posture. But this is bad posture too. Good posture is natural and relaxed; with your spine properly aligned, the weight of your torso is supported by your hips, legs, and feet, not solely your spine.

Good posture is natural, but not automatic. This is because poor posture is the result of years of bad habits, which must be "unlearned" before good posture can be learned. A good start is not to slump or twist to accommodate your furniture; adjust chairs, desks, and word processors to accommodate you. To improve the strength and flexibility of the muscles that contribute to good posture, try the stretching and strengthening exercises on pages 104–105. Mild aerobic exercise (walking, jogging, cycling, swimming, or rowing, for instance) can also help improve posture.

STANDING TALL

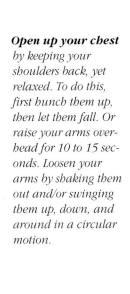

Keep your head up *and aligned over your neck (don't push it forward past your neck). Imagine that a silken thread attached to the top of your head is being gently pulled upward, and let your head move up with it. This helps straighten your neck and lengthen your spine. Think of your head, neck, and torso moving easily as one unit, cradled in the hips and supported by the lower body.*

Open up your chest *by keeping your shoulders back, yet relaxed. To do this, first hunch them up, then let them fall. Or raise your arms overhead for 10 to 15 seconds. Loosen your arms by shaking them out and/or swinging them up, down, and around in a circular motion.*

Don't throw yourself off balance *by locking your knees when you stand. Instead, keep your knees flexed very slightly and tilt forward very slightly from the hips. Notice that when you do this, your weight is centered mostly on the balls of your feet. This reduces the burden on your lower back and makes your upper body feel looser and lighter.*

GOOD AND BAD STRETCHES

Proper stretching helps maintain flexibility, develop the full range of motion in joints, and prevent injuries and soreness. How you stretch matters; stretching incorrectly (facing page) may do more harm than good.

SOME POINTERS FOR BETTER STRETCHING

■ ***Always stretch briefly when you warm up*** for a strenuous exercise session. Stretch again after cooldown, when your muscles are tight from exertion.

■ ***Stop if you feel pain.*** Stretching gradually elongates muscle and connective tissue fibers; it shouldn't hurt.

■ ***Concentrate on slow or static stretches.*** Move slowly into the stretch position and hold it firmly without bouncing. Start by holding each stretch for 3 to 5 seconds and work up to 10 or 15 seconds. Stretch the major muscles of the legs, abdomen, chest, and back first; then stretch the smaller muscles of the neck, arms, hands, and feet.

■ ***Be consistent and patient.*** Flexibility gains take time — months, not weeks. The increased activity of a new fitness program may tighten muscles at first. In general, men are less flexible than women and may need more stretching.

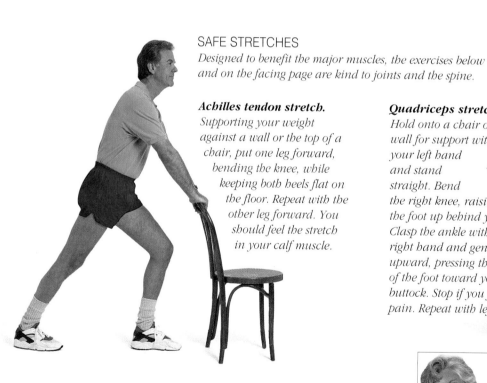

SAFE STRETCHES
Designed to benefit the major muscles, the exercises below and on the facing page are kind to joints and the spine.

Achilles tendon stretch. *Supporting your weight against a wall or the top of a chair, put one leg forward, bending the knee, while keeping both heels flat on the floor. Repeat with the other leg forward. You should feel the stretch in your calf muscle.*

Quadriceps stretch. *Hold onto a chair or wall for support with your left hand and stand straight. Bend the right knee, raising the foot up behind you. Clasp the ankle with your right hand and gently pull upward, pressing the bottom of the foot toward your buttock. Stop if you feel knee pain. Repeat with left leg.*

Side neck stretches. *Gently lean your head to the right. Return to an erect position. Lean your head forward and return to an erect position. Lean your head left. Always return to an erect position between stretches and never simply rotate the neck.*

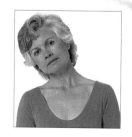

UNSAFE STRETCHES

Unsafe stretches that can damage muscles and connective tissue are shown below. Avoid these exercises. Safe stretches are shown in photographs on the facing page and below.

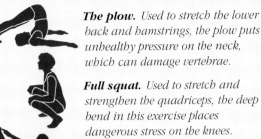

Swan stretch. *Lying on your stomach and simultaneously raising your legs, arms, and chest strains the lower back.*

Locked-knee toe touch. *A common stretch for lower-back muscles and hamstrings, this movement is especially harmful when you bounce up and down.*

Hurdler's stretch. *Designed to stretch the quadriceps and hamstrings, it can damage knee ligaments.*

The plow. *Used to stretch the lower back and hamstrings, the plow puts unhealthy pressure on the neck, which can damage vertebrae.*

Full squat. *Used to stretch and strengthen the quadriceps, the deep bend in this exercise places dangerous stress on the knees.*

Ballistic kick. *Kicking the leg, Rockette-style, can pull—or even tear—hamstring and gluteal (buttocks) muscles.*

360-degree neck rotation. *Rolling the head in full circles or vigorously bending it back and forth (or up and down) can hurt vertebrae.*

Lower back/buttocks stretch. *Lie on your back with both legs straight. Using your hands, bring one knee toward your chest, keeping the other leg straight. As you hold, press your back to the floor. Switch legs and repeat movement.*

Shoulder stretch. *Stand straight with your arms at your sides. With palms facing forward, move both arms as far behind you as you can. You should feel a pull across the shoulders.*

Sit-and-reach stretch. *To stretch the lower-back, hamstring, back-of-knee, and calf muscles, sit on the floor with your legs straight out in front of you, toes pointed upward. Move your hands toward your feet as far as you can. Hold, then try to lengthen the stretch slightly without straining or locking your knees.*

Cobra stretch. *To stretch and strengthen abdominal and lower-back muscles, lie on your stomach and use your arms to raise your upper body 10 to 20 degrees. Keep hips on the floor throughout, particularly if you have lower-back problems.*

DESIGNING YOUR OWN BALANCED EXERCISE PROGRAM

Just as true fitness is a mix of different physical qualities (cardiorespiratory capacity, muscle strength, muscle endurance, ratio of muscle to fat in the body, and flexibility), a good exercise program should be a careful balance of activities that suit you.

CONSIDER THE BASICS

To maintain complete adult fitness, the American College of Sports Medicine suggests a weekly program of three to five 20- to 60-minute sessions of aerobic exercise plus two or more strength-training sessions.

The chart on the facing page lists physical activities that contribute to the various components of fitness. Luckily, many forms of exercise—particularly aerobic activities like walking and dancing—promote fitness in several areas. Walking, for example, develops lower body muscle strength and endurance and increases metabolism (which can help you burn off extra fat) at the same time that it increases cardiorespiratory fitness. Stretching during warmups and cooldowns (pp.104–105) increases flexibility. By adding a couple of weekly weight-training sessions for upper body muscular strength and endurance, you can address all five components of fitness with basically two activities. For many people, that is the simplest way to get fit and stay fit.

CROSS-TRAINING

You may not want to confine yourself to just two activities. Too much repetition can strain muscles and increase your risk of injury. It can also make exercise sessions monotonous. Consider cross-training, or building your fitness program around more than one aerobic activity. Several activities, in addition to being more fun, condition a greater variety of muscles. Cross-training can involve a main exercise activity augmented by one or more supporting activities, or it can reflect an equal commitment to two or three types of exercise.

PICKING YOUR SPORTS

Good cross-training works different sets of muscles. Popular cross-training combinations are walking or jogging, cycling, and swimming, which complement one another well. Walking or running conditions muscles at the back of the legs; cycling builds up the quadriceps at the front of the thigh; swimming, especially free-

WHEN TO PASS UP CERTAIN EXERCISES

The exercises described in this chapter are designed for healthy people of any age or fitness level. If you have a health problem, check with your doctor before trying any new vigorous physical activity. The conditions below may put some exercises off-limits.

■ *High blood pressure.* Sprinting, vigorous calisthenics, and weight training for strength can raise blood pressure. So can holding your breath during the exertion phase of exercise.

■ *Overweight.* Jogging, rope jumping, and other high-impact aerobic activities may put excessive pressure on the joints and increase the risk of injury.

■ *Recent surgery or a serious illness.* Follow your doctor's advice about physical activity during your recovery and later. Prepare yourself for a gradual return to your former fitness level.

■ *Arthritis.* Regular moderate workouts may improve symptoms. High-impact activities, however, may aggravate pain and inflammation. Swimming and other low-impact water exercises are ideal.

style and breaststroke, tones the muscles of the upper body.

You can pick your own cross-training activities based on what you like to do and the season. If you live in a snow belt, for example, you may want to consider cross-country skiing or ice skating in the winter. Summer by a lake suggests rowing or swimming. Or, for convenience, you may want to combine walking or jogging outdoors with working out at a gym or on home equipment.

If you are exercising seriously for the first time, begin with walking. Then when you reach a comfortable fitness level, add a second activity. Begin slowly to avoid soreness or injury.

CUSTOMIZING YOUR OWN PROGRAM

For exercise to have a lasting benefit, it has to become a life-long habit. Making good on the commitment will be easier if you center your exercise around activities that you enjoy. People who love to go cycling in the park, for example, shouldn't make themselves jog around a track. A couple who has a wonderful time practicing ballroom dancing steps shouldn't sign up to swim laps.

If you have never been active, don't let self-consciousness or shyness hold you back. Fitness doesn't depend on athletic skills. Start with walking and then sample other possibilities for variety. If you've never learned how to swim, ride a bicycle, or dance, taking lessons may be a treat.

Set short-term fitness goals with measurable results; seeing progress on a weekly chart will motivate you. Whether you want to reduce your blood pressure or increase your metabolism to lose

MIX-AND-MATCH TRAINING MENU

Each of the sports below can contribute to a balanced exercise program. Choose complementary activities for total body fitness.

Sport	Body Benefits
Aerobics (low-impact)	Excellent for aerobic fitness and overall body toning.
Bicycling	Excellent for aerobic endurance and weight control. Develops strong legs and thighs.
Golf	Excellent for eye-hand coordination. May enhance aerobic fitness if you walk course briskly.
Jogging	Excellent for leg endurance, aerobic fitness, and weight control.
Rowing	Excellent for upper-body and leg strength and endurance and for aerobic fitness.
Stair climbing	Excellent for aerobic fitness, leg and buttock strength, and overall toning.
Stationary bicycling	Excellent for aerobic fitness, weight control, and leg strength and endurance.
Swimming	Excellent for developing arms and shoulders and great for aerobic endurance. Also good for overall flexibility and stress relief.
Tennis/ Racquetball	Excellent for eye-hand coordination, balance, leg and arm toning, and flexibility. Moderately good for aerobic fitness and weight loss.
Walking	Excellent for leg endurance, aerobic fitness, and weight control.
Weight training	Excellent for overall muscle, tendon, and bone strength. Can improve performance in sports.
Yoga	Excellent for flexibility, relaxation, and reducing stress.

EXERCISE ACTIVITIES FOR FITNESS GOALS

Aerobic (cardiorespiratory) fitness. Brisk walking, jogging, swimming, water aerobics, aerobic dancing, cycling, stair climbing, cross-country skiing, rowing, dancing (ballroom or square), rope jumping, skating.

Muscular strength. Calisthenics (push-ups, abdominal curl-ups), weight training (using heavy weights and few repetitions).

Muscular endurance. Any aerobic activity, calisthenics, weight training (using light weights and many repetitions).

Body composition (ratio of muscle to fat). Any activity that burns calories can make some contribution to weight (and fat) loss; moderate aerobic activities that can be sustained for longer periods of time (see above) are better than short bursts of high-intensity aerobic or anaerobic activity.

Flexibility. Any activity that requires full range of movement and stretches muscles and connective tissue (tendons and ligaments), such as calisthenics, yoga, rowing, swimming, all done at a moderate pace. Water exercises, which eliminate stress on joints, are especially effective.

HOME EXERCISE VIA VIDEO

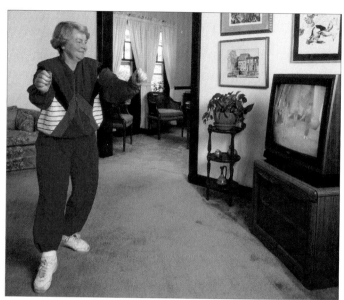

SIGNS OF A GOOD VIDEO

Clear instruction. The instructor should explain each exercise carefully, identifying the muscles it involves, telling you how to breathe, and describing how you should feel as you do each movement.

Safety cues. The instructor should give you reminders ("keep your back flat to the floor"; "watch how your leg is aligned") throughout the tape. There should be a heart rate check during the aerobic phase of the exercise regimen.

Completeness. The tape should start with a warmup and safe stretches (pp.104–105), include a progression from simple to more difficult movements, and end with a cooldown and safe stretches.The instructor should also explain how to increase the intensity of the workout.

If you prefer exercising at home, use an exercise videotape. Be choosy. Many are ineffective, and some are potentially harmful. Make sure the instructor is certified by one of the following: the American College of Sports Medicine, the American Council on Exercise, the Aerobics and Fitness Association of America, or the Cooper Institute for Aerobics Research.

Try out several videos. Match the program to your fitness level. If you are new to exercise, pick a beginning program. For strength training, look for a video featuring equipment like rubber bands, small dumbbells, or weights. For aerobic fitness, be sure the program gives you at least 20 minutes of exercise that raises your heart rate into your training zone (p.97).

GETTING STARTED

Clear enough room in front of your television set so that you can move comfortably without hitting anything. You may want to use an exercise mat. In any case, never exercise on a nonresilient floor (concrete or tile, for example), even if it is carpeted. A hard floor won't absorb impact and is likely to cause injuries.

Start slowly and don't overdo.You don't have to keep up with the pace of the video until you are ready. If any moves cause pain, skip them.

weight, noting positive changes will keep you going during the critical 3 months that it often takes to integrate regular exercise into your everyday life.

Also set long-term goals—6 months, 9 months, or a year from now. These will keep you from expecting instant results in fat loss or gains in strength and endurance, which take longer.

Suit your own style. Some people like solitude and keeping an independent exercise schedule.

Others prefer exercising with a partner or group. If a companion makes workouts more fun for you, enlist a spouse or friend to accompany you. Alternatively, sign up for an exercise class or join a walking or jogging group.

HOW TO STAY WITH YOUR FITNESS REGIMEN

■ *Build up your activity level slowly* (see *Fitness Program for Beginners,* p.110). Running a mile or taking a 2-hour aerobic dance class on your first day won't improve your fitness. If such excesses don't injure you, they will make you tired, sore, and likely to drop out.

■ *Make exercise convenient.* If you can walk briskly half an hour to get to work, you don't have to make time during the day for an aerobic workout. Think twice before joining a health club that is miles out of your way. If your program is centered on outdoor activities, have indoor alternatives for days when the weather is bad.

■ *Give exercise priority in your schedule.* "Not having time" to exercise is an evasion. A survey shows that exercisers and nonexercisers have the same amount of leisure time—about 24 hours a week. During busy periods, save time by increasing the intensity of workouts instead of skipping them.

■ *Maintain what you achieve.* You can't store the benefits of exercise for very long. Missing a day or two won't hurt, but skipping too many successive workouts will put you back where you started. Even professional athletes lose a portion of their fitness if they don't exercise for a few weeks.

■ *Find a comfortable fitness level.* You don't need to keep intensifying your program once you have met your fitness goals. Research shows that you can maintain fitness with less activity than it took to become fit. In fact, continuously increasing your workout time raises your risk of hurting yourself.

■ *Accept temporary setbacks.* Then pick up your regimen again as soon as you can. An illness, an injury, or a personal crisis will inevitably interrupt your exercise program. If you miss a few days of exercise, you can probably start again at the level where you left off. With a break of a week or more, you should re-evaluate your fitness (p.97) and work back to your former level very slowly.

■ *Make other healthful changes.* Smokers and people who are overweight are the most likely candidates to quit exercising. Let exercise help you give up smoking and unhealthful eating.

■ *Keep a support network.* You can benefit from staying in touch with other exercisers. You may be inspired by what you see other people accomplish. Or you may enjoy mentoring a spouse, child, or friend.

■ *Consider competing.* Participating in a race, swim meet, golf tournament, or tennis match may give a focus to your fitness regimen.

■ *Reward yourself.* Getting fit and staying fit are achievements. Treat yourself periodically to a special evening out, new clothes, or a trip.

WARMUPS AND COOLDOWNS

To prevent injuries and the soreness associated with strenuous exercise, nothing is more effective than warming up before you start and cooling down before you stop. Warming up prepares your body for the demands of your workout. Cooling down allows your body to recover from the strenuous exertion and return to a resting state.

During warmup, your heart rate, body temperature, and blood flow to the muscles all increase. The work load and oxygen requirements of the heart also are increased, preparing it to cope with sudden high-intensity exercise. Muscles stretch and become more flexible. Your whole body revs up to function more efficiently, preventing unwelcome shocks to its systems.

Suddenly stopping a high-energy activity without a cooldown causes blood to pool in the muscles you have been using, which can cause dizziness as well as later pain, swelling, and stiffness. Cooldown also helps the body remove waste products created during a workout.

The best way to warm up for many activities is to do a gentle version of the exercise for 5 to 10 minutes. Walkers should start with a stroll, joggers with a walk or slow jog, swimmers with a few slow and easy laps. As part of the warmup, slowly stretch the muscles that you will be using.

For your cooldown, simply spend the last 5 to 10 minutes of your workout performing your activity at a low level, just as you did during the warmup. After cooldown is the most effective time to schedule a longer, more thorough stretching routine for yourself (pp.104–105).

STAYING FIT ON THE GO

Long, confining trips can make your body feel cramped and sluggish. If you are driving, stop every 2 hours and get out of the car for 5 minutes of stretching exercises (pp.104–105) and, if possible, a 10-minute walk. In a bus, boat, train, or plane, walk up and down the aisle when you can. If there is enough space near the rest rooms, try exercising there. Confined to a seat, you will feel better after a round of in-seat stretches. Repeat each exercise (or set) three to five times and the whole sequence every hour or so.

■ *Arm-shoulder stretch.* Clasp your hands behind your head; push your elbows back as far as they will go. Hold 10 seconds.
■ *Back stretch.* Sit with your knees together and feet flat on the floor. Hold your left knee with your right hand and turn your shoulders as far to the left as you can (as if you were looking behind you). Hold the right knee with the left hand; turn to the right.
■ *Leg stretch.* Draw one knee to your chest with both hands. Hold 10 seconds. Repeat using the other knee.
■ *Toe circulation.* With your foot several inches off the floor, alternately point and flex your toes 10 times for each foot.
■ *Seat relief.* Tighten your buttock muscles; hold for a full minute. Relax; repeat.

SAMPLE FITNESS PROGRAMS

The three exercise regimens outlined below and at right address separate fitness goals. The first program offers a safe introduction to regular exercise, the second concentrates on aerobic endurance, and the third emphasizes muscle strength. Follow the program that is most appropriate to your needs.

FITNESS PROGRAM FOR BEGINNERS. When you are new to regular exercise, you must start slowly and work up to full fitness gradually to avoid injury and excessive muscle soreness. This 10-week regimen readies you for a maintenance program (right). Walking is the most accessible aerobic activity for most beginners, but you can substitute other aerobic activities. To build aerobic fitness, work out at a pace that keeps your heart beating in the lower end of your target heart-rate, or training, zone, gradually raising it to the mid-range as you gain fitness (p.97). Calisthenics should include abdominal curls and modified push-ups (p.98). Consult a fitness trainer for weight-training exercises. Alternate aerobic exercise and calisthenics or weight-training from day to day. Take 1 day a week off from exercise to allow muscles to repair themselves.

	Walk	Weight Training or Calisthenics
Week 1	20 minutes (3 sessions)	10 minutes (2 sessions)
Week 2	20 minutes (3 sessions)	10 minutes (2 sessions)
Week 3	25 minutes (3 sessions)	10 minutes (2 sessions)
Week 4	25 minutes (3 sessions)	15 minutes (2 sessions)
Week 5	30 minutes (3 sessions)	15 minutes (2 sessions)
Week 6	30 minutes (4 sessions)	15 minutes (2 sessions)
Week 7	30 minutes (4 sessions)	20 minutes (2 sessions)
Week 8	35 minutes (4 sessions)	20 minutes (2 sessions)
Week 9	35 minutes (4 sessions)	20 minutes (2–3 sessions)
Week 10	40 minutes (4 sessions)	20 minutes (2–3 sessions)

MAINTENANCE PROGRAMS FOR KEEPING FIT. Once you have achieved fitness, you can keep yourself in shape with a less intensive exercise program. The aerobic regimen (below left) focuses on sustaining top cardiovascular fitness with a minimum of strength building; the muscle strength program (below right) increases your muscle power while keeping you aerobically fit. In either program you may substitute other aerobic activities from the list on page 107 for the aerobic slots. You should get guidance for weight training at a gym or fitness center. If you don't feel comfortable doing your own calisthenics, sign up for a class at a Y or fitness center.

	Program for Building Aerobic Endurance	*Program for Building Muscle Strength*
Monday	Walk briskly for 30 minutes, then do 20 minutes of weight training or calisthenics.	Walk at any pace for 20–30 minutes, then do 20 minutes of weight training or calisthenics.
Tuesday	Day off.	Day off.
Wednesday	Cycle (indoors or out) for 30–45 minutes. Include some hills or sections of harder riding to build aerobic fitness.	30–45 minutes of a game or sport that uses the major muscles, such as tennis, racquetball, squash, golf, or softball.
Thursday	Swim for 30–45 minutes. Vary your strokes; if you wish, use a kick board or flotation vest to build leg endurance, a pull buoy to work on arms.	Swim for 20–30 minutes, then do 20 minutes of weight training or calisthenics.
Friday	Day off.	Day off.
Saturday	Walk briskly for 45 minutes.	Walk at any pace for 20–30 minutes, then do 20 minutes of weight training or calisthenics.
Sunday	Day off or walking or other light aerobic activity if you wish.	Day off or light muscle-strengthening activities if you wish, such as raking, vacuuming, chopping wood, or washing the car.

WARNING SIGNS

Everyone has occasional muscle soreness during exercise or moments when they feel the strain of their exertion. But regular exercise should never cause you serious pain or distress. While you are working out, if you experience any of the following symptoms, stop immediately and check with your doctor before you exercise again.

- **Chest pain**
- **Nausea**
- **Shortness of breath**
- **Severe joint or muscle pain**
- **Irregular heartbeat**
- **Faintness**
- **Noticeable pallor**
- **Excessive fatigue**

Outdoor Exercising in the Heat and Cold

. . . .

Whenever the temperature creeps way up or inches way down, adjust your exercise program to ensure your health and safety. Since your body works harder in both very hot and very cold weather, your first adjustment involves not exercising as intensely. Go by your pulse rate (p.97), and don't exceed your target zone.

BEATING THE HEAT

To protect yourself in the heat, always drink plenty of water, avoid working out when it's too hot and humid, and stay as cool and comfortable as possible. Increasing your fluid intake and accommodating the humidity are crucial. Drink water before, during, and after workouts. Avoid alcohol and caffeine; they have a diuretic ef-

HOT WEATHER DANGERS

Heat Exhaustion. *Fatigue, weakness, nausea, headache, clammy skin, lightheadedness, and irritability can all be symptoms. Treat heat exhaustion by cooling off, increasing fluid intake, and taking a few days' rest.*

Heatstroke. *A medical emergency, heatstroke can occur suddenly. Warning signals are a high fever, burning in the muscles and lungs; hot, dry skin; dry mouth; labored breathing; dizziness; weakness; nausea; and disorientation. Get victims out of the sun at once and cool them off with cold drinks and by pouring water on their bodies (or applying ice packs). Some victims can become irrational. Keep them quiet, lying down with feet elevated, and quickly summon medical help.*

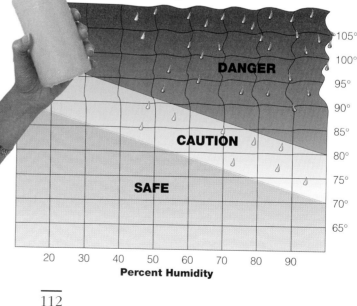

DANGER

CAUTION

SAFE

105°
100°
95°
90°
85°
80°
75°
70°
65°

20   30   40   50   60   70   80   90

Percent Humidity

fect that increases water loss. When heat and humidity are high, sweat cannot evaporate, your body begins to overheat, and your heart is increasingly stressed — you are at risk of heatstroke. Consult the hot weather chart (below left) and never exercise when conditions are in the danger zone.

You can stay cooler (and avoid more pollutants) by exercising in the morning or evening, when temperatures are lower. For comfort, wear as little clothing as you can and nothing that chafes or binds. Deflect sun with white or light colors and a hat. Use water-resistant sunscreen (reapply it hourly). Work out in shaded areas as much as possible. And remember to drink plenty of water.

STAYING WARM IN THE COLD

The secret to exercising in cold weather is dressing properly, preferably in lightweight layers you can add or remove as needed and as weather conditions shift. A thermal layer next to your skin will wick moisture away. Add a wool layer for insulation, then one that resists wind and water but "breathes" so that perspiration doesn't build up. Clothes with zippers let you cool off during a workout as well as adjust to changes in the weather. A hat prevents loss of body heat through the top of your head. For warmth, mittens are better than gloves. On bitter cold days, you should also cover up your face.

Drink plenty of fluids—you perspire exercising in the cold too. But don't drink alcohol; it dilates your blood vessels, causing you to lose heat more rapidly.

Do your warmup, stretching, and cooldown inside. Start your workout facing into the wind so that you will work hardest when you are fresh and will avoid having it blow on your perspiring face and body on your return. Don't stand around in your damp clothes afterward; go inside right away. Finally, when it's icy underfoot, avoid the risk of a fall by working out indoors.

COLD WEATHER DANGERS

Frostbite. Loss of feeling is the major symptom; the skin turns white, red, then white again. Treat suspected frostbite by reheating the area rapidly in warm water (100° to 110° F). Never rub it with snow. See a doctor if you don't improve in 20 minutes. To prevent frostbite, check the cold weather chart (below) and dress accordingly.

Hypothermia. If you are wet and in the wind, you can suffer hypothermia at above-freezing temperatures. Signs include confusion, lethargy, slurred speech, and constant shivering. Get victims inside, into a hot shower or bath, and bundle them up. To prevent hypothermia, dress properly and stay dry and out of the wind.

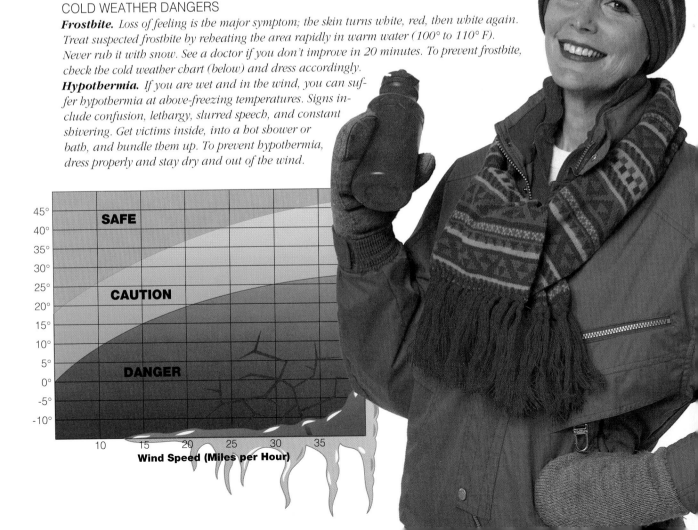

Avoiding and Overcoming Injuries

· ·

*I*njuries are a fact of life for many active people. Most are not serious, and many can be avoided entirely. Proper form and equipment; warmups, cooldowns, and stretching; and not overdoing it are the key factors in prevention.

WARNING SIGNALS

Stop or cut back on your workouts if you experience any of the following:

▪ *Muscle soreness* that lasts more than 48 hours after your workout.
▪ *A localized tingling* in your muscles.
▪ *Pain or discomfort that gets worse,* not better, the longer you exercise.
▪ *Pain first thing in the morning,* especially in your foot or lower leg.
▪ *Tight muscles* that don't loosen as you warm up and stretch them.
▪ *Redness or a warm feeling* that occurs in a localized area during or after your workout.

If any of these symptoms don't clear up within a reasonable amount of time, see your doctor.

THE COMMONEST PROBLEM

Virtually everyone has suffered a side stitch while exercising. A sharp pain in your side (usually the right), it is a form of muscle cramp you can experience just walking down the street.

Most muscle cramps, including side stitches, can be relieved by gentle stretching and massaging. If the pain persists or becomes severe, see a doctor. Decrease your risk of getting a muscle cramp by doing proper warmups and cooldowns, drinking plenty of fluids, and waiting a few hours after a meal or 1 hour after a snack before working out.

· ·

OVERUSE INJURIES

Anyone from a beginner to a professional athlete can suffer an overuse injury. Tiny tears in your muscles and/or ligaments and tendons can be caused by repeated striking or pounding (of the foot on pavement when jogging, for instance), repeated stretching and contracting of a muscle (in the shoulder when swimming), or constant joint use (of the elbow in tennis). To make repairs, your body increases its blood flow to the injured area, which causes pain and inflammation. Many overuse injuries will readily respond to the easy-to-remember RICE treatment: Rest, Ice (for 20 minutes at a time), Compression, and Elevation.

During the healing process, massage, heat, and rehabilitation exercises are often recommended. Heat can relieve stiffness and may speed healing; it should never be applied, however, until at least 48 hours after the injury or until the swelling has gone down. Be careful not to risk reinjury by rushing back and/or doing more exercise to "make up."

· ·

TRAUMA INJURIES

Mostly incurred during contact sports, a trauma injury usually will require medical help, sometimes on an emergency basis. Resulting from a blow, fall, twist, or other violent action, such injuries include broken bones, sprains, strains, twisted joints, bumps, and bruises. You should see a doctor if you have bleeding, intense pain, numbness, severely restricted movement, or swelling that doesn't abate in a few hours. Try to keep the area as immobilized as possible until you can get help.

COMMON SPORTS INJURIES

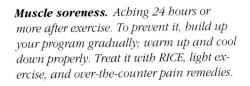

Muscle soreness. *Aching 24 hours or more after exercise. To prevent it, build up your program gradually; warm up and cool down properly. Treat it with RICE, light exercise, and over-the-counter pain remedies.*

Stress fracture. *A hairline bone break. You probably have one if pain persists after a few days' rest and there is inflammation. To prevent it, build up your program slowly and don't overdo. To diagnose and treat it, see an orthopedist. Usually you must rest the area for 6 to 8 weeks.*

Tennis elbow. *Inflammation of the elbow tendons. To prevent it, use correct form and the right equipment. Treat it with RICE and return to activity slowly. See a doctor if pain is severe or persistent.*

Runner's knee. *Pain in the knee area. To prevent it, strengthen those muscles, wear the right shoes, and use proper technique. For severe pain, or if mild pain persists after icing and rest, get medical help.*

Plantar fasciitis. *Pain in the heel and arch that can spread and become constant. To prevent it, wear shoes with good support and cushioning. Treat it with rest and ice. Heel pads and other orthotics will help prevent a recurrence.*

Shoulder bursitis. *Inflammation of the bursal sacs around the shoulder joint. To prevent it, warm up and stretch carefully. Strengthen the area with weight training. Treat it with rest and ice, and resume exercise gradually. For severe pain, see a doctor.*

Hamstring strain. *Pain in the back-of-thigh muscles. To prevent it, warm up, cool down, and stretch properly; build up your program gradually. Work on your flexibility. Treat it with RICE, and return to exercise slowly and carefully.*

Shin splints. *Tenderness or burning in the shin. To prevent it, strengthen and stretch front leg muscles. Work out on even surfaces, warm up slowly, and wear the right shoes. Treat it by cutting back or, with severe pain, taking several days off. Apply ice and elevate the legs.*

Achilles tendinitis. *Pain, stiffness, and swelling in the lower calf and heel. To prevent it, build up your program slowly, loosen calf muscles with stretching, and wear the right shoes. Don't suddenly shift types of surfaces. Treat it with RICE, and slowly resume activity under a doctor's care.*

Walking for Health

I f you want an exercise that improves your health, fits easily into your life, takes little or no time to learn, doesn't cost anything, requires no special equipment, and can be done almost any-where, anytime, with or without other people, then walking is for you. Hundreds of thousands of people have taken up walking for exercise in recent years, making it one of the country's most popular activities.

AN EXERCISE FOR EVERYONE

Any walking you are able to add to your daily schedule can help you control your weight, tone your muscles, and give you more energy. Walking can also lower your risk of heart disease. According to the latest research, walking—at any pace—helps the heart by increasing the levels of HDL cholesterol in your blood. HDL is the "good" cholesterol that helps protect you against heart disease.

Because of walking's growing popularity, many community organizations and recreation centers offer walking classes. These often include hikes in local historic or wooded areas, giving you the benefits of recreation as well as conditioning and instruction.

Heel. *The heel counter encases the heel, preventing side-to-side motion; it should be comfortable, yet rigid enough not to collapse when you squeeze it. Replace shoes with worn-down heels; they create an improper angle of foot, knee, and hip placement. Also replace shoes when they lose their support and cushioning, every 500 miles or so, sooner if you experience discomfort.*

Ankle. *The area around the top of the shoe (the heel collar) should be padded. Look for a notch or lowered section in the back of the collar to reduce pressure on the Achilles tendon.*

116

Correct technique is important to get the most out of any exercise. Even though you have been walking all your life, you may have acquired some bad habits. See page 118 to discover how you compare. Then turn to page 119 for help on setting up your own walking program.

WALKING VARIATIONS

Once you are walking properly and have embarked on a walking fitness program, you might want to consider other walking options. Here's a rundown of some possibilities.

Track Walking
Tracks are usually easier on your joints than concrete or asphalt and smoother than grass or dirt trails. Generally, walkers and slower joggers use the track's outside lanes, and fast runners the inside ones. When you walk on indoor tracks, which are often banked, you should make sure to reverse direction on alternate days because traversing a slanted surface puts more stress on the knees. Switching direction alternates the burden. In fact, you should periodically change your direction on any track.

Treadmill Walking
Treadmills let you walk in a small area; some are motorized and have computer programs to vary speed and simulate hills. Nonmotorized treadmills require extra effort to move the belt and may cause strain. Test a model before buying to make sure it allows you to walk with your natural stride.

(continued on page 121)

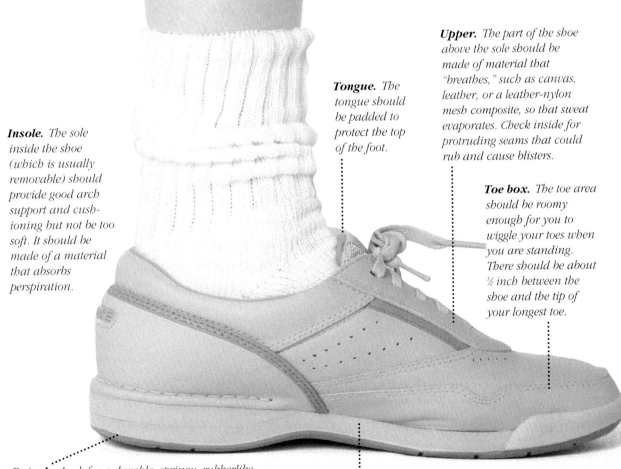

Tongue. The tongue should be padded to protect the top of the foot.

Upper. The part of the shoe above the sole should be made of material that "breathes," such as canvas, leather, or a leather-nylon mesh composite, so that sweat evaporates. Check inside for protruding seams that could rub and cause blisters.

Insole. The sole inside the shoe (which is usually removable) should provide good arch support and cushioning but not be too soft. It should be made of a material that absorbs perspiration.

Toe box. The toe area should be roomy enough for you to wiggle your toes when you are standing. There should be about ½ inch between the shoe and the tip of your longest toe.

Outsole. Look for a durable, springy, rubberlike material that will wear well but is not so hard that it completely resists pressure from your finger or thumb. It should be patterned for traction and to prevent slipping.

Midsole. You need cushioning but also firmness for support; the midsole should flex at the ball of the foot but be hard to bend at the arch and heel.

How to Walk: The Basics

Head. *Look ahead, not down; keep your head level, relaxed, and gently balanced at the top of your spinal column. Don't lean your neck forward; this can disrupt your posture and strain your neck and back. Relax your face and jaw; tense facial muscles contribute to tight muscles elsewhere in the body.*

Shoulders. *Keep your shoulders back and relaxed.*

Back and abdomen. *Stand tall (p.103). Don't bend forward from the waist or arch backward; both stances can strain back muscles. Keep your buttocks tucked in to prevent lower-back pain, and flatten your lower back to make this position—called the pelvic tilt—easier to maintain.*

Chest. *Keep the chest up but in a natural position, not thrust out, military style.*

Arms. *The arms should swing naturally and coordinate with the opposite leg—that is, the left arm should come forward with the right foot. This is a natural movement most people make without thinking. Swinging your arms across your chest throws you off balance and wastes energy. As you walk faster, bend your elbows more and pump your arms harder, but keep them relaxed, with wrists straight.*

Hands. *Keep your hands loosely cupped; clenching them tenses your whole upper body.*

Hips. *As you step forward, the hip motion is forward, not side to side. This natural, relaxed movement allows an effortless lengthening of your stride.*

Feet. *The feet should land in parallel tracks, with the toes pointed straight ahead. Land first on your heel, flexing your foot just before you do, then roll forward across the ball of the foot and push off with the toes. Flexing may cause pain in the shins of new walkers; avoid it by tilting your foot slightly to the outside edge and trying to keep your ankle flexible.*

Legs/stride. *Stride length should feel natural, not strained. If you are overstriding, your head bobs up and down with each step. Don't lift your legs; rather, picture yourself gliding along, as if on skates.*

BEGINNING AND INTERMEDIATE WALKING PROGRAMS

Do at least three exercise sessions during each week of the programs. If you experience any strain or fatigue as you advance, drop back to the previous level until you feel ready to advance again. Once you finish the last week of the Intermediate Program, you can go on to build the length and intensity of your walks or stay at the same level. The important thing is to exercise in your target heart-rate zone.

BEGINNING PROGRAM. Walk on flat ground; if hills are unavoidable, slow your pace.

	Warmup	*Target Zone* Exercising*	*Cooldown*	*Total*
Week 1	Walk slowly 5 minutes	Walk briskly 5 minutes	Walk slowly 5 minutes	15 minutes
Week 2	Walk slowly 5 minutes	Walk briskly 7 minutes	Walk slowly 5 minutes	17 minutes
Week 3	Walk slowly 5 minutes	Walk briskly 9 minutes	Walk slowly 5 minutes	19 minutes
Week 4	Walk slowly 5 minutes	Walk briskly 11 minutes	Walk slowly 5 minutes	21 minutes
Week 5	Walk slowly 5 minutes	Walk briskly 13 minutes	Walk slowly 5 minutes	23 minutes
Week 6	Walk slowly 5 minutes	Walk briskly 15 minutes	Walk slowly 5 minutes	25 minutes

INTERMEDIATE PROGRAM. Gradually add hills. Be careful not to strain yourself.

	Warmup	Target Zone Exercising	Cooldown	Total
Week 1	Walk slowly 5 minutes	Walk briskly 18 minutes	Walk slowly 5 minutes	28 minutes
Week 2	Walk slowly 5 minutes	Walk briskly 20 minutes	Walk slowly 5 minutes	30 minutes
Week 3	Walk slowly 5 minutes	Walk briskly 23 minutes	Walk slowly 5 minutes	33 minutes
Week 4	Walk slowly 5 minutes	Walk briskly 26 minutes	Walk slowly 5 minutes	36 minutes
Week 5	Walk slowly 5 minutes	Walk briskly 28 minutes	Walk slowly 5 minutes	38 minutes
Week 6	Walk slowly 5 minutes	Walk briskly 30 minutes	Walk slowly 5 minutes	40 minutes

See page 97 to learn how to estimate your target zone.

SAFETY ON THE ROAD

 Be on the alert for potential trouble. Pay attention to cars, cyclists, pedestrians, possible assailants, and animals, as well as your footing. Avoid high-traffic areas whenever you can. They are less safe, more polluted, crowded, and noisy.

 Obey the rules of the road. If you can't use the sidewalk, walk or jog on the left side of the street, facing traffic, and switch sides as you go around a blind curve. Cross only at crosswalks and never against the light. If you are cycling, stay on the right side, with traffic; use signals to indicate a right or left turn.

 Make yourself visible at night. White or light-colored clothing can be seen for only about 200 feet—a driver might not be able to stop in time. Increase your visibility with a reflective vest or strips of reflective tape on your clothes—and on your feet, ankles, and legs, which attract attention as they move. On your bike, use halogen head and tail lights powered by rechargeable batteries or a generator. If you walk or jog, carry a small flashlight or strap a blinking light to your arm or leg. No matter how visible you think you are, stick to sidewalks and paths as much as possible.

 Don't get lost. Always familiarize yourself with an area beforehand. Take a map if you don't know an area well. Carry identification and money for a telephone call and/or transportation home. If you do get lost, ask for directions if you feel safe doing so. Otherwise, proceed calmly and confidently, as though you have a destination, until you reach a safe area.

 Don't become a crime victim. Avoid deserted places. Never exercise at night in an area you have not visited in daylight or in one that is questionable. Vary the route, length, and timing of your workouts (some criminals spy on potential victims to learn their routines); be wary of strangers; and carry a small alarm or whistle. And never assume crime can't happen to you.

 Allow your eyes to adjust at night. When you first step out or head into an especially dark spot, give your eyes time to adjust. Never look directly at headlights (they can temporarily blind you); look sideways instead to pick up the car in your peripheral vision. If a car seems not to see you or swerves toward you, get off the road as quickly as possible.

 Avoid wearing headphones. It's safest not to wear headphones; if you do, lower the volume so that you can hear noises around you—cars, joggers, cyclists, barking dogs. Headphones make you a more likely crime target too.

 Watch out for dogs. If you stay off their property, most dogs won't bother you. Never approach a strange dog. If one comes at you and acts unfriendly, don't run; slowly and calmly move away sideways. Keep your arms down, don't move suddenly, and don't look the dog in the eye—it will take this as a threat. If the dog attacks, don't fight back; the dog will become more aggressive. If you are knocked down, roll onto your stomach and cover your face. If you are bitten, rinse the wound with water, wash it with soap, and see a doctor at once. Have the dog's rabies immunization records checked.

Snowshoeing

Try snowshoeing if you want to keep walking outdoors even when deep snow covers the ground. Most people have no trouble mastering the technique, which is basically walking with the toes pointed slightly outward. If you use ski poles with your snowshoes, you will also give your upper body a workout. It's a good idea to rent your equipment at first to see how you like the sport. Practice snowshoeing in a flat, open area before you attempt hills and obstacles, and keep your first few excursions brief and close to shelter. Later you can venture out on several-hour or even some all-day rambles.

Race Walking

While race walking is not difficult to do, the technique does not come naturally to most people. It is a good idea to obtain instruction. You can work one-on-one with a personal trainer, take a class, or watch an instructional video. Race walkers modify the walking technique to achieve maximum speed with a fluid, low-to-the-ground motion that uses as little energy as possible and minimizes the risk of injury. While race walkers appear to be swinging their hips from side to side, careful observation will reveal that all motion is direct-

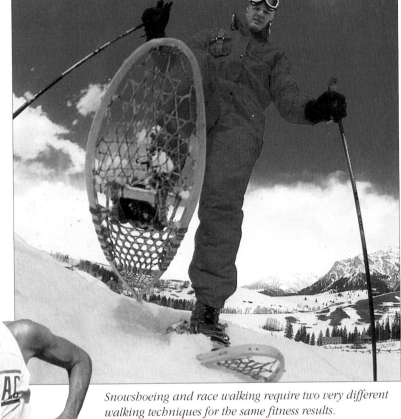

Snowshoeing and race walking require two very different walking techniques for the same fitness results.

ed forward. Arms are held at a 90-degree angle and pumped from the shoulder, never the elbow.

If you find that race walking is definitely the sport for you, you might consider inquiring about competitions at your local walking or running clubs. The sport is an Olympic event, and many running races have race-walking divisions. However, Olympic rules require you to straighten the weight-bearing knee with each stride, which many people find too strenuous. A new kind of race-walking event is evolving, called competitive fitness walking, which does not require you to do this.

> **❝Take a two-mile walk every morning before breakfast.❞**
>
> *—Harry S. Truman (1884-1972), advice on how to reach the age of 80, given by him on his 80th birthday, May 5, 1964*

Profile

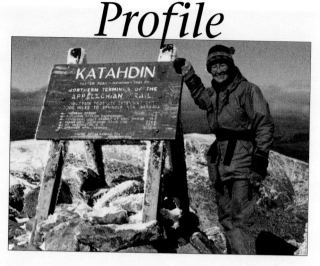

AGE AND EXPERIENCE HELP MOMMA JO REYNOLDS FULFILL A LIFELONG DREAM

As a country girl, Jo Reynolds often came across markers for the Appalachian Trail and fantasized trekking its 2,000-plus miles from Georgia to Maine. She was 54 when she took a career break and turned her "romantic idea into rugged reality." Her grown children lent her much of her equipment: the genesis of her trail name, Momma Jo.

Nearly 4 million people, half over 40, hike the trail annually. Reynolds was a "through hiker," one of the 1,300 who try to walk the entire trail in one season. About 220 finish. The 5-foot 4-inch, 117-pound Reynolds, toting a 35- to 40-pound backpack, finished in 5 1⁄2 months. She was never injured, never even got a blister, and credits her feat to "good luck, age, and experience."

The younger hikers gave Reynolds a unique perspective. "At 28, I was the mother of three. Talking to people who were my age then gave me an incredibly rich sense of freedom at doing the hike at this age." On September 30, 1991, she hiked the trail's last section with family, friends, and a 24-year-old through hiker who had dreamed of hiking the trail since she was 9. "We had that in common—30 years apart!"

Hiking

An enjoyable way to explore the world around you, hiking can take you from the trails of your local city park to wilderness areas. To hike comfortably, raise your fitness level to the point where you can walk 4 to 5 miles on level ground without undue fatigue or strain. Then start walking up and down hills. (Going downhill is actually harder on your muscles than going up.) Take along a knapsack to get used to carrying extra weight.

For short hikes, almost any pair of previously worn, comfortable, sturdy shoes will do, except sneakers, which do not provide ankle support or traction. For longer hikes, wear hiking boots. Ask a knowledgeable salesperson at a camping and outdoor equipment store to help you select a suitable pair. Dress defensively; take along a poncho and sweaters to protect you from weather changes such as sudden rainstorms and from the colder air (which can be up to 30 degrees lower) on mountaintops. In areas where hunting is permitted, you should always wear bright colors.

If you are hiking for more than a couple of hours, be sure to take food and water. Hiking burns about 300 calories an hour and can dehydrate you quickly. Drink ½ cup of water at least every 20 minutes, more if it's hot or you are sweating profusely.

Respect your environment: don't litter, trample plants, or disturb animals. Don't drink untreated water, overextend yourself, or take chances. In remote areas, it's a good idea to know first aid.

Orienteering

An increasingly popular sport that appeals to people of all ages, abilities, and fitness levels, orienteer-

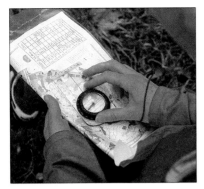

Turn the map so that it is oriented in the direction you are going.

ing gives you both a physical and mental workout. Using a map and compass, you traverse an outdoor area unknown to you.

To participate, contact a local club to find out when and where meets are held. In most cases, you can just show up with a compass (or rent one there), register, and get a map of your chosen route. The larger A meets, however, are more formally organized than the smaller B and C meets, and you must sign up ahead of time. There are usually six routes, ranging in difficulty from beginner to expert. Instruction for beginners is generally available.

At the signal, you head off walking (or running if you want to be competitive) between various control points to the finish line. The route that you travel may be from 1 to more than 7 miles. Most meets involve only walking or running, but some also utilize bicycles, canoes, or cross-country skis.

WALKING WITH FRIENDS—AND TO MEET THEM

Joining a walking club is a great way to stay motivated and meet other walkers. Most clubs offer group walks; walking instruction; talks on health and fitness; walking competitions, tours, and vacations; and social activities.

One of the newest and fastest-growing types of walking club is the mall walking club. Your local mall has many attractions: safety, relative quiet, cleanliness, convenience, protection from the elements, the companionship of other walkers, and even discounts and freebies from store proprietors eager to attract new customers.

Mall walking became popular in the 1980's, particularly among middle-aged and retired people. It is now a well-organized movement with more than a million hard-core adherents. Mall owners have responded by opening earlier, measuring out routes, and even offering club members maps and special deals. Some malls offer health screenings, fitness seminars, and instruction on warming up and stretching.

To find out about walking clubs (mall or other types), ask other walkers or try health clubs, Y's, running clubs, local hospitals, senior citizen groups, universities or colleges, or the management of your local mall. If there are none in your area, consider starting one yourself.

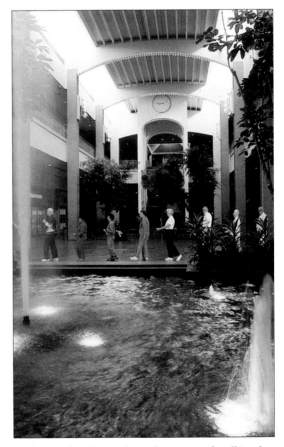

At the local mall, you have the option of walking by yourself, with a friend, or with a group.

SWIMMING:
THE KINDEST SPORT

Topped only by walking and biking in popularity, swimming is an ideal aerobic exercise. It uses all the major muscles—upper body and lower body —and, depending on your stroke and speed, burns between 300 and 1,000 calories an hour (jogging at 6 miles for an hour burns about 600 calories).

SOMETHING FOR EVERYONE

Swimming, in addition to its cardiovascular benefit, increases muscle flexibility and strength without jarring bones or joints. Swimming is a low-impact activity that, because of water's buoyan-

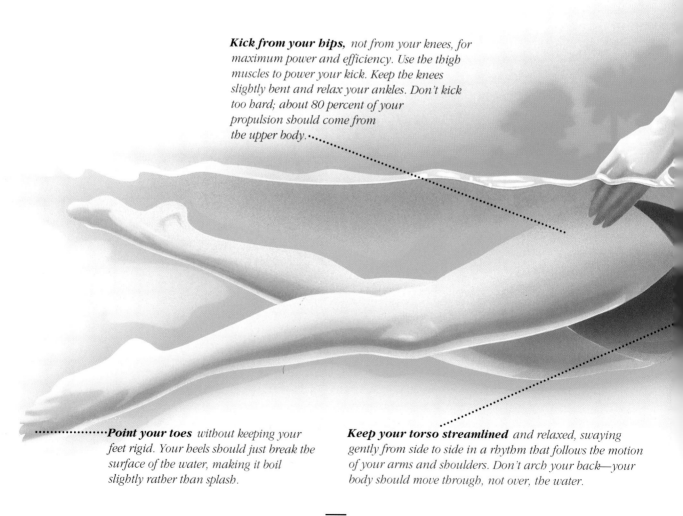

Kick from your hips, *not from your knees, for maximum power and efficiency. Use the thigh muscles to power your kick. Keep the knees slightly bent and relax your ankles. Don't kick too hard; about 80 percent of your propulsion should come from the upper body.*

Point your toes *without keeping your feet rigid. Your heels should just break the surface of the water, making it boil slightly rather than splash.*

Keep your torso streamlined *and relaxed, swaying gently from side to side in a rhythm that follows the motion of your arms and shoulders. Don't arch your back—your body should move through, not over, the water.*

cy, is also therapeutic for people who have hurt themselves in other sports or who suffer from heart disease, arthritis, or back problems. Obese people, for whom jogging or cycling is risky, can safely swim for fitness. Swimmers find their sport relaxing and exhilarating at the same time, a boon to both body and spirit.

SWIMMING TECHNIQUE

If you know how to swim, you can start the Beginning Swimming Program (p.126) as soon as you locate a suitable pool. First, however, you may want to have a swimming teacher observe and critique your form. Techniques that were developed for competitive swimmers have made freestyle swimming (the crawl), the breaststroke, and the backstroke more efficient.

Mastering proper swimming technique is important because bad form is wasteful and wears you out, taking the pleasure out of the sport and preventing you from reaching your fitness goals. The drawing below illustrates the best freestyle form.

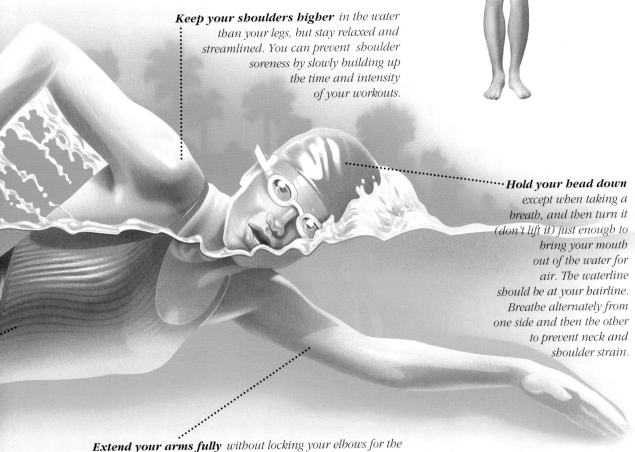

In the S-pattern *stroke, you get more thrust because your arms push against still water, not against their own choppy wake.*

Keep your shoulders higher *in the water than your legs, but stay relaxed and streamlined. You can prevent shoulder soreness by slowly building up the time and intensity of your workouts.*

Hold your head down *except when taking a breath, and then turn it (don't lift it) just enough to bring your mouth out of the water for air. The waterline should be at your hairline. Breathe alternately from one side and then the other to prevent neck and shoulder strain.*

Extend your arms fully *without locking your elbows for the catch phase, the point at which the hand enters the water (fingertips first). Pull downward in an S-shaped curve across your torso (above right). Your elbow should be higher than your hand as your arm comes out of the water.*

BEGINNING SWIMMING PROGRAM

This regimen lets you work up gradually to exercising in your training zone. To calculate your maximum heart rate for swimming (p.97), subtract your age from 207 rather than 220. (The water's buoyancy and temperature keep your heart rate 10 to 13 beats slower.) Use the stretches on pages 104–105 to limber up. If you experience any of the warning signs on page 111, get out of the pool at once. A pool length is assumed to be 25 yards.

	Warmup	Target Zone Exercising	Cooldown	Total
Weeks 1 and 2	Stretch and limber up for 10 minutes.	Swim 1 length and walk back. Continue for 5–8 minutes.	Walk slowly in the water and stretch for 10 minutes.	25–28 minutes
Weeks 3 and 4	Stretch and limber up for 10 minutes.	Try swimming 2 lengths before walking a length. Continue for 8–10 minutes.	Walk slowly in the water and stretch for 10 minutes.	28–30 minutes
Weeks 5 and 6	Stretch and limber up for 10 minutes.	Try 3 lengths before pausing. Continue for 10–12 minutes.	Walk slowly in the water and stretch for 10 minutes.	30–32 minutes
Weeks 7 and 8	Stretch and limber up for 10 minutes.	Try 4 lengths without stopping. Continue for 12–15 minutes.	Walk slowly in the water and stretch for 10 minutes.	32–35 minutes
Weeks 9 and 10	Stretch and limber up for 10 minutes.	Try 5 lengths without stopping. Continue for 15–18 minutes.	Walk slowly in the water and stretch for 10 minutes.	35–38 minutes
After week 10	Stretch and limber up for 10 minutes.	Work up to a swimming distance that you can cover in 20 minutes at a pace that enables you to achieve 60 percent of your maximum heart rate.	Walk slowly in the water and stretch for 10 minutes.	40 minutes

LOCATING A GOOD POOL

You can usually find a pool suitable for lap swimming at a local school, a Y, a public park, or a sports club. You need a pool with defined lap lanes that are at least 20 (preferably 25) yards long.

When selecting a pool, check that the areas around the water and the locker rooms are clean and that the pool water is clear enough to see the drain at the bottom of the deep end. Water temperature should be between 78 and 84 degrees. A beginner should choose a pool with a shallow section for safely practicing strokes. At any pool, make sure that a qualified lifeguard is on duty at all times—even good swimmers can get cramps or hit their heads while in the water and should never swim alone.

WORKING OUT IN WATER

Swimming is not the only form of aquatic exercise. Because water offers many times more resistance than air, doing other kinds of exercise in water builds extra strength and endurance while also lowering the risk of injury. Water calisthenics work pairs of muscles (such as hamstrings and gluteals in the thigh or triceps and biceps in the upper arm) better than land-based routines. You can also get full aerobic benefit if the workout includes at least 20 minutes of continuous exercise—walking or jogging against water resistance, for example—that raises your heart rate into the training zone (p.97).

You can do aquatic routines in a shallow pool. But, in deep water, wear a flotation vest to keep your body erect so that you walk or jog naturally instead of just treading water.

Many pools offer water exercise classes, or you can use a book or video (see p.108) to design a routine to do with a friend (you shouldn't exercise in water alone). Always stretch and warm up for 5 to 10 minutes before starting and cool down and stretch afterward.

Golfers and tennis players have discovered training benefits in swinging old clubs and racquets under water. Water resistance strengthens the muscles used in the swing, giving it more power. Slowing the movement reveals flaws in your technique.

. . . .

EQUIPMENT

Unless you are in a serious competition, you can wear any swimsuit that is comfortable and stays in place while you move. Nylon or Lycra racing suits are simple, sleek, and reasonably priced.

A rubber bathing cap protects your hair from the chemicals used to disinfect pool water and keeps long hair out of your eyes. Gog-

gles improve underwater vision and, if they are properly fitted and sealed, protect your eyes from pool chemicals, which often cause redness and stinging.

Training devices may look like toys, but they allow you to concentrate on individual parts of your swimming technique while also varying your workouts. A kickboard, for example, rests your upper body while you practice different kicks. Gripping a pull buoy between your legs keeps your lower body afloat while you strengthen arm strokes. Swim fins, which make you go much faster, also reinforce proper freestyle kicking technique and offer a good workout for the hamstring, quadricep, calf, and abdominal muscles. Using hand paddles gives your arms and shoulders a vigorous workout.

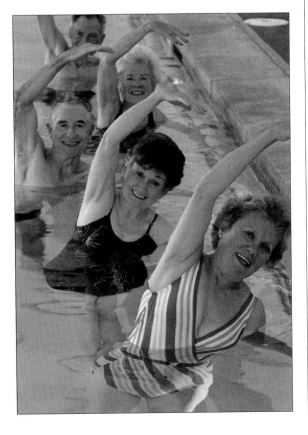

Members of a water aerobic exercise class stretch during the warmup period before their regular aquatic workout. Both men and women find water exercise fun and refreshing.

FAST FACTS

■ You cool off two to five times faster in water than in air of the same temperature. So it's a good idea to swim or exercise in water when it's too hot and humid to work out on land.

■ While women walkers prefer to follow complex routes, men choose straight and direct walking paths. Men, however, are more likely than women to give strangers complex directions to a location.

■ Laughter is good for your body as well as your psyche. Scientists have found that sustained laughter is a form of aerobic exercise. While you chortle, your stomach, neck, and shoulder muscles rapidly contract and relax, your heart rate goes up, and you take deep breaths. A researcher suggests that 100 laughs equal 10 minutes of rowing.

■ Both relaxation techniques and exercise reduce your level of anxiety with equal efficiency. Several tests show, however, that the calming effects of a good workout last longer.

■ According to a recent study, each additional mile a sedentary person walks or runs can lengthen his life by 21 minutes.

BICYCLING: GOING THE DISTANCE

Bicycling is a calorie-burning, heart-rate-raising activity that lets you cover far greater distances than walking or jogging and is gentler on your joints.

THE RIGHT BIKE

Your outdoor bike should fit properly and be in good working order. A salesperson at a reputable bike shop can help you select one with the correct frame size (which is not adjustable) and set the seat and handlebars at the right height for you. Take your bike in for a yearly tune-up, and check brakes, gears, and tires before every outing.

If the weather prevents biking outside or if you prefer indoor safety and comfort, you can get just as good a workout on a stationary bike (p.132).

ON THE ROAD

Cyclists must obey the rules of the road; keep to the right and stay in single file. Don't ride in dirt or gravel, which can be dangerous. Avoid hugging the curb; drivers can't see you as well and you have no room to maneuver.

Try to anticipate hills, bumps, turns, and obstacles. To go up a hill, shift to a lower gear. Don't wear or carry anything that can get caught in the bike's moving parts. Above all, stay balanced; don't wear a heavy pack, and leave both your hands free to steer, brake, and change gears.

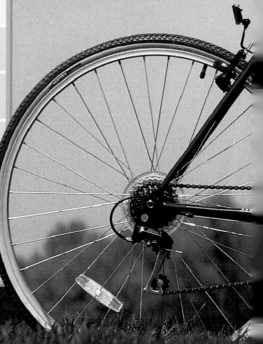

Raise your buttocks off the seat when going over bumps *to minimize soreness over the long haul.*

BEGINNING OUTDOOR BICYCLING PROGRAM

Do at least three exercise sessions during each week of the program. Work in comfortable gear and stay on flat terrain for the first few weeks. If you feel overstressed at any point, drop back to a previous level until you feel ready to advance. Lower your target heart-rate zone when you bike for longer periods. For instance, if you cycle between 40 and 90 minutes, aim for a target zone of 60 to 70 percent.

	Warmup	Target Zone* Exercising	Cooldown	Total
Weeks 1 – 4	Slow cycling for 5 – 10 minutes	10 – 15 minutes	Slow cycling for 5 – 10 minutes	20 – 35 minutes
Weeks 5 – 8	Slow cycling for 5 – 10 minutes	15 – 20 minutes	Slow cycling for 5 – 10 minutes	25 – 40 minutes
Weeks 9 – 12	Slow cycling for 5 – 10 minutes	25 – 35 minutes	Slow cycling for 5 – 10 minutes	35 – 55 minutes
After week 12	As you become better conditioned and need to work harder to reach your target zone, consider speeding up, increasing your bike's gear tension, or including more hills in your route. Only add one of these factors at a time. Your aim is to reach your target zone, not to overextend yourself.			

* See page 97 to learn how to estimate your target zone.

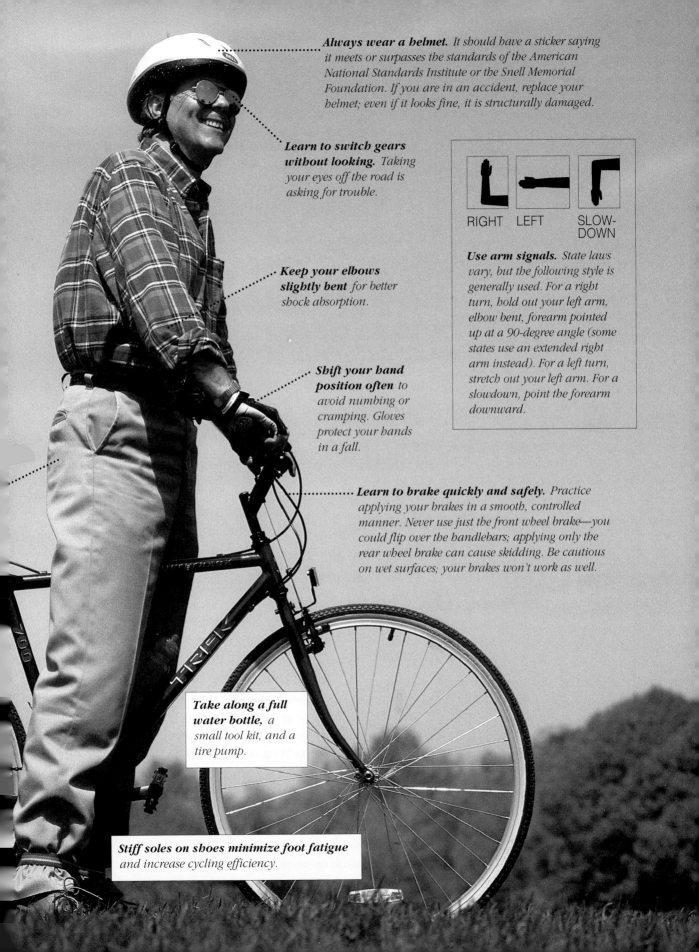

Always wear a helmet. *It should have a sticker saying it meets or surpasses the standards of the American National Standards Institute or the Snell Memorial Foundation. If you are in an accident, replace your helmet; even if it looks fine, it is structurally damaged.*

Learn to switch gears without looking. *Taking your eyes off the road is asking for trouble.*

Keep your elbows slightly bent *for better shock absorption.*

Shift your hand position often *to avoid numbing or cramping. Gloves protect your hands in a fall.*

RIGHT   LEFT   SLOW-
DOWN

Use arm signals. *State laws vary, but the following style is generally used. For a right turn, hold out your left arm, elbow bent, forearm pointed up at a 90-degree angle (some states use an extended right arm instead). For a left turn, stretch out your left arm. For a slowdown, point the forearm downward.*

Learn to brake quickly and safely. *Practice applying your brakes in a smooth, controlled manner. Never use just the front wheel brake—you could flip over the handlebars; applying only the rear wheel brake can cause skidding. Be cautious on wet surfaces; your brakes won't work as well.*

Take along a full water bottle, *a small tool kit, and a tire pump.*

Stiff soles on shoes minimize foot fatigue *and increase cycling efficiency.*

JOGGING: AEROBICS IN A HURRY

*J*ogging, like walking, is an aerobic activity that appeals to people of all ages, requires no special skills, costs no more than a pair of good shoes every 500 miles, and can be enjoyed almost anytime, anywhere, indoors or outdoors.

THE ADVANTAGES—AND DISADVANTAGES—OF RUNNING

Jogging appeals to busy people; you can maintain aerobic fitness with only 20 minutes of work three or four times a week. Dedicated joggers and runners (a jogger's pace is usually 5 to 8 miles an hour, and a runner's is generally that speed or more) also claim that jogging keeps them trim, improves sleep, and reduces stress.

Jogging and running have one drawback: a high injury rate. Each time your foot hits the ground, a force equivalent to almost three times your weight pounds through your body while the muscles in the lower body work to propel you through the stride. This pounding and driving may make the muscles, connective tissues, and bones of the lower body vulnerable to injuries, from inflammation and muscle strains to sprains and stress fractures.

REDUCING RISKS OF INJURY

To lower your chances of getting hurt, follow safe running rules. Buy running shoes that fit properly (your toes shouldn't be cramped), support your feet, and absorb shock. Wear socks (synthetics or blends) that wick perspiration away from your feet.

Pay attention to form; wasteful motion can tire you. Find your own natural stride. Maintain good posture while you jog, and keep your arms swinging at waist level, not across your chest.

Pick a forgiving running surface such as a cushioned synthetic indoor or outdoor track, a grassy field, or a dirt road. If you run on a banked track, alternate directions so that your body gets equal time on both sides of the

BEGINNING JOGGING PROGRAM

Don't start a jogging program until you can comfortably walk 3 miles in 30–45 minutes. As a beginning jogger, your goal should be to walk/jog for 20 minutes without stopping. If you find this too strenuous, continue to walk. (See a doctor if you experience any of the danger signs described on page 111.) If you feel excessively tired at any point, go back to the previous week's level. Don't worry about your pace. Once you've established a 20-minute routine, you can jog for longer periods if you wish or try to jog a little faster to keep in your target heart-rate zone (p.97).

	Warmup	Target Zone Exercising	Cooldown	Total
Week 1	Stretch and walk for 5–10 minutes.	Alternate 1 minute of jogging with 2 minutes of walking for 20 minutes. Three sessions, skipping a day between each.	Walk 5 minutes, then stretch 5 minutes.	35–40 minutes
Week 2	Stretch and walk for 5–10 minutes.	Alternate 1 minute of jogging with 1 minute of walking for 20 minutes. Three or four sessions, skipping a day between each.	Walk 5 minutes, then stretch 5 minutes.	35–40 minutes
Weeks 3 - 10	Stretch and walk for 5–10 minutes.	Over 8 weeks (or more if you need it), gradually increase the length of the jogging segments and cut the walking times until you are jogging comfortably for the full 20 minutes without a break. Three or four sessions, skipping a day between each.	Walk 5 minutes, then stretch 5 minutes.	35–40 minutes

slant. Try not to run straight down a steep hill (it distorts your form); walk or run down in a zigzag pattern instead.

Limit your jogging to four 30-minute sessions a week (or 20 miles) with a day off after each session. Injury rates go up steeply after 20 miles a week.

. . . .

GETTING STARTED

If you are new to exercise, follow the Beginning Walking Program on page 119. When you can walk briskly for 45 minutes three or four times a week, you are ready for a jog/walk regimen (facing page). If you play tennis, soccer, or softball regularly, you can't assume you are fit enough to jog the full distance immediately. The running you do in such sports comes in short bursts, which don't develop your aerobic capacity or the muscle power needed for jogging.

HOW FAST DO YOU JOG?

To find out how fast you are jogging, time yourself running a mile. Find your minutes for completing a mile in the left column; your speed will be in the right column.

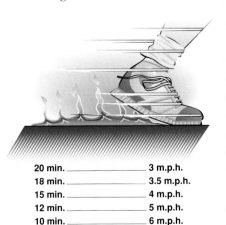

20 min.	3 m.p.h.
18 min.	3.5 m.p.h.
15 min.	4 m.p.h.
12 min.	5 m.p.h.
10 min.	6 m.p.h.
8 min.	7.5 m.p.h.
6 min.	10 m.p.h.

Profile

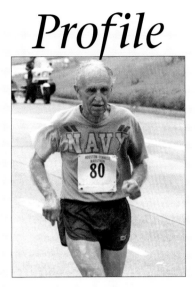

CLYDE J. VILLEMEZ: IN IT FOR THE LONG RUN

Clyde J. Villemez was 60 years old and had just retired from an army career when his son, a college runner, challenged him to come to the track for some exercise. "I hadn't run since high school," Villemez recalls. "But I tried it a few times and liked it. I got friends together on weekends to run. We would meet in Houston's Memorial Park and frequently would finish with a family picnic."

Running became a passion for Villemez. He entered local races. "We'd run cross-country, and often we didn't know what the distance was," he says. "I never thought of it as work. A run was an adventure." In 1972, Villemez entered his first marathon. He completed the 26.2 miles in 4 hours 18 minutes. "I wasn't trying to run fast; I just wanted to see what it was like to run that far," he says.

That was the first of more than 50 marathons Villemez has run, making him a local hero in Port Arthur, Texas, where he lives with his wife, Lillian, a walker. Villemez now has more than 31,000 miles of running and 450 races to his credit. He still covers 50 to 60 miles a week (more before a marathon).

EXERCISING AT HOME

I f home exercise appeals to you, you are not alone. Most Americans who work out do so at home. It's convenient, private, and protected from the weather. And you can exercise by yourself or with a friend or family member.

CHOOSING A MACHINE: BE REALISTIC AND PRACTICAL

Buying a home exercise machine is no guarantee that you will use it. You should be committed to regular exercise, and your choice should reflect your interests, needs, and abilities. Remember, too, no single machine can lead to total fitness.

Never buy a machine without trying it out. It should be comfortable, easy to use, and sturdy. Instruction is important to prevent injury. Ask your salesperson to instruct you or, better yet, take lessons at a health club.

Stationary bicycles, the most popular home machines, come in three models: single action, dual action, and recumbent. The first and third work only your lower body; the second also works your arms. A recumbent has a chairlike seat with the pedals out in front. Or attach an outdoor bike to a training stand.

If you want to simulate stair climbing, buy a home stair climber. Single-action machines work only the lower body; dual-action ones, the upper body as well.

All rowers and cross-country ski machines work both the up-

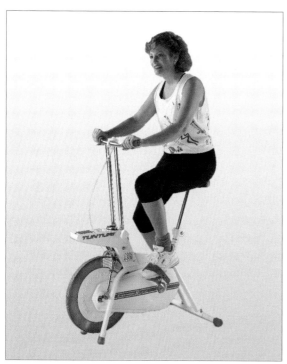

Stationary bicycle. *Set the seat of your stationary bicycle (single-action model above) to allow your legs to be almost fully extended. The tension, seat, and handlebars should be easy to adjust.*

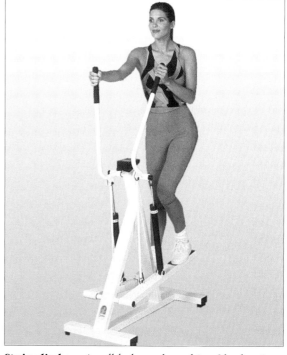

Stair climber. *A well-balanced machine (dual-action model above) has a smooth action and adjustable resistance. On single-action models, don't lean on the handrails (and lose fitness benefits) when you get tired.*

per and lower body. In one type of rower, you pull a bar secured to a chain attached to a flywheel or fan. In another, you pull one or two poles against hydraulic tension. The flywheel type is bigger and costlier; most hydraulics can be put in a closet. A rower with a contoured seat that moves on a track is best for comfort.

There are two types of ski machines. In one, you pull ropes attached to a pulley; in the other, you pull and push poles attached to its base. In both, your feet move back and forth on sliding tracks. Practice with your arms first, then add the leg motions.

Treadmills, another increasingly popular machine, come in electronic or self-powered models. Those with arm handles also exercise the upper body.

SETTING UP YOUR HOME EXERCISE AREA

Make your exercise area comfortable and appealing. You'll hardly be motivated to work out on a machine stuck in a dank corner of your basement. Place your machine on a flat surface so that it won't rock, jump, or slide. Protect your floors with a rubber or plastic mat. Leave space to do your stretches, and make sure children and pets can't be hurt by the machine's moving parts.

Keep yourself entertained while you work out. Watching television, reading, listening to music or books on tape, and having other people around can take the tedium out of exercise and make you more likely to stick with your program.

> **❝The Wise, for Cure, on Exercise depend.❞**
>
> *—John Dryden, 17th-century English poet*

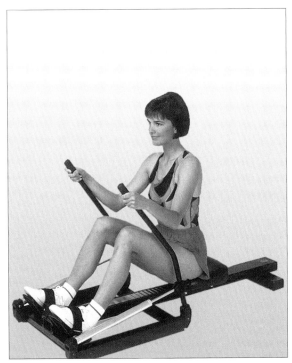

Rowing machine. *With your feet strapped to a panel or footrests, you push back at the start of a stroke and slide forward at the end (hydraulic model above). Tension, foot straps, and pole length should be adjustable.*

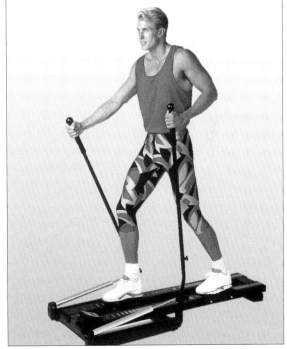

Cross-country ski machine. *The machine should fit you exactly (pole model above) or have adjustable pole length and (for a pulley model) stomach cushion height. Leg and arm tensions should be adjustable.*

WEIGHT TRAINING FOR STRENGTH

*L*ong *associated with body-building competitions or the transformation of the 98-pound weakling in the old Charles Atlas ads, weight training is actually the most effective way for men and women to increase muscle strength and endurance.*

WHY YOU NEED STRENGTH

Life is easier if you don't have to strain to do such ordinary tasks as lifting a child or pushing a mower. Strong muscles stabilize joints and improve balance and coordination, protecting you from injuries while you do chores or other kinds of exercise. Muscle strength gives you greater athletic prowess (a stronger golf swing or tennis serve). Muscle-building exercises help build bone density, reducing your risk of fractures.

FREE WEIGHTS VS. MACHINES

There are two types of weight-training equipment: free weights (barbells and dumbbells) and weight machines. Whichever you choose, you need expert instruction in the beginning to prevent hurting yourself. Find a reputable health club with knowledgeable trainers who can spend a few sessions with you to design a program and teach you technique.

Some experts consider weight machines safer for beginners be-cause there is less risk of injury from dropping the weights. But you can minimize this danger by using correct form, working within your limits, and having a partner "spot" the weights—that is, stand nearby to catch them if they start to fall. Free weights cost less and are easier to use in limited home exercise space.

Women need not worry about developing massive muscles from weight training. It is biologically harder to "bulk up" a woman's muscles, and the process requires hours of daily training.

Muscular fitness involves both endurance and strength. Most weight training builds both, but you can emphasize one. Working against light resistance, or weight, with many repetitions builds endurance. Lifting heavier weights a few times builds strength.

WEIGHT MACHINE LEG CURL
Working on the hamstring muscles at the back of the thigh, an exerciser lifts both legs together from the knees against a weight machine's preset resistance level. It's important in this exercise not to raise your hips off the bench. A trainer should show you how to do the exercise and help you set a safe resistance level.

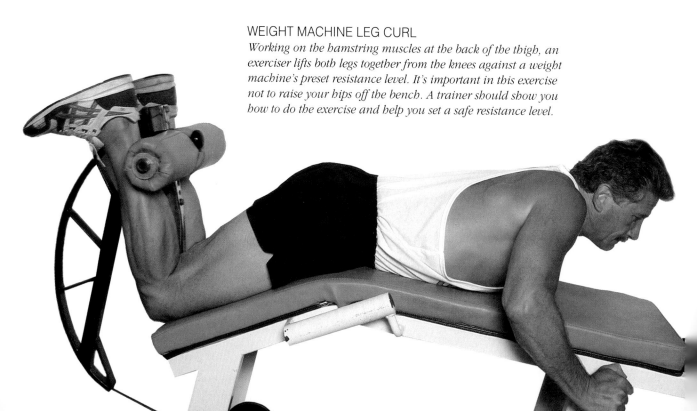

HEALTH CLUBS

To receive instruction from qualified trainers, learn new exercises, and meet other active people, you may want to join a health club. Clubs vary in cost, facilities, and atmosphere; you should choose carefully, using the guidelines below.

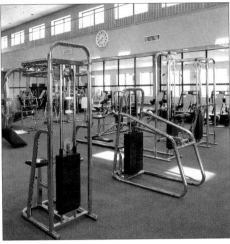

▨ Go for convenience. Pick a club near your home or office. Know what you want in the way of equipment, facilities, classes, personnel, and services.

▨ Visit the club at the time of day you plan to work out to see how crowded it is then, what equipment is available, and how you like the other members. Talk to the members.

▨ Ask about medical clearance. If the club requires a doctor's OK or a stress test, the staff values health and safety.

▨ Check staff qualifications. Trainers should have a background in exercise physiology, kinesiology, or physical education, and be certified by the American College of Sports Medicine, the American Council on Exercise, the Aerobics and Fitness Association of America, or the Cooper Institute of Aerobics Research. Someone trained in emergency medical care should be on duty at all times.

▨ Check the club's longevity. Older clubs are more likely to be financially stable and to stay in business.

FREE WEIGHT ARM CURL
To strengthen her biceps, an exerciser raises two barbells simultaneously (she could also alternate arms). With her feet apart and knees slightly bent, she completes the curl by slowly lowering the barbells to thigh level. Never lock your elbow joint in this exercise.

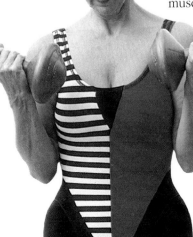

GUIDELINES FOR WEIGHT-TRAINING WORKOUTS

Wear comfortable clothing and supportive shoes. Warm up and cool down (p.109).

Never hold your breath during weight training—it can cause your blood pressure to rise dangerously. Instead, exhale as you lift the weight and inhale as you bring the weight down.

Lift and lower weights slowly, using a smooth, controlled motion. If you depend on a weight's momentum to move it, you won't get strengthening benefits.

Start with weights that you can lift comfortably 10 to 15 times (a "set"). As you get stronger, you may either increase the number of repetitions or the amount of weight (not both at once). When a set of 15 repetitions of an exercise feels easy, try increasing the weight 5 percent. Let your muscles recover between sets.

Work the large muscle groups (legs, back, chest, arms) first, but include all muscles in your total workout plan. Also equally work the muscles in opposing pairs—hamstrings on the back of the thigh and quadriceps on the front of the thigh, for example.

To maintain strength, train with weights at least twice a week, but never work the same muscles on consecutive days; muscles need 24 hours to recover.

EXERCISING AS YOU AGE

The need for regular physical activity increases with age. Exercise holds off the body's physical deterioration, helps maintain its metabolic rate, and allows you to live more fully and independently. Luckily, it's never too late to start a fitness program.

SUITING YOUR NEEDS

An exercise program for older people should be tailored to individual fitness levels and take into account any orthopedic, cardiovascular, musculoskeletal, visual, or balance problems that may have come with age.

Those who have been inactive for years will tire more easily at the beginning but ultimately may

CHAIR EXERCISES

If you must spend a lot of time confined to a chair, you can stay flexible and strong by doing the traveler's exercises on page 110, the neck stretch on page 104, and the exercises below. Repeat each 4 to 6 times.

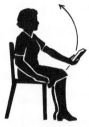

Arm strengtheners. *Hold a book or can of soup in one hand. Lift it overhead and bring it down; extend it in front of you (shoulder level) and back. Repeat with the other hand. As you get stronger, use a heavier object.*

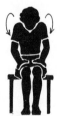

Shoulder stretch. *Shrug both shoulders up to your ears, rotate them backward, and then lower them to their original position.*

Back stretch. *Lean forward and reach for your knees, calves, ankles, and the floor, holding each position for 1 to 2 seconds.*

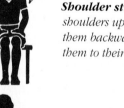

Arm-shoulder stretch. *Extend your arms to either side at shoulder height. Rotate your arms in small circles, first clockwise and then counterclockwise.*

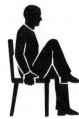

Hip flexor strengthener. *Bring one knee as close to your chest as you can. Repeat with the other knee. Alternate your legs as if you were doing a high-stepping march.*

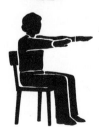

Arm-wrist-hand stretch. *Extend your arms in front of you, parallel to the floor. While you open and close your hands and rotate your wrists, move your arms in an arc to meet over your head. Return to the original position and repeat.*

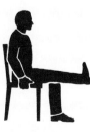

Quadricep strengthener/ankle stretch. *Sitting straight with both feet flat on the floor, lift one leg from the knee so that it is parallel to the floor. Hold the position, flex your foot, and rotate the ankle. Repeat with the other leg.*

show the greatest gains. Such people, however, should undergo a complete physical examination, including a stress test, before starting an exercise program. Older individuals—both beginners and those who have stayed fit—should follow the rules below.

GENERAL GUIDELINES

Keep a regular exercise schedule and follow a well-rounded program that includes aerobic, strength-building, endurance-building, and flexibility-enhancing exercises. If you want to build up the intensity of your exercise, do it very gradually.

If you have sore joints, avoid or limit activities such as running and other high-impact aerobics that put stress on those joints. Stick to walking, swimming, and other water exercises.

Warm up and cool down for longer periods (10 to 15 minutes) than you would at a younger age. A longer transition into and out of exercise allows your body more time to adjust to and recover from the exertion of exercise.

During the aerobic part of your workout, maintain a heart rate of between 50 and 85 percent of your maximum rate (p.97). When you are ready to exercise more, it is safer to lengthen a session than to raise its intensity. Remember, however, that the lower the heart rate, the longer you need to exercise to get the benefit. In most cases, you should limit your total workout time to an hour.

Exhale during the exertion part of an exercise and inhale during relaxation. If you have high blood pressure, don't engage in high-intensity or isometric exercises, such as lifting heavy weights, downhill skiing, and sprinting.

GOING FOR THE GOLD IN THE GOLDEN YEARS

Participants in the biennial U.S. National Senior Sports Classic—The Senior Olympics—come from all over the United States and range in age from 55 (the minimum) to 99. Their backgrounds are as diverse as their ages. Almost 40 years after winning the state championship, a high school girls' basketball team reunites and wins gold. A cancer survivor in his mid-eighties, who played 2 to 4 hours a day during 7 weeks of radiation therapy, continues to compete nationally in senior men's tennis.

Some of these athletes took up sports as youngsters and never stopped playing. Others started exercising later in life, liked it, and became

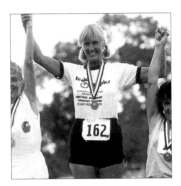

Sprinter Jane Clarkson won three gold medals at the age of 60. Coached by her son, she started running at 55.

competitive. Senior athletes who have placed first, second, or third in state Qualifying Senior Games compete nationally in 18 different sports—archery, badminton, basketball, bowling, cycling, track and field, golf, horseshoes, racquetball, shuffleboard, softball, swimming, table tennis, tennis, 10K road race, race walking, triathlon, and volleyball.

For more information, write to the U.S. Senior Sports Organization, 14323 South Outer Forty Road, Chesterfield, Missouri 63017.

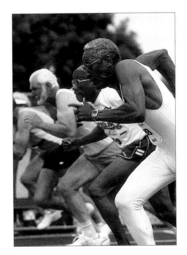

Race winner Jim Law (far right in picture at left) began running again in his sixties— after a 40-year hiatus.

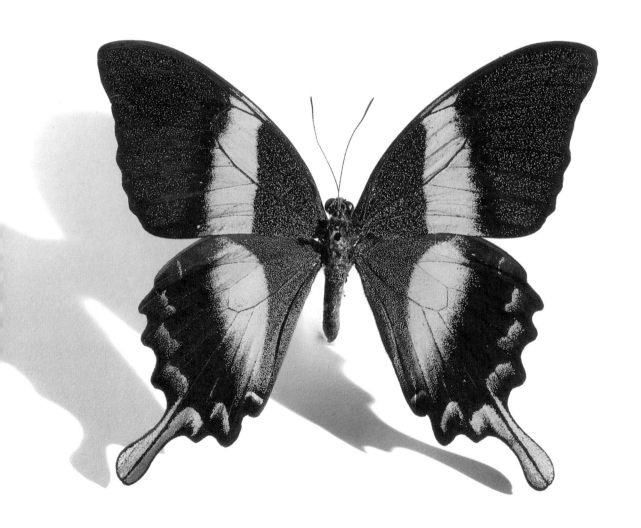

Chapter 4

LOOKING YOUR BEST

▨ CARING FOR CHANGING SKIN *140*

▨ CONSIDERING PLASTIC SURGERY *148*

▨ MINOR PROCEDURES,
MAJOR RESULTS *150*

▨ MAJOR PROCEDURES FOR
MAXIMUM RESULTS *152*

▨ MODIFYING HAIR CARE *156*

▨ DEALING WITH GRAY HAIR *158*

▨ FACING UP TO HAIR LOSS *160*

▨ FOR HEALTHY TEETH *162*

▨ FOR THAT PERFECT SMILE *164*

▨ TAKING CARE OF
HANDS AND FEET *166*

▨ MAKING THE MOST
OF YOUR APPEARANCE *168*

CARING FOR CHANGING SKIN

Because your skin changes throughout your life, you can't adopt a single care regimen and stick with it forever. Understanding how skin ages, decade by decade, helps you to anticipate when and how to treat it differently.

HOW NORMAL SKIN IS ALTERED BY AGING

Most people outgrow acne by the age of 20. By 30, you may see tiny crow's-feet around your eyes, your first wrinkles. You also start losing the cells that produce the pigment melanin, leading to a paler complexion and less protection from the sun's ultraviolet rays; melanin loss proceeds at the rate of 6 to 8 percent a decade.

At about the age of 40, the fat in the innermost layer of your skin starts to shrink. In the middle layer, or dermis, the collagen that forms the skin's fibrous supporting structure gradually decreases, as do the elastin fibers that make your skin flexible. Cell production in the epidermis, or outer layer of skin, slows. Your skin becomes thinner, less supple, and more prone to wrinkles.

In your fifties, wrinkles become deeper and cheeks may sag. Although blood vessels in the skin become sparser, on sun-damaged faces, near-the-surface blood vessels may make a pattern of red lines called telangiectasia. Glands in the dermis secrete less oil, leading to drier skin. In your sixties and seventies, your skin becomes more parched, thinner, paler, and more wrinkled.

PREVENTING SKIN DAMAGE

How your skin ages is essentially dictated by genes, which you can't control, and sun exposure, which you can control (p.147). You can't undo a lifetime of over-exposure, but further sun damage can be avoided.

Wrinkles, the most obvious sign of aging, generally appear earlier in women than in men because men's skin is thicker. Black or dark skin, protected by higher concentrations of melanin, stays smooth longer than fair skin.

But wrinkling, too, is partly under your control. Along with the sun, smoking is a major cause of wrinkles. The chemicals in tobacco constrict blood vessels, and thus promote wrinkles by reducing blood flow to the skin. Squinting through the haze hastens the formation of crow's feet.

Bags and rings appear under the eyes because this area has the thinnest skin in the body. As the skin loses resilience, fluid collects

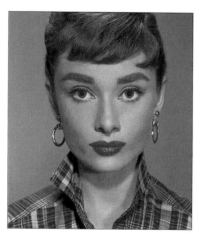
Actress Audrey Hepburn in her twenties played beguiling ingenues.

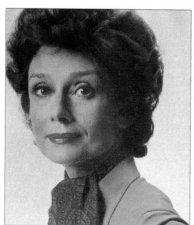
Hepburn in her forties had a more sculptured face and smile lines.

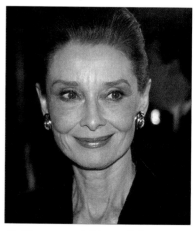
At 60, more wrinkles and thinner skin didn't diminish Hepburn's glow.

under it, making it bulge and sag. Veins near the surface show through as dark circles. Although a tendency to develop these conditions is hereditary, fatigue and eye irritation exacerbate them. Raising the head of your bed (put blocks under the legs) may reduce puffiness by letting fluid drain away. Don't rub your eyes; you may stretch the fragile skin beneath them. And get plenty of sleep. Some researchers believe that body tissues replenish themselves during sleep.

. . . .

PAMPERING BODY SKIN

Soothing as a long hot bath may feel, soaking dries aging skin. A lukewarm bath of 15 minutes or less is better. And think twice about bath oil; it can make the tub slippery. Use ½ cup of salt in the bath water instead.

Taking a brief shower is less drying than bathing in plain water. In winter, when your skin is exposed to harsh weather and dry heat, dermatologists suggest limiting showers to three or four a week. In warm, humid climates, no restriction is necessary.

If your skin is dry, choose a mild nondrying body soap (for faial cleansers, see chart, p.143). Deodorant soaps, which work by killing the germs that cause perspiration to smell bad, are sometimes harsh on sensitive skin.

After your bath or shower, pat—don't rub—yourself dry and use a moisturizing lotion right away to lock in the water your skin has absorbed.

> **❝***Nature gives you the face you have at 20; at 50, you get the face you deserve.***❞**
>
> —*Fashion designer*
> *Coco Chanel*

This cross section of skin *shows three layers. As skin ages, the connective tissue (collagen and elastin) in the middle layer, or dermis, and the fat cells in the lower subcutaneous layer (hypodermis) decrease, making skin thinner, less resilient, and more prone to wrinkles. The oil glands slow their production, and the skin becomes drier and more delicate.*

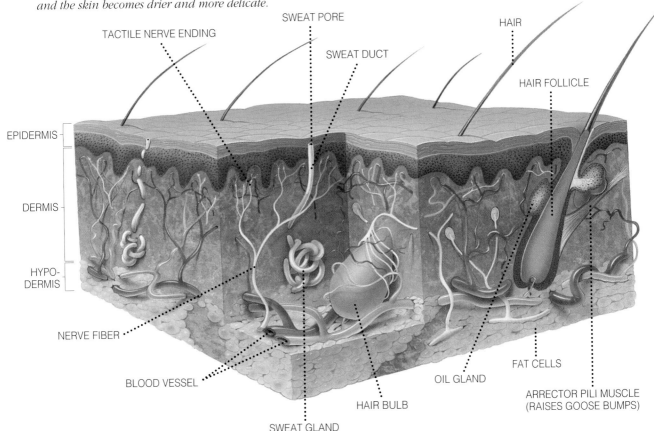

TACTILE NERVE ENDING
SWEAT PORE
SWEAT DUCT
HAIR
HAIR FOLLICLE
EPIDERMIS
DERMIS
HYPO-DERMIS
NERVE FIBER
BLOOD VESSEL
SWEAT GLAND
HAIR BULB
OIL GLAND
FAT CELLS
ARRECTOR PILI MUSCLE
(RAISES GOOSE BUMPS)

A MATURE WOMAN'S FACIAL REGIMEN

Washing your face too often with soap wears away the protective film that holds in natural moisture. Women with dry skin may prefer to clean their faces with creams or other special products (see chart on facing page). Limit face cleanings to once or twice a day. Apply soap with your fingertips instead of a washcloth, rinse thoroughly, pat dry, and follow up with a moisturizer.

Toners—astringents, skin fresheners, and clarifying lotions, which are formulated to clean up after cleansing

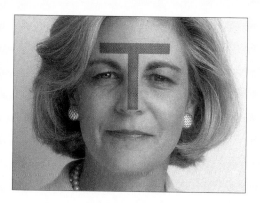

The T-zone is the area of the face most likely to be oily and to harbor enlarged pores, blackheads, and other blemishes. It often requires special cleaning.

creams—often rob your skin of moisture. Many have a high alcohol content and are only appropriate for use on oily areas such as the T-zone (above). Sloughing products, or exfoliants, which re-

move dead skin cells, are controversial. Some dermatologists feel that they are too harsh for aging skin; other experts think that sloughing speeds up skin-cell replacement in older skin and refines skin texture.

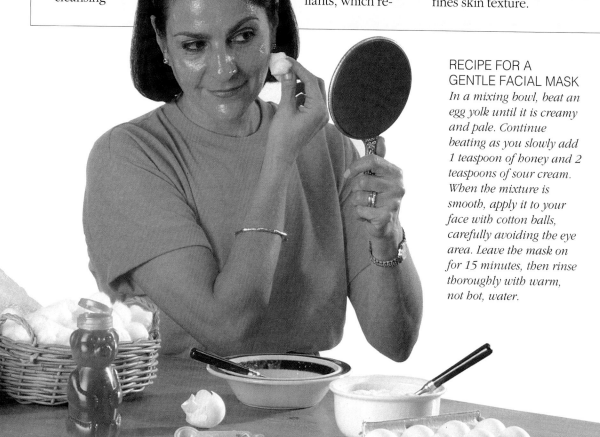

RECIPE FOR A
GENTLE FACIAL MASK
In a mixing bowl, beat an egg yolk until it is creamy and pale. Continue beating as you slowly add 1 teaspoon of honey and 2 teaspoons of sour cream. When the mixture is smooth, apply it to your face with cotton balls, carefully avoiding the eye area. Leave the mask on for 15 minutes, then rinse thoroughly with warm, not hot, water.

FACIAL TREATMENTS

Beauty salons and spas offer a variety of facial treatments for both men and women. Such pampering is relaxing and good for the psyche, but not all the offerings benefit aging skin.

■ *Facial sauna.* Luxurious at a salon, a refreshing facial sauna can also be enjoyed at home. Using steam to moisturize, cleanse, and soften your skin every 6 weeks may give your face (and your spirits) a lift. Buy an inexpensive electric facial sauna appliance or simply fill a basin with boiling water. Drape a towel over your head and shoulders to form a tent and lean over the steaming water for 5 to 10 minutes. While your skin is soft and your pores are open, remove any blackheads with a tissue and dab the pore with antiseptic. Apply a moisturizer to the whole face. As an extra treat after the sauna, lie down with your feet elevated and place cool wet tea bags or cotton pads moistened with witch hazel on your eyes. Rest for 10 minutes.

■ *Masks.* Dermatologists differ on the subject of facial masks. Some claim they clear away dead surface skin, deep-cleanse, and stimulate circulation. Others fear they are too drying for aging skin. Certainly the traditional clay mask or mud pack made of fuller's earth is very drying. Perhaps more suitable for mature skin are gels, which form a clear film on the face that can later be pulled or rinsed off. You can make a mask suitable for dry skin by using a few kitchen staples (see recipe on facing page).

■ *Massage and exercise.* Dermatologists advise against vigorous massaging of the face, which can damage delicate skin. Facial exercises, promoted by some

CHOOSING A FACIAL CLEANSER

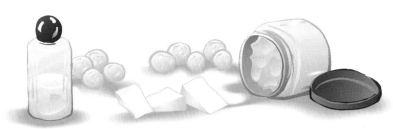

Product	Skin Type	Pros/Cons	Suggestions
Soapless soap	Normal, dry, or sensitive	Not irritating, contains moisturizers, and leaves no film, but expensive.	Look for soapless soaps at a pharmacy.
Superfatted soap	Normal to dry	Not irritating, contains moisturizers, but may leave residual film.	Rinse thoroughly.
Toilet soap	Oily	Inexpensive but harsh; may be irritating.	Choose an unscented soap with few ingredients. Rinse thoroughly in hard water.
Transparent soap	Sensitive but oily	Not irritating, but lathers poorly and melts easily.	To counteract melting tendency, dry after use.
Cleansing cream and lotion	Extremely dry and sensitive	Removes makeup effectively and contains moisturizers, but cleans poorly and leaves film.	After wiping off, wash face with gentle soap.
Astringent	Normal to oily	Removes excess oil and temporarily tightens pores, but may be irritating; some products that claim to be astringent are not.	Check ingredients; true astringents contain tannin in such forms as witch hazel, birch, and nettle.
Clarifying lotion	Normal to oily	Removes dead cells for smoother skin, but may be irritating.	Use no more than once or twice a week.
Skin freshener	All skin types	Provides further cleansing; temporarily tightens and refreshes skin, but may be drying and irritating.	For dry or sensitive skin, use products with little or no alcohol only in the oily T-zone (facing page).
Sloughing cream	Sensitive and dry	Removes dead cells in least abrasive way, but may be harsh and drying.	Apply lightly and moisturize afterward.
Sloughing grains	Normal to oily	Removes dead cells and excess oil, but may be harsh and drying.	Scrub lightly with fingertips; moisturize afterward. Do not use if skin is inflamed.
Sloughing pad	All skin types	Removes dead cells for smoother skin, but may be harsh and drying or cause dilated blood vessels in extreme cases.	Use with care once a month or every 3 weeks with soap or lotion; make soft circular motions.
Gel mask	Normal to oily	Helps restore moisture and removes dead cells gently, but often expensive.	Check ingredients or make your own out of egg yolk, honey, and sour cream (facing page).
Paste mask	Normal to oily	Smooths skin and absorbs impurities, but may be drying.	Use infrequently; once every 3–4 weeks is safe.

beauty consultants, are also controversial. Some experts think that they actually aggravate wrinkles. Exercise that keeps your body fit (see Chapter 3), however, also improves circulation to the skin and makes it look glowing.

. . . .

CARING FOR A MAN'S FACE

A man's skin, which is usually oilier than a woman's, will eventually need moisturizers too, especially if the skin is sensitive. If your skin feels dry, consider switching to an after-shave balm, which is less drying than an alcohol-based lotion or astringent.

If you shave every day, you can damage your skin simply by shaving incorrectly. Dermatologists suggest that before you shave with a safety razor, you soften your beard for several minutes with a warm washcloth and plenty of shaving cream or foam. Proceed as shown above right. Take the time to avoid nicks while you shave. If you do cut yourself, stop the flow of blood with a styptic pencil, available at any drugstore.

Before shaving with an electric razor, weaken your whiskers with a product designed for use with electric shavers. If you are subject to ingrown hairs, always move the razor in the direction the beard grows. You won't get as close a shave, but you will help prevent the painful condition. Be firm, but gentle. Shaving too vigorously with an electric razor can irritate sensitive skin.

Whichever kind of razor you prefer, don't shave just before exercising; newly shaved skin is especially vulnerable to the salt in perspiration, which stings, and to sunburn. Exercise first, then shower and shave afterward.

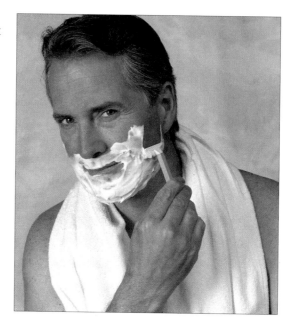

Proper shaving can protect a man's skin. If you prefer a safety razor, use one with a sharp blade (dull blades drag across your skin). Shave only once over each part of the beard area, moving the razor in the direction that the beard grows. Try to avoid stretching your skin to get a better razor angle.

SKIN SENSITIVITIES TO COSMETIC INGREDIENTS

Some ingredients in soaps and other cosmetics cause an allergic response on sensitive skin—usually an itchy rash called contact dermatitis. A dermatologist or allergist can test to determine the culprit. Among the ingredients most likely to provoke allergies are fragrances, preservatives, emulsifiers, and lanolin. Fragrance ingredients are difficult to identify. Some scents have as

To test a new cosmetic before using it on a large area of skin, rub a small amount onto your inner arm. Cover the area with a bandage for 24 hours, then check your skin. If there is no redness or irritation, the product is probably safe to use.

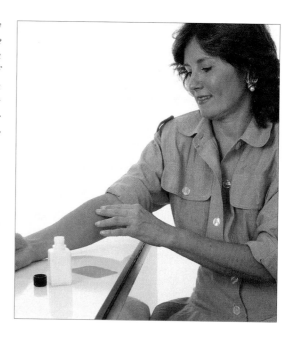

many as 300 components, which manufacturers are reluctant to name for patent reasons. Some fragrances found in men's after-shave products are photoaller-genic—that is, allergic reactions occur only when a treated face is exposed to the sun.

As you grow older, your skin becomes more sensitive, so it's a good idea to patch-test new products before using them (facing page). You can suddenly develop an allergy to an ingredient you have used your whole life. Also, a manufacturer may change an ingredient in a product that you have used safely for years.

Once you know that you are sensitive to a cosmetic ingredient, you can stop using products that contain it. Always read cosmetic labels before buying (right).

Among cosmetics, skin care products are most likely to cause an allergic reaction because they often contain lanolin, emulsifiers, and preservatives. Makeup also frequently has these ingredients, plus fragrances and red and yellow dyes, which can be irritating. Many people are sensitive to the para-aminobenzoic acid (PABA) used in many sunscreens. You can find PABA-free sunscreens at department store cosmetics counters or drugstores.

If your skin is sensitive, look for lines of cosmetics labeled fragrance-free, hypoallergenic, or allergy-tested. Such products are formulated with fewer common allergens and may be less irritating to your skin.

Most rashes caused by cosmetic products are mild and clear up in a few days after you stop using the product. If the itch becomes annoying, a nonprescription cortisone ointment will usually relieve it. See your doctor when a rash persists or is severe.

HOW TO READ COSMETIC LABELS

Cosmetics manufacturers are required by the Food and Drug Administration (FDA) to test a product for safety but not to prove its effectiveness. Ingredients must be listed on the product's container in order of the quantity used (major ingredient first), but exact amounts need not be given.

Some common ingredients you are likely to see on cosmetic labels are shown on the lotion bottle at right. Active ingredients include emollients (which help seal in moisture) such as lanolin, mineral oil, and petrolatum (petroleum), and humectants (which attract water to the skin surface) such as glycerin, lactic acid, and urea. Inactive ingredients include preservatives, fragrances, and emulsifiers (which keep the product from separating).

INGREDIENTS

WATER, MINERAL OIL, PETROLATUM, PROPYLENE GLYCOL, GLYCERIN, MICROCRYSTALLINE WAX, LANOLIN ALCOHOL, PARABENS, FRAGRANCE

The word *natural* on a label connotes no special benefit. So-called natural ingredients are often so denatured in processing that their scent is added artificially. Expensive natural additives of dubious value are cucumber, egg, honey, milk, placental extract, royal bee jelly, mink oil, and turtle oil.

Products that are labeled fragrance-free may still contain some masking fragrance to hide unpleasant odors (check the list of ingredients). For people with a sensitivity to fragrance, such products may still be off-limits.

Preservative-free products such as many mascaras and some moisturizers are less likely to irritate eyes or sensitive skin than other products, but they won't have the same safe shelf life. Preservative-free products ought to be replaced every 3 months (or sooner if they smell strange).

SKIN PROBLEMS THAT AFFECT OLDER PEOPLE

Inflamed bumps and broken or enlarged blood vessels on the face indicate rosacea. The disease can be aggravated by sun, heat, smoking, alcohol, and emotional stress. Prompt treatment by a doctor prevents the condition from spreading or getting worse.

In seborrheic dermatitis, a reddish scaly rash develops in the scalp, eyebrows, folds of the nose, corners of the mouth, behind the ears, over the breastbone, or under the arms. The rash, which is very common, may be triggered by severe stress (it can appear after a heart attack, for example). If using an antidandruff shampoo doesn't clear up such a rash, see a doctor.

Another rash, intertrigo, usually develops during hot, humid weather and affects parts of the body that rub against each other, such as the inner thighs of overweight people or under pendulous breasts. Keep the affected area uncovered at night and dry it with powder during the day. In severe cases, consult a doctor.

Aging skin is also subject to benign tumors such as skin tags (small fleshy lumps) and seborrheic keratoses (dark, pebbly nodules), often found on the face, neck, or torso. These benign growths can be removed for cosmetic reasons in your doctor's office. More serious precancerous growths should be checked immediately and removed promptly by your doctor.

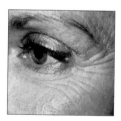

Before Retin-A treatment, a woman's face shows deep lines around the eyes.

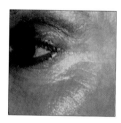

After 6 months of regular Retin-A use, the eye area looks much smoother.

REJUVENATION FORMULAS

Scientists have yet to come up with a magic youth cream. Tretinoin, or retinoic acid, the vitamin-A derivative known commercially as Retin-A, however, has raised hopes. Developed to treat severe acne, tretinoin has been shown to smooth out some fine lines and wrinkles in older adults and also to fade age spots. However, it has little effect on deep lines or wrinkles.

Many users suffer skin irritation in the first few weeks. Tretinoin-treated skin is very sensitive to the sun and should be covered with a strong sunscreen outdoors. The Food and Drug Administration has not approved tretinoin as an antiwrinkle salve, although doctors can legally prescribe it for these purposes.

Safer, albeit somewhat less effective, are nonprescription exfoliants and moisturizers containing alpha hydroxy acids. These acids are thought to dissolve the bonds that hold surface skin cells together, allowing dead cells to slough off.

CAN HORMONES HELP?

It's well-known that estrogen replacement slows aging of a woman's skin. But what about other hormones? A study published in 1990 described the benefits of giving genetically engineered human hormone to 12 elderly men who had low levels of natural growth hormone. The treatment, which lasted 6 months, induced, among other improvements, thicker, younger-looking skin. Still, this study has raised more questions than hopes.

Some people continue to produce growth hormone well into old age; how would the treatment affect them? Would the benefits last? Are there adverse side effects? While none showed up during the study, excess growth hormone in other situations has caused a variety of serious illnesses. Clearly, more study is needed.

SEASONAL CONSIDERATIONS

Winter calls for special skin protection. Cold weather can chap exposed skin outdoors, while dry heat saps skin of moisture indoors. Use moisturizers often and cut down on lengthy showers and baths. Outside, cover up with a hat, gloves, and a scarf that you can draw across your face when winds are bitter. Remember that the sun can be harmful even in winter, especially when reflected by snow; protect exposed skin with sunscreen. Inside, keep heat low, if possible, to preserve humidity. Consider a humidifier if you can't control the heat.

In summer, protect your skin from the sun (facing page). Air-conditioning dehumidifies the air; set the thermostat high enough (80°F) to keep moisture in the air.

THE SUN AND YOUR SKIN

The power of the sun to damage your skin is sometimes underestimated. Ultraviolet radiation injures the cells that produce elastin and collagen fibers, causing wrinkles. It also overstimulates pigment cells, creating irregular coloring, including the brown blotches, erroneously called liver spots, that appear on faces, forearms, and hands.

The damaging effects of sunlight on skin go far beyond wrinkling, toughening, and discoloring. Sun exposure accounts for roughly 90 percent of skin cancer and is considered a major cause of cataracts. Ultraviolet radiation is also believed to impair the skin's immune responses by damaging skin cells' genetic material. As the earth's ozone layer thins, the sun's rays—which penetrate clouds—are becoming more intense and more dangerous.

HOW TO PROTECT YOURSELF

Always use a sunscreen with a sun protection factor (SPF) of at least 15. To determine how long you can stay out, multiply the SPF listed on the label by the length of time it takes your unprotected skin to burn. If you are fair, you probably start to redden after 12 minutes. Multiplying 12 (minutes to redden) by 15 (SPF) gives you 180 minutes, or 3 hours, to stay safely outdoors wearing a liberal amount of sunscreen on all exposed skin. Reapply sunscreen after swimming or perspiring heavily. (Reapplication doesn't allow you to stay out longer; it simply restores the protection you had when you first put on sunscreen.)

The SPF factor refers to protection against only one kind of ultraviolet rays, those called UVB. UVA rays also cause skin damage. Only sunscreens labeled "broad spectrum" give full UVA and UVB protection. Look for the ingredient Parsol 1789 (avobenzone), which has

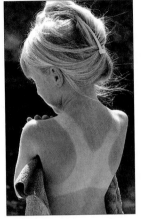

been proven effective against UVA.

If your skin is sensitive to chemical sunscreens, use titanium dioxide ointment, which blocks ultraviolet rays by reflecting sunlight. For particularly sensitive areas—the nose, the tips of the ears, the top of a bald head—use titanium dioxide ointment or another sun block such as zinc oxide. Or cover the area with opaque clothing (denim is good) that is dry—sun can penetrate a wet T-shirt. A wide-brimmed hat can protect your face and eyes from direct sunlight but not from reflected light bouncing off sand, snow, or water, so always wear appropriate sunglasses too.

Sun strength varies with the season and time of day. Many doctors suggest staying indoors between 11 A.M. and 3 P.M. in summer. Elevation and distance from the equator are also important. Shorten your daily sun time in the tropics and on mountains.

Finally, you should be aware that certain medications (some antibiotics, for example) make your skin more sun sensitive. Ask your doctor about any drugs that you are taking.

CONSIDERING PLASTIC SURGERY

Millions of Americans have undergone plastic surgery, seeking to repair defects or damage from illness or injury or to make already presentable faces or figures even better. Some hoped to better their chances for jobs or romance; others simply wished to regain a more youthful appearance.

THE PROS AND CONS

Before you consider plastic surgery, you should know what it can and cannot do for you. No surgical wizardry can turn a 60-year-old face into one that looks 20. A face lift can make you look younger and more rested; it cannot postpone aging forever. Nor can you repeat a procedure indefinitely; too many face lifts, for example, can result in a stretched look and more visible scars. Plastic surgery is not a cure-all for life's problems either. A cosmetic operation may raise the self-esteem of someone with a noticeable defect, but it cannot guarantee either a spectacular social life or a brilliant career. Then, too, the surgery is not without risk. The complications are comparable to those from other major operations. Relatively minor consequences include scars, distorted features, and skin discolorations. Possible serious aftereffects include excessive bleeding, infection, or, in extreme cases, permanent nerve or eye damage.

Plastic surgery for the body is riskier than for the face. General anesthesia, which has dangers for the heart, lungs, and kidneys, is often required; you may take months to recover. The older and less healthy you are, the greater the risk and the slower the healing. Smoking can delay healing too. If you can't quit, at least stop smoking for 2 weeks before and 2 weeks after your surgery.

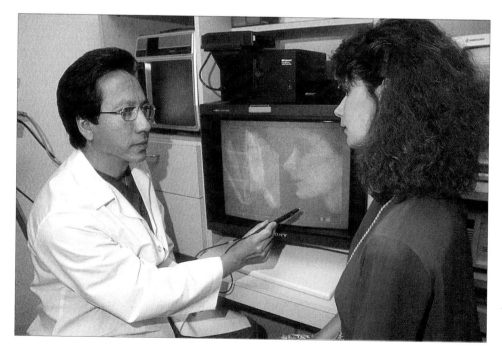

With computer imaging, the surgeon can give you a two-dimensional preview of the possible results of a plastic surgery procedure by drawing the desired changes onto your picture with a "mouse" pen. There is no guarantee, however, that the actual result with three-dimensional living tissue will resemble the picture exactly.

HOW TO FIND THE RIGHT PLASTIC SURGEON

It's not a good idea to rely on advertisements or magazine articles to find a plastic surgeon. In this very commercial and highly competitive field, the most highly publicized practitioners may be more concerned with their profit than with your well-being.

A better source is a friend or co-worker who has had a positive experience. You should realize, however, that since no two individuals are exactly alike, there is no guarantee that you will have a similar outcome. A family physician who knows the plastic surgeons in your area may have some recommendations. Or you can secure a list from your county medical society or from the American Society of Plastic and Reconstructive Surgeons (444 East Algonquin Road, Arlington Heights, IL 60005), whose members are all certified by the American Board of Plastic Surgery (ABPS), the only official certifying group for this specialty.

Check the credentials of any plastic surgeon you are considering in the *Directory of Medical Specialists,* which is available in most libraries, or else contact the relevant specialty board. Doctors certified by the ABPS have the most complete training in all kinds of plastic surgery, but other medical specialists may be qualified to perform cosmetic operations in their areas of specialization. These include otolaryngologists (ear, nose, and throat doctors); ophthalmologists (eye doctors); and dermatologists (skin doctors). Each specialty includes training in plastic surgery and has its own certifying board. Always be sure to ask exactly what special training and experience the doctor has had.

Your doctor should also have privileges at a reputable hospital because you may have to be an in-patient for major surgery or if you have complications. If you are to undergo your operation at an independent clinic or in a doctor's office, find out if the place has passed muster with one of the groups that inspect or evaluate such facilities. These groups are the American Association for Accreditation of Ambulatory Plastic Surgery Facilities; the Accreditation Association for Ambulatory Health Care, Inc.; and the Joint Commission for the Accreditation of Healthcare Organizations.

Before you decide on any plastic surgeon, make an appointment for a consultation. Feel free to discuss your expectations and ask about risks and complications as well as benefits. If you are shown before and after photos of other patients, keep in mind that they can be misleading because much of their effect may be created by lighting, camera angle, and hair style. Beware of any doctor who promises you an instant, total transformation or one who urges you to undergo more surgery than you feel is necessary. Above all, avoid any doctor who makes you feel demeaned, ugly, or humiliated.

The doctor or one of his staff should clearly explain the costs of treatment. Generally, you must make full payment in advance, and surgery that is purely cosmetic will not be covered by your insurance; nor, in most cases, will it be tax-deductible. But many plastic surgeons accept credit cards or participate in the special loan program established by the American Society of Plastic and Reconstructive Surgeons.

FAST FACTS

■ Doctors routinely examine your nails for clues to your general health. Bluish nails, for example, can indicate heart or lung problems or simply be a side effect of your medication; pale nails can indicate anemia; pitted, spooned nails or a nail separated from its bed, psoriasis, anemia, hypothyroidism, or a number of other chronic illnesses.

■ Commercial products can't shrink pores in the skin for more than an hour or two. Pore size is determined by genes, not astringents.

■ Cellulite, the lumpy clusters of fat cells in the skin of the thighs, hips, and buttocks, can't be dissolved or broken down by any cream or salve. Despite the claims of numerous products on the market, there is no remedy for cellulite other than diet and exercise—and even these may not work entirely.

■ Frequent shampooing can cause hair loss if you scrub so vigorously that you damage the hair shaft. Gentle shampooing and massaging the scalp, however, stimulates blood flow to the hair follicles and improves hair health.

Minor Procedures, Major Results

M*ajor operations such as face lifts are not the only kinds of cosmetic surgery available. You can also improve your appearance with several minor surgical procedures, some of which can be done in your doctor's office.*

ELIMINATING BLEMISHES AND SMALL GROWTHS

You can have blemishes and small growths removed in a plastic surgeon's or dermatologist's office under local anesthesia (or with none at all). The doctor can scrape off a growth such as a keratosis with a small surgical instrument called a curette. Skin tags can often be snipped off painlessly with special scissors. Your doctor may use an electric needle to dry up unwanted tissue (electrodesiccation) or to "boil" it with a hot electric current (electrocoagulation). Electrosurgery can often be effective on age spots, skin tags, overgrown oil glands (sebaceous gland hyperplasia), and tiny dilated ("broken") blood vessels on the face (telangiectasia).

Laser treatment is expensive, but it can often fade port wine stains, smooth out small wrinkles above the mouth, and eliminate facial spider veins. Lasers have not proved effective for spider veins in the legs.

DERMABRASION — NOT JUST FOR ACNE

To smooth out fine lines and wrinkles in aging skin, your doctor may decide on dermabrasion.

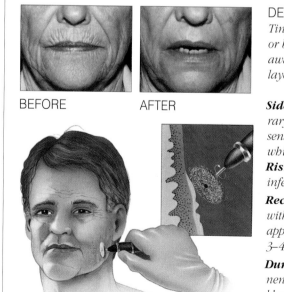

BEFORE   AFTER

DERMABRASION
Tiny rotating wheels or brushes shave away the topmost layer of your skin.

Side effects. *Temporary swelling, sun sensitivity, redness, whiteheads, itching.*
Risks. *Scarring, infection.*
Recovery. *3–14 days, with normal appearance in 3–4 weeks.*
Duration. *Permanent (but new wrinkles may develop).*

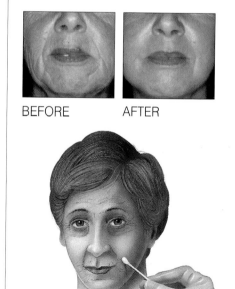

BEFORE   AFTER

You usually undergo the procedure in an outpatient surgical clinic or a hospital operating room under local or general anesthesia. Afterward, you must avoid direct exposure to the sun for several months and wear sun block and a hat whenever you go out.

Dermabrasion won't help deep wrinkles, and because the new skin is lighter in tone, the procedure is more effective on fair skin than on dark skin.

CHEMICAL PEELS

Painful and sometimes risky, chemical peels inflict a controlled chemical burn on the face. Depending on the extent of the peel, the procedure can be done in a hospital, an outpatient surgical facility, or the doctor's office.

The less caustic TCA (trichloracetic acid) is often combined with other products to produce a "light" peel similar to a sunburn.

The outer layer of skin flakes off after 3 or 4 days, leaving a pink complexion free of noticeable fine lines or blemishes. You may need several treatments because the effects of one peel may last only 3 or 4 months. Some doctors find that pretreatment with retinoic acid (Retin-A) several weeks before the peel improves results.

"Deep" peels, which are effective for removing wrinkles at the corners of the eyes and around the lips, usually involve the caustic phenol. Patients liken the experience to having liquid fire applied to the skin, but sedatives can alleviate some of the pain. The face is usually wrapped in adhesive tape for a day or two to maximize penetration. After the tape is removed, a protective crust forms that dissolves a few days later with the application of soap and water and then ointment or moisturizers. You must avoid or protect against sun exposure for several months.

COLLAGEN INJECTIONS

Another widely used antiaging treatment involves collagen, a fibrous body protein that is derived from cowhide. The collagen is combined with a local anesthetic and injected into the skin on your face or neck to fill out hollows formed by wrinkles or scars. It supplements your own skin's collagen (which deteriorates as you age) and helps to smooth and firm your skin.

The procedure is usually done in a doctor's office over two or more sessions. The injection itself takes only minutes and causes little discomfort. Collagen injections work best on deep lines in the forehead and at the corners of the eyes and the mouth. They are also effective for plumping up thin vertical lines (rhides) above the upper lip. Injections directly into the lips, however, do not have the approval of the Food and Drug Administration (FDA).

CHEMICAL PEELS
For a full face peel, the solution is applied everywhere except the lips, eyelids, and brows.

Side effects. *Temporary itching, throbbing, swelling, redness, sun sensitivity, whiteheads.*
Risks. *Scarring, infection, permanent lightening of the skin.*
Recovery. *7–14 days, with normal appearance in 3–4 weeks for a "deep" peel, 1 week for a "light" peel.*
Duration. *Permanent (with the possible exception of "light" peels), though new wrinkles may develop as your skin ages.*

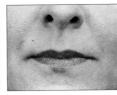
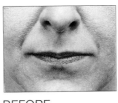

BEFORE   AFTER

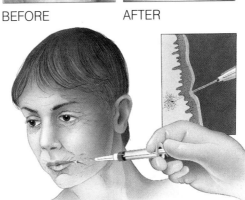

COLLAGEN INJECTIONS
The collagen is injected under the wrinkle.

Side effects. *Temporary stinging, redness, swelling, throbbing, excessive fullness.*
Risks. *Allergy to collagen (a pretest can usually determine), irregular appearance.*
Recovery. *1 day, with normal appearance in 10 days.*
Duration. *Usually 9 months or less.*

Major Procedures for
Maximum Results

*C*elebrities who openly discuss their plastic surgery make it seem almost routine. But no matter how happy the result you see, plastic surgery is a serious affair. Never undergo it without knowing exactly what is involved and what your risks are.

FACE LIFT

Technically known as a rhytidectomy, a face lift removes sagging skin, wrinkles, and perhaps some underlying fat from the face and neck. During your consultation, the surgeon may use sketches to

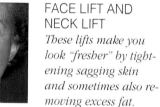
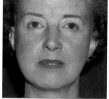

BEFORE   AFTER

FACE LIFT AND NECK LIFT
These lifts make you look "fresher" by tightening sagging skin and sometimes also removing excess fat.

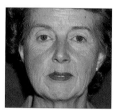

1. *The incision begins at the temple and goes down. If necessary, loose neck muscles are cut and tightened.*

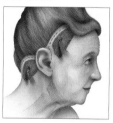

2. *The surgeon separates the skin from the underlying fat and muscle, then pulls it up and back.*

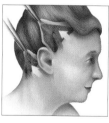

3. *The excess skin is cut away, and the remaining skin is sutured into place.*

Side effects. *Temporary "tight" sensation, bruising and swelling, numbness, dry skin, thinned hair at temples; for men, permanent need to shave behind ears.*

Risks. *Scarring, patches of permanent numbness, nerve injury that causes abnormal muscle function, infection.*

Recovery. *7–14 days, with normal appearance in 10–21 days.*

Duration. *Usually 5–10 years.*

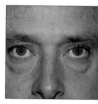
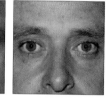

BEFORE   AFTER

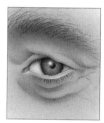

1. *Incisions are made in each eyelid, often extending into the crow's-feet at the corners of the eyes.*

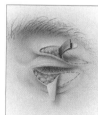

2. *The surgeon removes excess fat deposits from each lid and cuts away the extra skin.*

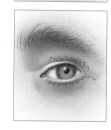

3. *The remaining skin is sutured back into place.*

help you understand the procedure. Some doctors take photographs of your face and draw on them; others simulate the desired changes by using computer imaging (p.148). These are valuable exercises, but they cannot guarantee that the results with actual living tissues will be identical.

The operation is usually performed under local anesthesia with sedatives, although sometimes general anesthesia will be used. The surgeon works on one side of the face first, then on the other. The operation generally takes between 2 and 4 hours. The surgeon may perform it in his office, in an independent clinic, or in a hospital.

There is a newer, more extensive variation of the face lift in which the doctor also trims and tightens the underlying muscles and connective tissue. Some surgeons believe this procedure gives better results, but others caution that it may increase the risk of nerve damage.

After the surgery, your face and head are loosely bandaged, and a drain may be inserted in back of the ear to carry away any blood accumulating under the skin. Your face will be bruised and swollen, and you will probably need medication for pain.

EYELID TUCK

Sometimes combined with a face lift, an eyelid tuck, or blepharoplasty, is usually done to remove pouches under the eyes as well as drooping folds of skin on the upper lid, which can make a person look tired and in some cases interfere with vision. You can have either the upper or lower lids operated on, or both at the same

---

EYELID TUCK

This procedure removes the excess skin and fat that age sometimes brings to the cushioned eye sockets designed to protect the eyes.

Side effects.
Temporary tightness, throbbing, bruising and swelling, numbness, eye dryness.
Risks. *Temporary vision problems, long-term eye dryness, infection, excessive white showing beneath the eyeball, temporary or permanent difficulty in closing the eyes to sleep.*
Recovery. *5–14 days, with normal appearance in 5–14 days.*
Duration. *Usually 5–10 years.*

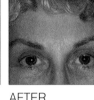
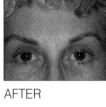

BEFORE   AFTER

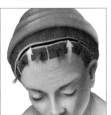

1. The surgeon makes the incision behind your hairline to hide the scar.

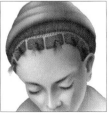

2. After strips of muscle under the skin that cause wrinkling are cut out, the skin is pulled upward.

3. Excess skin is removed and the surgeon closes the incision with stitches or staples.

FOREHEAD LIFT

Not only can this lift smooth your forehead, but it can sometimes raise your upper eyelids too.

Side effects.
Temporary swelling, numbness, bruising, headaches, inhibited hair growth.
Risks. *Scar that widens, permanent numbness, muscle weakness, infection, accumulation of blood beneath the skin that may require drainage.*
Recovery. *7–14 days, with normal appearance in 10–21 days.*
Duration. *Usually 5–10 years.*

time. Before the surgery, besides discussing the hoped-for improvements and possible risks with the surgeon, you may need to consult an ophthalmologist to discuss any vision problems that might complicate or even preclude the operation.

After the operation, the doctor puts ointment on your eyes and may also apply a pressure bandage for a few hours. During your recovery, keep your head elevated, especially when you sleep, and use cold compresses to reduce swelling and bruising. (If you have ever had a black eye, you know what you will look like.) You will need painkillers at first. Hairline scars will usually nearly disappear within 6 months to a year; most are in the natural lines and creases around the eyes and thus are virtually invisible.

OTHER PARTIAL LIFTS

The neck and forehead can also be "lifted." The neck surgery is often part of an overall face lift (see p.152), although it can be done separately. A forehead or brow lift is usually done as a separate operation (see p.153); it relieves sagging eyebrows, a deeply furrowed forehead, or drooping tissue around the eyes. The procedure may not be recommended if you have already had surgery on your upper eyelids, because further stretching may make it impossible for you to close your eyes completely.

NOSE SURGERY

People undergo most other kinds of plastic surgery on the face and head fairly early in life, usually for cosmetic reasons. These include such procedures as pinning back too-prominent ears (otoplasty) or changing the size and shape of the nose (rhinoplasty). Nose jobs are sometimes performed later in life too, although after the age of 40, your nasal tissues are thicker and harder to shape.

Surgery to trim just the tip of the nose can be performed up to the age of 70 on a person who is healthy. Since the incisions are generally made inside the nostrils, there are no visible scars. Because of residual swelling, however, you may not be able to enjoy the full benefits of a newly shaped nose for a year.

BREAST SURGERY

Women who feel their figures are unattractive may decide to undergo breast surgery. Many want to increase their bust size; others seek to do just the opposite.

Breast reduction. Oversized breasts can be a physical and a psychological burden. Their weight can even cause chronic backache. Breast reduction surgery (reduction mammoplasty) may alleviate the problem. It is a major operation requiring general anesthesia and a hospital stay of several days. After the surgery, you will need pain medication for perhaps as long as 10 days and will have to avoid lifting heavy objects or doing any strenuous activity for several weeks.

Breast lift. An alternative to a breast reduction is a breast lift (mastopexy), which removes only skin, not underlying tissue. The scarring is permanent, but the results are not; large breasts will sag again. The procedure is most successful on women with small breasts, who sometimes have implants inserted at the same time.

Breast enlargement. Surgery to increase breast size (augmentation mammoplasty) has been the subject of controversy. An estimated 2 million American women have had silicone gel implants inserted in their breasts since the implants went on the market in the early 1960's. The use of silicone implants has been restricted by the FDA because of claims, disputed by some, that complications may be more frequent and severe than had been thought.

If you already have silicone implants, the experts urge that you undergo frequent breast examinations (including self-examination), as well as regular mammograms by a specially trained radiologist, to check for an unsuspected rupture or leak or early breast cancer, which may be harder to detect with an implant.

You can opt for other methods of increasing breast size, such as implants filled with saline solution. Also, to reconstruct a breast after a mastectomy, a flap of skin, muscle, and fatty tissue can be taken from your abdomen, thigh, or buttock and sutured into place. This is a complex operation that requires general anesthesia and a long period of recuperation.

THE TUMMY TUCK

An operation designed to shore up a sagging middle, the "tummy tuck" (abdominoplasty) is often performed on middle-aged women who have had several children or on people who have large deposits of fat that won't respond to diet and exercise. The operation requires general anesthesia, a hospital stay of 3 to 5 days, and 4 to 6 weeks of convalescence. It leaves you with a permanent hip-to-hip scar.

LIPOSUCTION

Another popular operation, liposuction (suction lipectomy) involves sucking out fat from such areas as the chin, abdomen, thighs, or buttocks through a thin tube. It is not recommended for people over 45 because their inelastic skin tends to sag over the areas of missing fat. Liposuction does not cure obesity because no more than about 6 pounds of fat can safely be suctioned away. Skin with "cellulite" may actually look worse after treatment.

· ·

POSTSURGERY SUGGESTIONS

After any major cosmetic operation, it will take some time before you feel well and look your best. Be sure to get plenty of rest and don't rush back to your regular schedule. When you go outside, wear sunscreen and a hat and avoid direct sunlight; this will prevent darkening or uneven pigmentation in the scarred areas. A hat can also hide healing facial scars, as can scarves, tinted glasses, or a longer hair style. Some doctors employ cosmetics experts to provide patients with "camouflage counseling."

Men should use electric razors on their temporarily numb skin or perhaps grow a beard to camouflage their skin discoloration. Women should follow their surgeons' directions about when to resume using cosmetics. Eye makeup should be avoided for 7 to 10 days after eyelid surgery. Opaque concealing creams can hide the facial bruises of both sexes. Hypoallergenic moisturizers are helpful, but harsh cleansers are not. Blow-drying your hair on a cool setting is safer than toweling it dry.

Profile

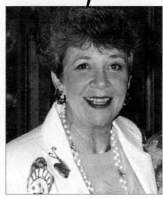

JEANNE APPLE'S EYELID SURGERY MADE HER "FEEL REALLY GOOD."

Many mornings Jeanne Apple's eyes were so swollen that she had to place cold washcloths on them to reduce the swelling. Both upper and lower lids had been puffy for years, and allergies aggravated the condition. In 1976, the year she turned 50, the Houston woman underwent eyelid surgery. When the doctor removed her bandages, he warned that she might be shocked by the bruising. But Apple was thrilled: "I can see!" She hadn't realized how much her puffy eyelids had interfered with her vision. Today she remains just as pleased with the surgery. "It's supposed to last 10 years, but it's lasted longer."

What about the pain and discomfort? "It's kind of like having a baby; you forget. I would never tell someone not to do it because of the pain. I think the doctor's attitude is very important. Mine was so kind. He explained exactly what would be done and answered a lot of questions. I felt good about that."

Always an active person, Apple recently opened a clothing boutique with her daughter. She regards her eyelid surgery as one of many turning points in her life. "It made me feel really good, and then I went on to the next thing."

Modifying Hair Care

Hair, like skin, changes on a genetic timetable that differs from person to person. If you know what to watch for, you can adjust your care regimen to accommodate the changes and keep your hair healthy and looking its best.

SIGNS OF CHANGE

Sooner or later, you will start to see gray in your hair (actually hairs with no color) as the production of pigment at the roots of your hair follicles slows. Graying can begin as early as your twenties or as late as your sixties.

Your hair may seem thinner. In women, hormonal changes cause some hair follicles to shut down, resulting in sparser growth. The hair that is produced becomes finer. In men, the hairline may begin to recede in a gene-determined pattern (see p.160).

In both sexes, the oil-producing glands of the scalp slow down, making both the scalp and the hair drier and more brittle.

HOW TO COPE

As it becomes more fragile, your hair needs gentler handling. Use a wide-toothed comb, particularly on wet hair; a brush can pull wet strands out of the scalp. Choose a brush with natural bristles that have rounded ends; nylon bristles have sharp tips that can crack or split hair. Brush your hair to distribute scalp oil and remove dirt, but fewer than the traditional 100 strokes a day. Don't pull your hair back severely, use rubber bands, or roll it tightly on curlers; the tension may break strands of hair.

Shampooing every few days, rather than daily, helps preserve your hair's moisture and shine. For gentle cleansing, dilute your shampoo by half. Lather up only once, using your fingertips to scrub the scalp.

SHAMPOOS AND RINSES

Even experts can't be definitive about shampoos and conditioning rinses; there are too many variations on the market, and each individual's hair can respond quite differently to particular ingredients. Buy trial sizes and experiment. Once you find several products that work for you, rotate them every few shampoos to avoid a buildup of conditioning substances, which can leave your hair sticky and dull.

Look for mild pH-balanced, or neutral, shampoos (acidic is better for damaged hair). A protein formula will temporarily add volume. Frequent shampooing may be all you need to keep dandruff in check. If not, use a mild dandruff shampoo containing zinc pyrithione. A stronger tar formula may be used once a week if you need it. If the tar shampoo causes bumps on the scalp, however, stop using it and consult a dermatologist about your dandruff.

Cream rinses or conditioners are generally a good idea for dry hair, although they can leave fine tresses limp. Shampoo and conditioner mixes neither clean nor

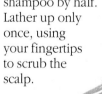

condition as well as separate shampoos and conditioners.

Hair damaged by dyeing, straightening, or permanent waving can benefit from deep-conditioning treatments once or twice a month. Apply a commercial product or rub vegetable oil into your hair, cover with plastic wrap, and cover with a hot towel for 20 to 30 minutes. Afterward, rinse your hair thoroughly.

STYLING PRODUCTS

Hair mousses, gels, and sprays help style and hold a hairdo. Many of these products, however, contain alcohol, which dries the hair. They also leave a sticky coating that attracts dirt.

Try to find a becoming hairdo that doesn't depend on styling aids. An experienced hairdresser can help you. If you do use styling products, stick to alcohol-free or low-alcohol ones.

High heat can damage your hair, so avoid using a dryer, curling iron, or electric rollers every day. To minimize dryer damage, use a low heat setting. Work the dryer back and forth at least 6 inches from your head, starting at the nape of the neck. Concentrate on the bottom layers of hair; the top layer, more exposed to the sun, is more vulnerable to injury. Drying from underneath also gives your hair added volume.

PROTECTING YOUR HAIR

Sun and harsh weather dehydrate your hair. An easy and becoming shield is a hat. If you swim, always wear a bathing cap. After swimming, wash and condition your hair. And if, despite these precautions, you still spot split ends or brittle hair shafts, deep-condition once or twice a month.

Permanent waving and straightening, which use the same chemicals, destroy the protective cuticle of the hair shaft. To limit the damage, ask your hairdresser to use the mildest type of solution that is appropriate for your hair. Another option is treating—curling or straightening—only part of your hair. Schedule your appointments for repeating either process as far apart as possible.

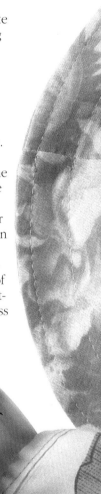

Hair protection starts with a hat, which acts as a sun block in summer or a windbreak in winter. A bathing cap limits damage to a swimmer's hair from chlorine or saltwater.

DEALING WITH GRAY HAIR

*S*ome men and women panic at the first signs of *gray hair, believing that it brands them as being prematurely old. Others enjoy the look of distinction—and perhaps even authority—that a little gray at the temples can project.*

PERSONAL CHOICES

However you feel about your graying hair, you have many options. You can accept your changing hair color gracefully and adapt your makeup and clothing colors to flatter it (p.169). You can hide the gray with a variety of products, both temporary and permanent. You can have your hair streaked by a hairdresser to make a virtue of your natural gray streaks. Or, if your hair is completely gray, you can glory in it and keep it from looking dingy or yellowed by using special rinses.

COVERING GRAY HAIR

If you want to hide gray hair, discuss it with your hairdresser first. Experts suggest going slightly lighter than your natural color to cover gray. The reason is that your skin, as well as your hair, tends to lose pigment with age. A lighter color is likely to be more becoming. A dark shade may look harsh against paler skin.

Gray hair can be handsome and distinctive on a woman (above), but it's fun to speculate on the effect of other hair colors. From blond to brunette to redhead, the model (right) shows an array of possibilities.

If your hair is healthy and not too porous, you can experiment with do-it-yourself temporary hair colorings. Because they wash out easily, you can undo mistakes. Beware of products, usually pitched to men, that promise to "progressively" restore color. Some comb-through color restorers contain small amounts of lead acetate. If lead is absorbed through the scalp, it can accumulate in the body and damage organs. Read labels carefully.

Temporary hair colorings are available in shampoo or mousse form. They coat the surface of your hair with water-soluble pigments that rinse out (and sometimes stain your pillowcase).

Semipermanent hair dyes are a popular choice for those just starting to go gray. The dye turns unpigmented hairs into subtle highlights but doesn't change the color of the rest of your hair. These hair colorings, which come in the form of shampoos or rinses, cover the hair with a waxy, pigmented coating that washes out over several weeks and adds thickness to your hair.

Permanent hair dyes, which thicken your hair by penetrating and swelling the hair shaft, last until your hair grows enough to reveal its true color at the roots (4 weeks or so). Men's preparations, formulated to cover gray rather than to change overall hair color, come in fewer shades and generally work faster than those marketed to women.

Have your first permanent coloring done by a professional, especially if you're thinking about a dramatic change. An expert can recommend the most flattering shades for you and spot such problems as porous hair that will color unevenly. Extensive highlighting or henna rinses (which can turn gray orange) are difficult to do yourself. Also, if you need color correction, it's best to let a professional hairdresser do it.

SAFETY GUIDELINES

Although used by millions, hair dyes can cause severe allergic reactions. Before each treatment, it is important to do a strand test according to the manufacturer's directions and wait 24 hours. Always apply the dye strictly by the accompanying instructions.

Many permanent hair dyes, particularly dark shades, contain chemicals that cause cancer in laboratory animals. Studies in humans are inconclusive, but a 1994 National Cancer Institute report of a long-term study involving more than a half-million women notes a slight increase in lymphoma and multiple myeloma among those who used black dyes for more than 20 years. Thus, it's prudent to space out your treatments or use lighter dyes.

Don't color and give your hair a permanent wave at the same time. All the chemicals from both processes will be too hard on your hair. Hairdressers suggest having a permanent first, since it can lighten your hair shade, then waiting a week to color.

TO GLORY IN YOUR GRAY

Prolonged sun exposure, tobacco smoke, the chemicals in some hair care products (such as resorcinol in dandruff shampoos), and even trace metals in water supplies can yellow gray hair.

Try first to eliminate the cause of the yellowing; then you can conceal it temporarily with a "gray enhancing" shampoo or mousse. Or try a wash-in toner (ask your hairdresser for suggestions) to increase the shine and add silvery highlights.

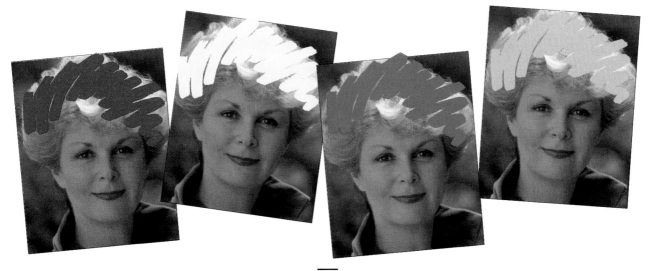

FACING UP TO HAIR LOSS

*A*s they grow older, two-thirds of all men experience some degree of balding—their hairlines recede and crowns thin. Women, too, may find their hair becoming thinner and finer, but they seldom actually become bald.

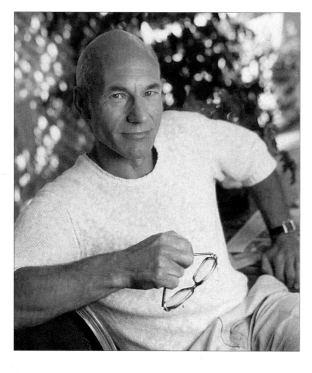

Baldness has not diminished the acting career—or the sex appeal—of Patrick Stewart, who has played, among other roles, Captain Jean-Luc Picard on the television series Star Trek: The Next Generation.

THE CAUSES OF BALDING

No one knows exactly what makes some men lose all their hair, but the genes from both parents play a part. It is known, however, that women can bring on a receding hairline with prolonged styling of their hair in tight buns or braids that put excessive tension on the hair root. (Loosen the coif to relieve the condition.)

The sudden appearance of bald patches in men or women may signal an autoimmune disease called alopecia areata, a usually temporary condition in which the body attacks its own hair follicles. Always see a dermatologist if you start to lose clumps of hair.

Radiation and chemotherapy also can cause temporary hair loss in cancer patients. In rare cases, physical trauma—even pregnancy—can cause a temporary hair loss in individuals.

THE SEARCH FOR A CURE

For all the patent medicines, salves, tonics, and massage machines hawked to the hopeful over the years, the first medication to treat hair loss effectively is a prescription drug called minoxidil (Rogaine), originally developed to treat hypertension. Its ability to stimulate hair growth was first noticed by hypertensive patients who were taking it orally.

Experiments using minoxidil in a 2 percent topical solution applied to the scalp have shown mixed results: 26 percent of 2,300 male subjects experienced moderate to dense regrowth after 4 months. After one year, 40 percent rated their regrowth as moderate, 8 percent as dense, 36 percent as minimal, and 16 percent as nonexistent. Treatment seems most effective in men just beginning to lose hair. (Recent studies involving women show 59 percent experience at least some regrowth.)

Researchers are exploring ways to make minoxidil more effective. Combining it with tretinoin (Retin-A) shows no increased efficacy. Other drugs under study include spironolactone (a diuretic), iamin (a wound healer), and finasteride (an antiandrogen).

If you are concerned about balding, consult a dermatologist. Only a doctor can tell if you are a candidate for minoxidil treatment. Be aware that if the drug works, you must continue to refill the prescription (average cost is $55 to $60 a month), and apply the solution twice a day. When the drug is discontinued, you lose whatever new hair you gained.

COSMETIC ALTERNATIVES

Some men live comfortably with balding—actor Yul Brynner, for example, made baldness a trademark, and Patrick Stewart (facing page) has been voted the "sexiest man on television" by loyal fans. Other men feel cheated and unhappy about losing their hair. For them there are ways to cover up balding: hairpieces or wigs, hair weaving, and hair transplants.

The easiest, safest, and least costly alternative to a bald head is a well-styled hairpiece (toupee) or wig. Human hair, which costs more and requires more upkeep than synthetics, generally looks more natural. You should have a hairpiece or wig individually fitted, trimmed, and, if necessary, tinted. You may want to buy two so that one can be cleaned and styled while you wear the other.

In hair weaving, a hairdresser attaches supplementary strands—natural or artificial—to your remaining hair. The new hair is then trimmed and styled to blend in naturally. As your hair grows out, the weave must be readjusted. You will probably need new weaving every 4 to 8 weeks. Look for a reputable hair-weaving specialist; an unskilled operator can put too much tension on the hair that is used as an anchor, causing further thinning and hair loss.

Hair transplants—moving skin plugs from thicker-haired areas of the scalp to bald spots—should be done by an experienced dermatologist or plastic surgeon to avoid medical complications and also to get natural-looking results that conform to how your hair grows. The total procedure is expensive and time-consuming. Transplants must be made in a series of sessions. The newly transplanted plugs then go into shock and lose hair before they produce new growth in the bald spots (100 days or so). Good transplants can, however, last a lifetime.

REMOVING UNWANTED HAIR

Hormonal changes associated with menopause in women sometimes cause hair growth in unwelcome places—the upper lip, the chin, or the bikini line. If such hair is fine, it can be camouflaged with an over-the-counter bleach solution. Otherwise, removal is the only satisfactory cosmetic treatment. Your choices are outlined below.

Tweezing, which removes hair by the root but doesn't stop regrowth, is best for plucking stray hairs from the eyebrows, chin, and upper lip.

Shaving your face with a safety razor and soap is no harder on the skin than using a depilatory (below), but shaving may encourage hair growth; repeat often to prevent stubble.

Depilatories are chemical preparations (creams or lotions) that weaken the hair so that it can be wiped away at the skin line. Some people are allergic to depilatories; do a patch test (p.144) before using one and never leave a depilatory on longer than the suggested time.

Waxing, which should be done by a professional, quickly but temporarily removes hair from large areas. A coating of hot wax is applied to the skin. As the wax cools, it hardens around the hairs on the skin. When the wax is peeled off, the attached hair is uprooted.

Electrolysis is the only permanent method of hair removal. A technician pulls individual hairs with a needlelike implement that sends an electric current into the follicle to destroy the hair bulb. As many as half of the treated follicles may regrow hair and require a second treatment, making electrolysis a long and expensive procedure. There is a danger of scarring and infection; look for a licensed and experienced practitioner who uses sterile equipment.

FOR HEALTHY TEETH

The key to healthy teeth is prevention: brushing and flossing, checkups at least twice a year, and good nutrition for healthy dental bone. As you grow older, you must prevent not cavities so much as gum disease, the main cause of tooth loss in adults.

THE RIGHT WAY TO BRUSH AND FLOSS

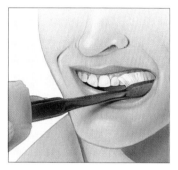 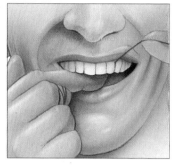

1. *Set the bristles against the teeth at a 45-degree angle. Using short strokes, brush gently but firmly back and forth as if massaging the gums. Don't scrub; that removes enamel.*
2. *Keeping the bristles at the same angle, slowly work all the way around your mouth, including the insides of your teeth.*
3. *Finish by lightly brushing the chewing surfaces and your tongue. If you are not sure that you are brushing correctly, ask your dentist or hygienist to give you instruction.*

1. *Take about 18 inches of floss (waxed or unwaxed) and wrap the ends around your index or middle fingers until only a 2- to 3-inch section remains in between.*
2. *Slip the floss between two teeth. Pull it partway around one tooth, and gently slide up beneath the gumline, then down again. Repeat this procedure two or three times on both sides of each tooth, using a clean piece of floss every few teeth.*
3. *Rinse vigorously to remove the loosened plaque.*

PROTECTING YOUR TEETH AND GUMS FROM PLAQUE

Your first line of defense against gum disease and decay is regular brushing to remove plaque, the sticky bacteria-filled coating that attacks the gums and turns into hard (and hard-to-remove) tartar. You should use a toothbrush that has rounded or tapered soft bristles, which are less likely to damage your gum tissue than hard bristles. Replace your brush regularly, especially after an illness or if the bristles become splayed.

Not all dental professionals agree on how often you need to brush. A general rule of thumb is twice a day, within a half hour of eating. Consult your dentist or hygienist on what's best for you. If you can't brush after eating, rinsing your mouth or drinking water will help. There is some evidence that chewing sugarless gum within 5 minutes after a meal helps to neutralize tooth-decaying acids in plaque. Chewing for more than 15 to 20 minutes regularly, however, can lead to jaw pain.

To prevent a buildup of tartar, also use dental floss daily to remove plaque between your teeth and under your gums. Brushing and flossing will help control plaque between checkups, during which the hygienist will remove any plaque you have missed or clumps of tartar that have formed.

HOLDERS
FOR DENTAL
FLOSS

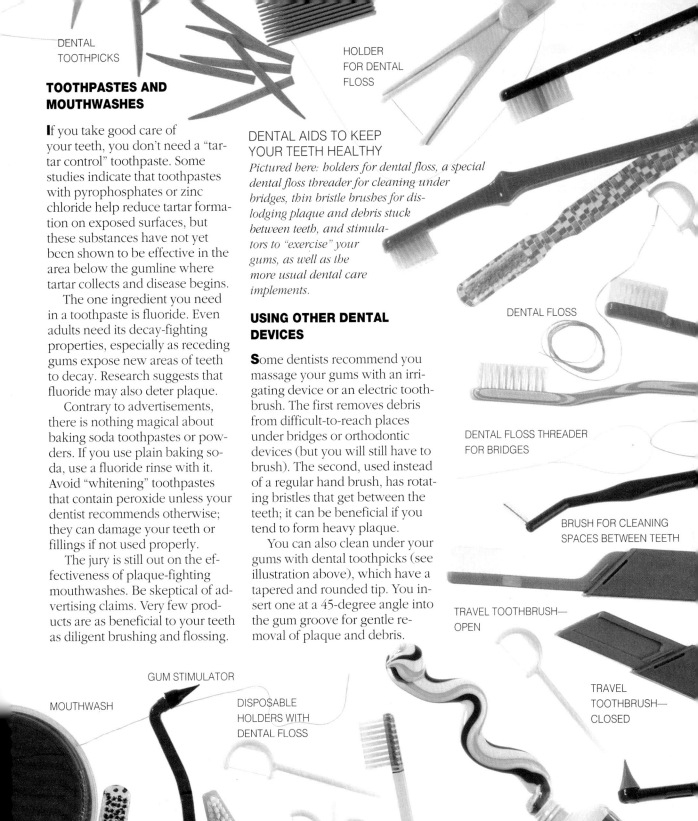

DENTAL TOOTHPICKS

HOLDER FOR DENTAL FLOSS

TOOTHPASTES AND MOUTHWASHES

If you take good care of your teeth, you don't need a "tartar control" toothpaste. Some studies indicate that toothpastes with pyrophosphates or zinc chloride help reduce tartar formation on exposed surfaces, but these substances have not yet been shown to be effective in the area below the gumline where tartar collects and disease begins.

The one ingredient you need in a toothpaste is fluoride. Even adults need its decay-fighting properties, especially as receding gums expose new areas of teeth to decay. Research suggests that fluoride may also deter plaque.

Contrary to advertisements, there is nothing magical about baking soda toothpastes or powders. If you use plain baking soda, use a fluoride rinse with it. Avoid "whitening" toothpastes that contain peroxide unless your dentist recommends otherwise; they can damage your teeth or fillings if not used properly.

The jury is still out on the effectiveness of plaque-fighting mouthwashes. Be skeptical of advertising claims. Very few products are as beneficial to your teeth as diligent brushing and flossing.

DENTAL AIDS TO KEEP YOUR TEETH HEALTHY

Pictured here: holders for dental floss, a special dental floss threader for cleaning under bridges, thin bristle brushes for dislodging plaque and debris stuck between teeth, and stimulators to "exercise" your gums, as well as the more usual dental care implements.

USING OTHER DENTAL DEVICES

Some dentists recommend you massage your gums with an irrigating device or an electric toothbrush. The first removes debris from difficult-to-reach places under bridges or orthodontic devices (but you will still have to brush). The second, used instead of a regular hand brush, has rotating bristles that get between the teeth; it can be beneficial if you tend to form heavy plaque.

You can also clean under your gums with dental toothpicks (see illustration above), which have a tapered and rounded tip. You insert one at a 45-degree angle into the gum groove for gentle removal of plaque and debris.

DENTAL FLOSS

DENTAL FLOSS THREADER FOR BRIDGES

BRUSH FOR CLEANING SPACES BETWEEN TEETH

TRAVEL TOOTHBRUSH— OPEN

TRAVEL TOOTHBRUSH— CLOSED

GUM STIMULATOR

MOUTHWASH

DISPOSABLE HOLDERS WITH DENTAL FLOSS

Fresh Mint Gel

FOR THAT PERFECT SMILE

I f you don't like the appearance of your teeth, modern dentistry offers options ranging from polishing, bleaching, and covering techniques (bonding, laminating, and capping) to such complex solutions as implants, dentures, and orthodontia.

POLISHING AND BLEACHING

Professional polishing can remove superficial stains caused by coffee, tea, or tobacco. Other types of stains need bleaching, a procedure that has to be repeated every few years. (Too many bleachings, however, can damage your fillings.) Over several office visits, the dentist applies a peroxide solution to each tooth. Or you may be fitted with a mouth guard containing bleaching gel that you wear a few hours a day for several weeks. Check with your dentist before treating minor stains with an over-the-counter do-it-yourself bleaching kit because misuse can damage your teeth.

BONDING AND LAMINATES

To cover discoloration too severe to be removed by bleach or to mask spacing and shape problems, bonding or laminates are used. In bonding, a puttylike resin is spread over the teeth, shaped, and then hardened. It is the less expensive method and lasts 3 to 5 years. Because the resin stains easily, if you choose bonding, cut down on tobacco and stain-producing foods and liquids, and have your teeth cleaned and polished more often.

Laminates (see below) last 3 to 8 years and may require maintenance and repair. Before you opt for either procedure, consult several specialists about the pros, cons, and costs in your particular case; ask to see before and after photos of other patients.

CROWNS

If your teeth are too decayed or damaged for the procedures just described, crowns can restore your smile; they're expensive, but they last about 10 years. The tooth is filed down to a peg onto which the hollow crown will be cemented. Then the dentist takes an impression of your mouth to ensure proper fit and bite. You wear a temporary crown while the permanent one is made.

DENTURES

All new dentures require adjustment as the underlying bone adapts to their pressure. Always tell your dentist of any discomfort; a poor fit can lead to many

---

LAMINATE VENEERS
Laminates can give you a beautiful smile, but because you lose some tooth enamel in the process, they are usually a permanent commitment.

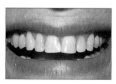
Before. *Dark teeth and an uneven smile.*

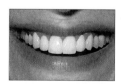
After. *A brighter, more even smile.*

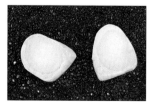
1. Porcelain laminate veneer shells are made from a mold of the teeth.

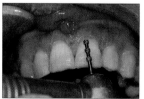
2. Some tooth enamel is removed so that the veneers will fit properly.

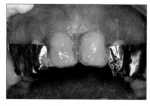
3. The teeth are prepared to receive the shells with an etching solution.

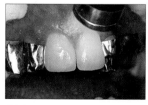
4. The veneers are cemented on, then cured with a high-intensity light.

problems, including mouth ulcerations and chronic canker sores.

Clean your dentures daily (or as your dentist instructs) with a denture brush and paste or powder. Brush your gums and any remaining natural teeth too. To avoid mouth sores or irritation, remove your dentures for a few hours daily or overnight. Put them in a denture-cleaning solution or plain cool or tepid water. Get an annual checkup to ensure that your dentures fit correctly and your gums remain healthy.

. . . .

IMPLANTS

A possible alternative to dentures or bridges is implants, artificial teeth attached to remaining bone or to a metal frame inserted over the jawbone and under the gum tissue. Implants look and feel like natural teeth, but the procedure is lengthy and expensive, and results may not be permanent. To be a good candidate for implants, you must be in good health and have healthy gums and adequate bone at the implant site. Check the feasibility of implants carefully and, most important, choose an experienced dentist.

. . . .

ORTHODONTIA

Although orthodontia is an expensive and lengthy process, a growing number of adults are resorting to it. Some wear braces to correct problems left untreated in childhood; others, to straighten teeth or treat bite-related problems. Braces have come a long way from the old "tin grin" standard. Some are made of tooth-colored plastic. More expensive ones, lingual braces, are inserted behind the teeth to be "invisible."

Profile

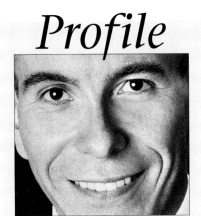

PAUL SLIMAK'S
NEW SMILE FOR HIS NEW LIFE

Paul Slimak can smile now—not the careful little smile he practiced for so many years, but a wide, happy one that shows off his dazzling teeth.

During his adolescence in Cleveland, Ohio, Slimak, now in his forties, became embarrassed about how crooked and crowded his front teeth were becoming and how long and pointed his eyeteeth were. But the expense of orthodontia kept him from doing anything about his situation until he began to pursue an acting career in New York.

For 7 long years, Slimak wore braces at least 5 hours a day and also while he slept. The braces were designed not only to shift his teeth (none were pulled or reduced) but also to reshape and bring forward his lower jaw to alleviate his TMJ (temporomandibular joint syndrome). As a result, not only did he look better, but he was able to breathe more fully. In addition, his periodic tinnitus (ringing in the ears) and neuralgic headaches diminished. "My orthodontist told me I was his most fanatical and disciplined patient," he says. "I was desperate for results." Slimak ended his 7-year odyssey by having laminates put on six top teeth, making them whiter and more even.

Was it worth it? Paul Slimak smiles. "It's the best thing I've ever done for myself!"

TAKING CARE OF HANDS AND FEET

It pays to give your hands and feet a little extra care. Rough hands can betray your age long before your face does. Aching feet can sour your expression, curtail your mobility, and affect how you feel about life in general.

KEEPING HANDS SOFT AND SMOOTH

For hand care, the first line of defense is a wardrobe of gloves. Keep a pair of cotton-lined rubber gloves next to the kitchen sink and gardening gloves beside your rake and trowel to prevent blisters and scratches as well as sun damage.

On cold days, warm gloves guard your skin against drying, cracking, and reddening. On hot days, cotton gloves shield your hands from the sun, the cause of freckles and the larger brown blotches of pigmentation that are misleadingly called liver spots.

Bleaching creams or gels, faithfully applied twice a day for 6 months, may lighten liver spots. For faster fading, ask your dermatologist for guidance. A more concentrated prescription bleach—if your skin shows no sensitivity to it in a patch test— may be more effective on your skin than an over-the-counter product. Be aware, however, that you must wear gloves or apply a sunscreen with an SPF of 15 or more to your hands every time you go outdoors—in winter as well as summer—to prevent the spots from recurring.

As hand skin gets drier and thinner, you should slather on cream or lotion more frequently, particularly after your hands have been soaked in water. Keeping your hands plumped up with moisture not only makes the skin softer but also makes the veins less noticeable.

REGIMEN FOR FINGERNAILS

Nails protect your fingertips, so you need to safeguard them. It may take 6 months to replace a damaged nail, and nails become more fragile with age.

Nails are porous and, like skin, dry out when exposed to hot water, detergents, and chemicals. Dryness makes them brittle and more likely to split.

To keep your fingernails healthy, don't use them as screwdrivers, pliers, lid openers, or pot scrubbers. Soak nails nightly in lukewarm water and generously apply a moisturizer to them. Every week or so, treat them to a manicure (facing page).

Lengthwise ridges on the nails are hereditary; you can brush on a liquid ridge filler or buff your nails to smooth them out. Crosswise ridges can be a symptom of diseases ranging from stress to heart trouble; see your doctor if they begin to form.

SECRETS OF HEALTHY FEET

Paying attention to your feet will keep them healthy and trouble free. Daily care should include washing them with soap, then rinsing and drying them well— especially between the toes. Dust them weekly with antifungal powder as a preventive measure.

Every other week, treat yourself to a pedicure (facing page). When your feet are tired, soak them in warm water and ½ cup Epsom salts for 10 to 15 minutes. Afterward, massage them and rest them in an elevated position.

Toenails are subject to fungal infections that cause yellowing and thickened or crumbling nails. Treatment entails using an antifungal cream or liquid containing either tolnaftate or clotrimazole. Apply cream or liquid to the toenails, between the toes, and to the sides and bottoms of the feet (not the tops) every night before going to bed. In addition, use an antifungal powder before putting on your shoes.

If friction and pressure have created calluses on your feet, soak them for about 10 minutes weekly in warm water and baking soda; then gently rub the calluses with a pumice stone. Never try to remove all of the dead skin in one treatment—the callus should be taken off gradually. If your calluses need cutting, see your podiatrist or dermatologist.

If aching feet are a persistent problem, check your shoe size— your feet may have widened. Shop for shoes in the afternoon, when your feet have spread, and pick shoes that feel roomy.

PAMPERING YOUR NAILS

Giving Yourself a Pedicure

1. Soak your feet in warm soapy water for 10 minutes. Clean the nails with a soft brush.

2. Dip a pumice stone in water and gently rub away rough, dead skin from your heels. Rinse your feet and dry them well.

3. Clip the nails straight across, level with the tips of the toes. Smooth out rough edges with an emery board; clipping or shaping the sides encourages painful ingrown nails.

4. Rub lotion into each foot, starting at the ball. Work the lotion around the toes and all along the soles and heels. Rotate the toe and ankle joints. Knead each foot with your fingers, massaging out kinks and sore spots.

5. Rub cuticle cream into each nail and gently push back the cuticle with a towel. Use cuticle clippers to remove loose bits of skin.

Applying Nail Polish

1. Remove old polish with non-acetone remover on a cotton pad.

2. Give the nails a manicure or pedicure (above and at right). To cover a damaged nail, use an acetate press-on, which is easily removed. More permanent artificial nails can cause infections and severe allergic reactions. If you are polishing your toenails, separate the toes with wads of cotton or tissue.

3. Starting at the white half-moon above the cuticle, apply an undercoat to each nail in three strokes: first down the middle and then down each side. Let it dry 4 or 5 minutes.

4. Apply two coats of color in the same way (let each coat dry before you start the next one) and finish with a fixative. Clean up smudges with polish remover.

5. Wait 15 minutes before using your hands or putting on hose and shoes.

Giving Yourself a Manicure

1. Shape your nails while they are dry. Using the fine side of an emery board, file each nail gently to follow the contour of your fingertips.

2. If your nails have ridges, stroke them lightly with a chamois-covered buffer. Rub back and forth across them for a few seconds.

3. Soak your nails in warm soapy water for a few minutes to loosen grit below the tips and to soften cuticles. Clean nails with a soft brush.

4. Gently push back the cuticle on each finger with the edge of a hand towel or an orange stick wrapped in cotton. With cuticle scissors, cut off any hangnail or jagged cuticle.

5. Rub buffing powder, paste, or cream into your nails. Buff crosswise until they shine. Massage cream or lotion around your cuticles.

6. To repair a split nail, use paper and adhesive from a nail-repair kit. Change the repair often to ward off infection.

MAKING THE MOST OF YOUR APPEARANCE

How you look often reflects how you feel—and it can easily turn into a self-fulfilling prophecy. You owe it to others—your family, friends, and co-workers—always to look your best. But most of all, you owe it to yourself.

FOLLOWING THE ABC'S OF GOOD GROOMING

Good grooming begins with basic hygiene—the daily routines of bathing, shaving, and using a deodorant. Give special attention to your hands and feet (pp.166–167). If you wear a fragrance, be careful how much of it you apply; your sense of smell diminishes as you grow older. Posture is important too (p.103); slouching or slumping detracts from your appearance, so be sure to stand tall and sit up straight.

To be certain that your clothes fit well, check yourself in a full-length mirror. Use a hand mirror to see how you look in back. Pants or skirts, for instance, should not cling or bag unattractively. If you see horizontal creases, the garment is too tight; vertical creases, too big.

When you shop for clothes, keep in mind that you don't have to be uncomfortable to be in style. Choose soft or thin fabrics, preferably natural ones that "breathe," such as cotton, wool, or silk. Pass up garments made of thick, stiff materials.

A good haircut is essential, so find a hairdresser who knows how to cut your kind of hair. Shorter styles are usually the best choice for a maturing face because they don't pull it down as longer styles do. Thinning hair looks fuller cut short and without a part that shows the scalp. A straighter style adds shine because smooth hair reflects more light than curly hair (see also pp.156–157).

> ## "*What is elegance? Soap and water!*"
>
> *— Cecil Beaton,*
> *legendary photographer*
> *and designer*

MAKEUP FOR MATURE SKIN

Your skin becomes lighter and drier as the years pass, so adjust your makeup accordingly. You can probably use the same colors as before, but softer, subtler shades may look better now.

On dry skin, cream blush is better than powder; spread it on the apple of your cheek for a younger look. Cream eye shadow minimizes crepey lines; the most youthful colors are muted or neutral browns, grays, and mauves. Try charcoal or brown mascara and eyeliner instead of black. Gently define your eyebrows at their natural arch, and make sure they are neither too heavy nor too thin for your face. Apply lip liner for definition and to prevent "bleeding," and use lip base coats with waxes and proteins to help mask vertical lip lines. To firm your chin, apply blusher and use a slightly darker foundation under your jawline. A combination cream and powder foundation will fill pores for a smoother look.

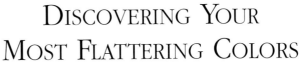

DISCOVERING YOUR MOST FLATTERING COLORS

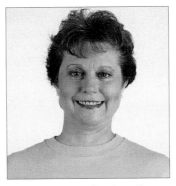 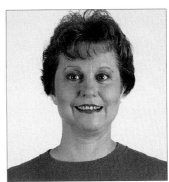

Unflattering. *A bright yellow jersey drains all the color from this woman's face.*

Flattering. *Her face comes to life in a bluish pink jersey that complements her skin tone.*

It's a good idea to review your color wardrobe periodically, discarding colors that no longer flatter you and adding new ones that do or simply getting rid of "safe" colors that may never have been right for you. Keep in mind that every basic color has a different effect depending on whether it's warm or cool—and also whether it's light or dark. There are orangish and bluish reds, yellowish and bluish greens. A color's undertone—its warmth or coolness—should complement your skin tone. For instance, a bluish red looks good on someone with a cool skin tone, provided its intensity—how dark or light it is—also looks right.

If primary yellow makes you look jaundiced, pastel yellow or tawny yellow may give your skin radiance. Or if a deep purple you have always worn looks harsh on you now, a lighter shade may look just right—and vice versa. If you have a dark complexion, rich colors will probably be flattering; if you are fair, you will usually look better in pastels.

To determine which colors are the most becoming on you visit a store on a quiet day and try on clothes in as many colors as possible. You will recognize the difference as soon as you look in the mirror. Flattering colors will brighten your skin tone, enhance your eyes, smooth your complexion, and even make you seem younger. The wrong colors will make your skin look dull or washed out (even sallow) and your eyes and hair lusterless, and you will look older.

DRESSING FOR YOUR BODY SHAPE—THE WELL-DRESSED WOMAN

Your body structure determines what styles look best on you. Review the current fashions and adopt those features that are flattering to you. Avoid both extreme styles and the fluttery, indistinct shapes and drab colors of "matronly" clothes.

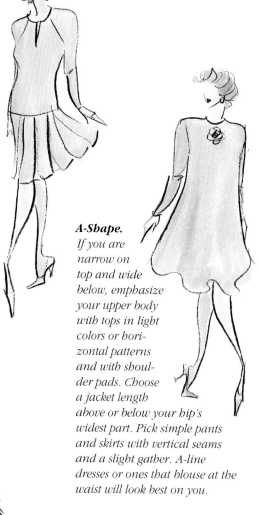

V-Shape. *If your bust and shoulders are wider than your hips, dress to minimize your upper body. Choose tailored blouses with straight or raglan sleeves, V-necks, or vertical closings that play down your bust. Skirts should be gathered or have wide pleats or a bottom flare. Drop-waisted dresses will flatter you most. Pick tailored pants with hip details.*

A-Shape. *If you are narrow on top and wide below, emphasize your upper body with tops in light colors or horizontal patterns and with shoulder pads. Choose a jacket length above or below your hip's widest part. Pick simple pants and skirts with vertical seams and a slight gather. A-line dresses or ones that blouse at the waist will look best on you.*

X-Shape. *If your bust and hips are the same width, and your waist is at least 9 to 10 inches smaller, you have the X, or hourglass, shape. If you are slender and average to tall in height, you can wear almost anything. If your figure is full or heavy, you will look best in clothes that elongate your figure with vertical lines.*

O-Shape. *If you have a wide body and thin legs, you will look best in outfits in a solid color or with thin vertical stripes. Pick long blousons and loose sweaters. Wear them with straight or slightly flared skirts and pants with full legs. Chemises and other dress styles with no defined waistline will flatter you the most.*

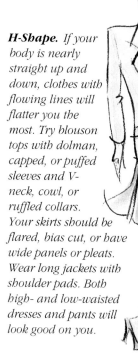

H-Shape. *If your body is nearly straight up and down, clothes with flowing lines will flatter you the most. Try blouson tops with dolman, capped, or puffed sleeves and V-neck, cowl, or ruffled collars. Your skirts should be flared, bias cut, or have wide panels or pleats. Wear long jackets with shoulder pads. Both high- and low-waisted dresses and pants will look good on you.*

DRESSING FOR YOUR BODY SHAPE—THE WELL-DRESSED MAN

Today men's clothes offer many more fashion choices than in the past. You can be well dressed in a variety of colors and fabrics, provided that you choose those styles that look best on your particular body structure.

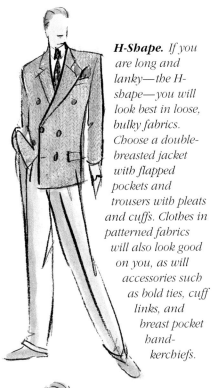

H-Shape. *If you are long and lanky—the H-shape—you will look best in loose, bulky fabrics. Choose a double-breasted jacket with flapped pockets and trousers with pleats and cuffs. Clothes in patterned fabrics will also look good on you, as will accessories such as bold ties, cuff links, and breast pocket handkerchiefs.*

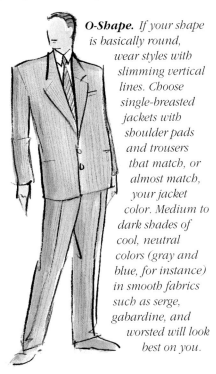

O-Shape. *If your shape is basically round, wear styles with slimming vertical lines. Choose single-breasted jackets with shoulder pads and trousers that match, or almost match, your jacket color. Medium to dark shades of cool, neutral colors (gray and blue, for instance) in smooth fabrics such as serge, gabardine, and worsted will look best on you.*

V-Shape. *If you are wide in the chest and shoulders but narrow in the hips, you can seem top-heavy. To look more balanced, wear sports jackets in dark or cool colors with cuffed trousers in light, warm colors. Avoid peaked lapels and jackets with flapped patch pockets. Pick flannel or serge for jackets, tweed or corduroy for slacks.*

A-Shape. *If you are narrow on top and wide below, dress to give a more vertical appearance. Combine jackets in light, warm colors and bulky fabrics with trousers in dark-colored gabardine or flannel. Pick a double-breasted jacket with inset pockets and a vent in the back to prevent riding up. Trousers should be plain—no pleats, no cuffs.*

171

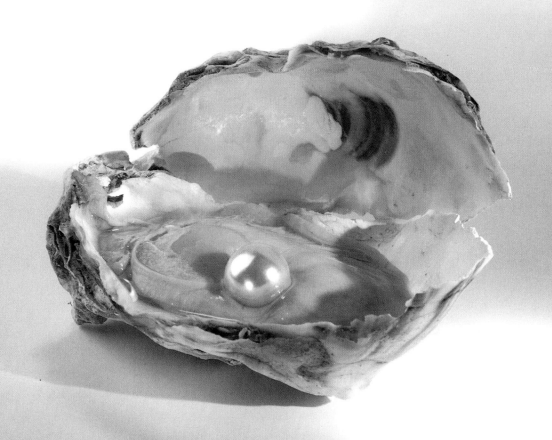

Chapter 5

COPING WITH LIFE'S CHANGES

. . . .

▨ STRESS IN THE MIDDLE YEARS *174*

▨ HANDLING MIDLIFE PASSAGES *184*

▨ CHANGING RELATIONSHIPS
WITH PARENTS *186*

▨ MAINTAINING YOUR MARRIAGE *188*

▨ DIVORCE: A MAJOR SHIFT IN STATUS *190*

▨ DEALING WITH LOSS *192*

▨ ALCOHOL AND MIDDLE AGE *196*

▨ STARTING A NEW CAREER *200*

▨ YOUR RETIREMENT YEARS *202*

▨ GETTING OLDER *210*

STRESS IN THE MIDDLE YEARS

Midlife, associated with crisis in many people's minds, can be a period of turmoil and change. But midlife also has unique satisfactions— increased self-knowledge, wisdom, and responsibility— to help you through difficult passages.

THE PRESSURES AT MIDLIFE

Middle-aged people face changing relationships and roles at a time when they are first encountering the limitations of their bodies. Career achievement can carry extra responsibilities. Job disappointment at midlife can lead to difficult career switches. Empty-nest mothers may look for recognition outside the home just as frail parents call for help.

Positive as well as negative events can be sources of tension. For some people, winning an award is every bit as stressful as losing a promotion.

HOW STRESS AFFECTS YOU

A certain amount of stress is unavoidable and actually helps you to live more fully (see below). Without some stress as stimulation, life would be pretty dull; handling a healthy level of stress —the amount varies from individual to individual—is even beneficial. But too much stress harms both your mind and body.

Like all animals, humans respond automatically to perceived threats in a process called the "fight or flight" response—a dynamic interaction of the brain and all body systems. This triggers a rise in adrenaline and other hormones. Your heartbeat accelerates, causing you to breathe faster and deeper. Muscles tense, blood vessels constrict, and blood pressure rises. Short-term, this response prepares you to escape from danger; long-term, it can provoke a host of symptoms.

THE CAUSES OF GREATEST STRESS

Major events—marriage, divorce, a death in the family, an illness or injury, losing a job or starting a new one—are recognized as stressful by most people. Doctors in several disciplines have developed systems for rating the degree of stress accompanying such events (facing page) and set

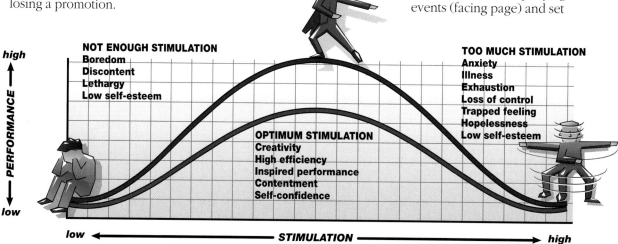

NOT ENOUGH STIMULATION
Boredom
Discontent
Lethargy
Low self-esteem

TOO MUCH STIMULATION
Anxiety
Illness
Exhaustion
Loss of control
Trapped feeling
Hopelessness
Low self-esteem

OPTIMUM STIMULATION
Creativity
High efficiency
Inspired performance
Contentment
Self-confidence

high / *low* — **PERFORMANCE**

low ← **STIMULATION** → *high*

How much stimulation—internal or external—constitutes harmful stress differs from individual to individual. Everyone needs some stimuli to function at all. More stimuli help you to achieve more and more important goals until an optimum level of stimulation is reached (blue line). You can—with practice and maturity—learn to handle more and more stimuli (red line), but each person has a limit—a point where too much stimulation, or stress, makes you first inefficient, and finally ill.

points at which stress becomes a health risk. The meaning—and stress level—of any event will differ from individual to individual.

Psychologist Richard Lazarus contends that life's little hassles may have an even greater impact on your well-being than bigger events. He suggests that the cumulative effect of such minor mishaps as getting caught in a traffic jam or losing your address book can cause more stress than a major trauma.

Without denying the impact of larger blows, Lazarus emphasizes the strong effect of chronic aggravations. What's encouraging about his view is that you can easily learn to anticipate and manage everyday irritants.

WHICH PERSONALITIES COPE BEST WITH STRESS?

Keeping your cool in a slow checkout line doesn't prove that you can cope with stress, although research suggests that people who can take such aggravating situations in stride stay healthier and live longer.

The Type A behavior of driven personalities, once believed to bring on heart attacks, is now seen in a somewhat different light. Some Type A traits—ambition and fierce competitiveness, for example—may help you handle stress because they motivate you to deal with the events and circumstances that cause you discomfort. So-called Type B personalities, people who appear to be relaxed and easygoing, may actually be suppressing a great deal of anger and internalizing the bad feelings brought on by stressful or irritating situations.

The issue may not be how you deal with anger—whether you

A MEASUREMENT FOR STRESS

Medical researchers at the University of Washington interviewed thousands of people to develop the Life Change Index Scale, a system for evaluating stressful events. The death of a spouse received the highest numerical rating of 100, but not all high-stress events are so painful or sad. Retirement, an expected event for which many people happily plan, rates almost as high in stress as getting fired, which often catches people unaware.

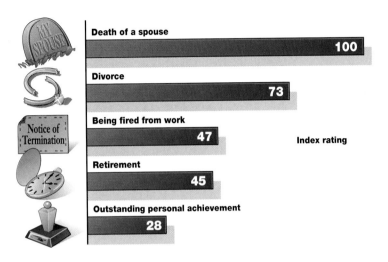

	Index rating
Death of a spouse	100
Divorce	73
Being fired from work	47
Retirement	45
Outstanding personal achievement	28

blow up or hold your tongue—but how *often* you experience hostile feelings. People who are always fuming, who are chronically cynical and mistrustful, cope least well with stress. Holding on to negative emotions such as anger or paranoia ("they" are out to get you) and letting aggravations accumulate—doing a slow burn—may put you at high risk for stress-related illness.

Most important, psychologists say, is whether you are able to do something about the sources of your negative feelings. Healthy anger can inspire you to make changes in your life that will improve it (quitting a job you don't like, for example). People who aren't able to make those helpful changes—who don't have control over what's making them miserable or who can't accept what they can't control—are most likely to suffer ill effects from stress.

THE HARDY PERSONALITY

Why some people thrive in high-stress situations while others fall to pieces has concerned psychologists for many years. One conclusion is that stress-resistant people have "hardy" personalities that enable them to cope more easily than others.

Such people, according to psychologist Suzanne Kobasa, believe they have greater control over their lives than the average person does. They tend to commit themselves strongly to whatever they do, to feel connected to the people around them, and to view change as a challenge. They actively try to solve the problems they come up against.

In contrast, people who succumb to stress most quickly feel powerless, alienated, threatened, and immobilized by change.

Some people seem to develop

hardiness naturally, without conscious effort. Others must work at it, cultivating the trait by monitoring their responses to stress and learning to replace self-defeating ones with more positive ones.

People who have long-term goals fare best in handling stress. The long view helps minimize the importance of everyday annoyances; problems become temporary setbacks in a lengthy process that is expected to have many frustrations.

HOW TO DEAL WITH STRESS

Traditional stategies for dealing with major stressful life events (see *Basic Coping Techniques,* facing page) are very effective.

Less understood but perhaps more important is how to keep an accumulation of mundane irritants from wearing you down.

The first step in beating day-to-day stress is to develop self-awareness. Everyone responds differently to different kinds of stress. You need to know your limits and the types of pressure that are most difficult for you.

LOOKING AT THE OPTIONS

Anything you do to initiate equilibrium in the face of a threat can be called coping. Coping can be conscious or unconscious, passive or active. Psychologists recognize several coping strategies, which generally fall into two

broad categories: problem-solving (facing problems and taking direct action to resolve them) and emotional resolution (altering how you perceive or react to stressful situations without trying to change the situations). No single method of coping works all the time, and people often use a combination of techniques to deal with their problems.

Relaxation techniques (pp.180-181) can be quite effective in reducing the effects of stress. Taking vitamin supplements, however, is considered ineffective. Although your body may need more vitamins and minerals during periods of physical stress (after surgery, for instance), mental stress does not appear to be relieved by vitamin formulas.

AVOIDING THE STRESS BAIT

A successful behavioral-therapy technique for dealing with stress urges you to think of tense situations in terms of "hooks." Imagine you are a fish swimming in a lake. Now and then a hook drops. The hook may be a traffic jam, a challenge from an argumentative spouse, or a rude clerk. Each day 30 or more hooks may come your way. You can decide whether to bite or not. When you bite, you react to the provocation with anger, aggravation, or impatience. When you don't bite, you swim around the hook, doing what you must without letting it get the better of you.

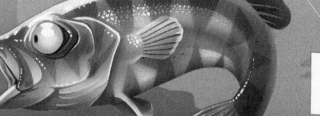

FIGHTING WITH YOUR SPOUSE

SLOW CHECKOUT LINE

LONG WAIT FOR THE DENTIST

SPILLING MILK ON THE NEWLY WAXED FLOOR

GETTING CAUGHT IN TRAFFIC

Many people seek refuge from stress in self-help groups. Support groups exist for people with all kinds of special problems. Many are patterned after Alcoholics Anonymous. The great value of these groups is the opportunity to share your troubles with people who have been through similar circumstances, who understand your feelings, and who can offer suggestions for coping.

THERAPEUTIC SOLUTIONS

Professional counseling can often help people deal with the stress in their lives. Seeking assistance from a certified social worker, psychologist, or psychiatrist is not a sign of weakness

BASIC COPING TECHNIQUES

When you are faced with a painful emotional experience, try one or more of the proven stress relievers listed below:
■ Talk to a trusted friend, family member, or religious counselor about what's troubling you. Express your anger. Neither holding anger in nor blowing up is constructive.
■ Cry if you feel like it. It may relieve tension.
■ Focus on action you can take—alone or with others—to resolve the situation or to make matters better.
■ Exercise on a regular basis and maintain a healthy diet.
■ Get all the sleep you need, but don't use sleep as an escape.
■ Avoid nonprescribed mood-altering drugs (including alcohol, which is a depressant).

or ineptitude. Instead, it suggests that you are willing and able to get the help you need to live the richest and happiest life possible.

Make a special effort to find a therapist who is right for you. Ask your friends or your doctors for recommendations and don't be

(continued on page 179)

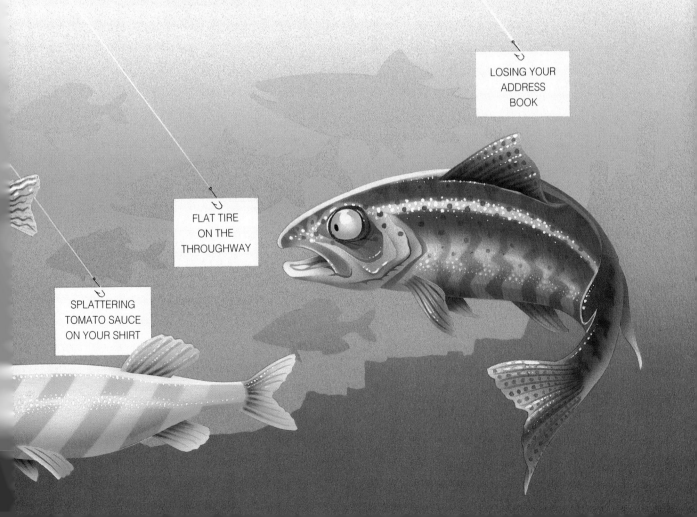

LOSING YOUR ADDRESS BOOK

FLAT TIRE ON THE THROUGHWAY

SPLATTERING TOMATO SAUCE ON YOUR SHIRT

THOSE FRIGHTENING ANXIETY DISORDERS

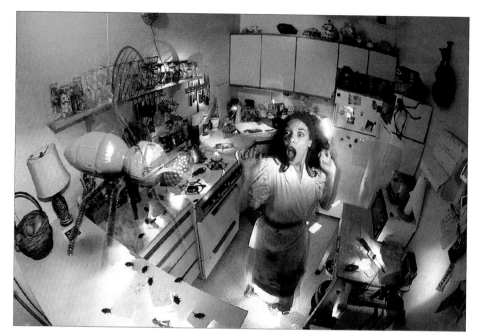

A victim of a phobia about bugs does not see insects realistically. To the phobic person, common household pests appear larger, more numerous, and more threatening than they do to others.

When you are threatened, you feel anxiety, or fear. Normal anxiety is a good survival instinct and helps you avoid danger. Some people, however, experience fear out of proportion to the actual threat confronting them. These exaggerated fears take the form of phobias, panic attacks, and other anxiety disorders.

Among the most widespread phobias are stage fright, fear of heights, fear of flying, fear of darkness, fear of dogs, cats, or snakes, fear of germs, and fear of enclosed or open spaces. The difference between a fear and a phobia is usually a matter of degree. A person who is afraid of snakes wears boots to hike through high grass where snakes might hide. Someone who is phobic about snakes simply won't go anywhere near the high grass.

In panic attacks, people feel fear so intense that they frequently experience physical symptoms resembling or interpreted as a heart attack. Accompanying the physical symptoms may be terror, a fear of going crazy or losing control, and a fear of dying.

In agoraphobia (fear of open spaces), a particularly difficult panic disorder, the individual fears being in places or situations from which escape might be difficult or in which help might not be available if he should suddenly develop incapacitating or embarrassing symptoms. This panic can be so extreme that the sufferer won't leave home unaccompanied.

Until recently people who suffered panic attacks were often misdiagnosed by doctors because their symptoms closely mimic those of other medical conditions. If you have panic attacks, be sure your doctor understands the condition. Effective treatment usually combines medications such as tranquilizers or antidepressants with cognitive-behavioral therapy aimed at changing the thoughts and habits that accompany attacks. Patients are encouraged to gradually face down the source of their fear.

afraid to interview several therapists before settling on one.

Cognitive-behavioral therapy, which combines talking with practical, behavior-changing techniques, can be quite successful. The purpose is to alter the negative thoughts ("I'm not smart enough" or "that's too difficult for me") that keep you from handling stressful situations.

If you are terrified of public speaking, for example, try imagining the audience all naked. You may laugh, but once you have changed how you see that audience, it becomes less fearsome.

Another example of a successful cognitive-behavioral therapy technique, *Avoiding the Stress Bait*, is shown on pages 176-177.

. . . .

ASSESSING YOURSELF

Learn to judge your own stress tolerances. Deadlines at work may be just your cup of tea—they get your adrenaline going and make you work better than ever. Spending a day with your 2-year-old grandson, however, may push you to the brink. You must recognize and acknowledge those situations that are most stressful for you. While you may not always be able to avoid them, you can learn to say no without feeling guilty and, if you can't escape, to anticipate and plan for dealing with the extra discomfort.

Listen to your body. It can tell you when you're fielding too much stress. You may get a headache or backache or feel increased muscle tension in your face, neck, and back. Your stomach may act up. Your mind may bubble over with a monologue of worries and angry thoughts, or you may not sleep well. These physical symptoms are warnings.

SOCIAL STRESSES

Society creates general social stresses that most people share. At midlife, such issues as growing older in a youth-oriented culture, owning up to long-term regrets and disappointments, and facing mortality form the backdrop for each person's woes.

Coping with these pressures takes ingenuity and resolve. By developing and relying on a solid, comfortable self-image, you're off to a good start. Then if you can replace societal prescriptions for happiness with your own internal measures of self-worth and accomplishment, setting your own standards becomes easier.

You can nurture your self-esteem by recognizing and cultivating your own talents and by also acknowledging to yourself the contributions you make to others. It always helps to maintain an active network of friends and relatives who respect and love you just as you are.

> **"***Man should not try to avoid stress any more than he would shun food, love, or exercise.***"**
>
> —*Dr. Hans Selye (1907-1982), Canadian endocrinologist and pioneer in studying the effects of stress on the human body*

. . . .

LEARNING TO BE A HEALTHY OPTIMIST

Optimism is the key to handling stress well, according to psychologist Martin Seligman. Fortunately for those who naturally take a bleak view, he believes that optimism can be learned. He suggests that you start by thinking about the way you habitually explain what happens to you.

A pessimist who loses a job says, "I always fail and I always will." An optimist, on the other hand, sees this bit of bad luck as a temporary setback that has happened in spite of good efforts and skill. Of course, optimists run the risk of denying responsibility for their problems. Pessimists, however, are more likely to become depressed and to suffer from illnesses associated with stress.

There is a healthy compromise. In a policy of "flexible optimism," you can see reality clearly while you hope for the best. Listen to how you explain events to yourself and try to filter out the pessimistic thoughts. As an experiment, consider more upbeat explanations. Look at them objectively and you may see that they aren't so outrageous. Work at changing the kinds of underlying assumptions that feed pessimism. Setting yourself unrealistically high standards, for example, unfairly diminishes some of your true accomplishments.

RELAXATION TECHNIQUES

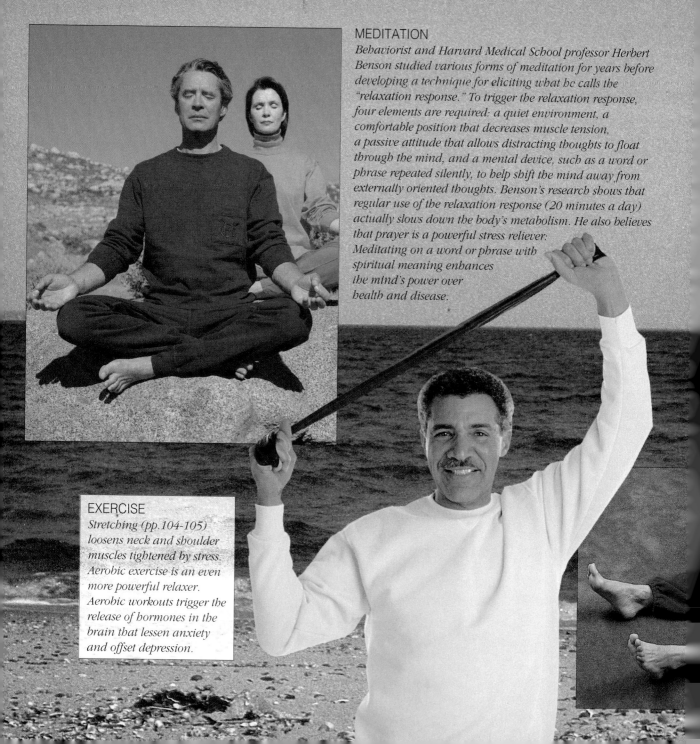

Handling stress well means taking action when it will help and letting go when action won't solve anything. Letting go is difficult. It means allowing yourself to relax, to stop worrying, and just to live from moment to moment. Letting go is a challenge for most people, but it may be the most rewarding discipline you'll ever develop.

Among the best-known and most effective techniques for quieting both mind and body are those shown below and on the facing page.

MEDITATION

Behaviorist and Harvard Medical School professor Herbert Benson studied various forms of meditation for years before developing a technique for eliciting what he calls the "relaxation response." To trigger the relaxation response, four elements are required: a quiet environment, a comfortable position that decreases muscle tension, a passive attitude that allows distracting thoughts to float through the mind, and a mental device, such as a word or phrase repeated silently, to help shift the mind away from externally oriented thoughts. Benson's research shows that regular use of the relaxation response (20 minutes a day) actually slows down the body's metabolism. He also believes that prayer is a powerful stress reliever. Meditating on a word or phrase with spiritual meaning enhances the mind's power over health and disease.

EXERCISE
Stretching (pp.104-105) loosens neck and shoulder muscles tightened by stress. Aerobic exercise is an even more powerful relaxer. Aerobic workouts trigger the release of hormones in the brain that lessen anxiety and offset depression.

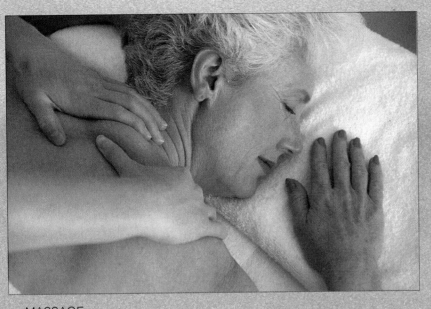

MASSAGE

A professional massage therapist gently but firmly works on stress-tensed shoulders, relaxing the muscles, relieving pain, and refreshing the recipient. You can take a class with a friend or spouse to learn safe and effective massage techniques to use on each other.

YOGA

An Eastern discipline, yoga combines physical exercise with meditative activity to stretch and strengthen muscles, relieve tension, and develop physical balance. Yoga requires instruction from a knowledgeable teacher.

PROGRESSIVE RELAXATION

This simple exercise, popular with actors and dancers, involves focusing on each part of the body individually and isolating tense spots. By alternately tightening each set of muscles, then loosening them, you can gradually relax your entire body from head to toe.

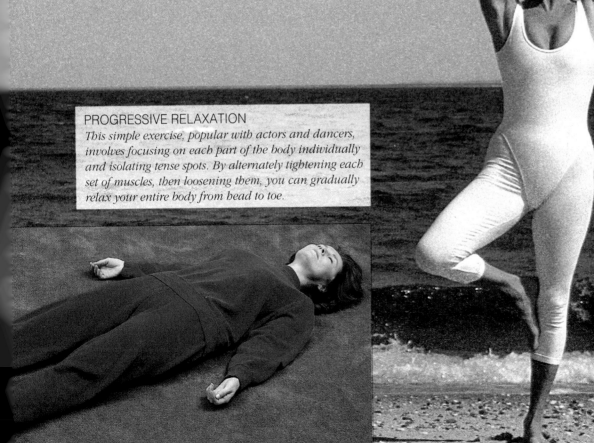

MANAGING YOUR TIME BETTER

According to recent data—and most people's experience—the work week is expanding and leisure time is evaporating, not only for top-level executives but for the average person as well. Most experts advocate organization as the key to getting a grip on time. They suggest you start by asking what your real goals are for yourself, your family, and your career. With goals established, break your time down into manageable segments.

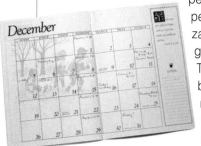

■ Use a monthly calendar for short-term scheduling and a 6-month calendar for long-range scheduling. Pencil in all the things that pertain to your goals, including classes you want to take (learning a computer program for your job or mastering the piano for fun), regular exercise sessions, social events, and family time.

■ On a daily action list, categorize tasks: those that need immediate attention (you had better do them yourself), those that can be delegated (you can hire a teenager to mow the lawn or to clean the garage, for example), and those that can be put off. To avoid procrastination, tackle the toughest jobs first, breaking them into smaller, less daunting components.

■ Free up time for the things you really want to do by simplifying your life. Let go of activities (your third church committee assignment or polishing the car *every* week, for example) that don't contribute to your goals.

■ Reduce the waste—and frustration—of everyday delays. Wherever you go, take reading material or a personal cassette player with a tape you want to hear. Then when you have to wait, you can make good use of or enjoy the time.

■ Set aside a half-hour toward the end of the day to worry. Psychologist Roland Nathan believes that having a formal worrying time cuts down on the amount of worrying you do.

THE VALUE OF LAUGHTER

Finding the humor in difficult situations has always broken the tension and helped people get some perspective on their problems. Now laughter researcher William Fry, professor emeritus in psychiatry at Stanford University Medical School, suggests that hearty laughter actually reduces the level of hormones associated with stress in the body. Earlier studies showed that laughter interrupts brain waves and reduces pain perception. Cultivating a sense of humor and learning how to laugh—even at yourself— gives you a powerful tool for healthy coping with stress.

HANDLING THE STRESSES OF THE WINTER HOLIDAYS

The winter holidays have their horrors—commercial cheer, too much rich food, extra demands on your time, and captive encounters with prickly relatives. But holiday blues are not as common—or as serious—as many psychologists used to believe. Holiday stress is greatly exaggerated, say researchers, who now believe that post-holiday letdown is a greater threat to emotional well-being for most people. Holiday blues typically exacerbate existing emotional problems, the experts say. Healthy people are likely to feel "up" for the holidays. The season has its benefits—paid vacation, special events, family visits, and gift giving. But the post-holiday season, when you return unwanted gifts, pay the bills, and work off the added pounds, can drag you down.

To prevent the blues during or after the holidays, maintain your exercise program (exercise is a great antidote for fatigue, depression, and overindulging). Don't drink too much (alcohol depresses the central nervous system). Make time for the special things you want to do. Share a holiday meal with someone who needs a surrogate family, or volunteer to help out at a shelter or hospital.

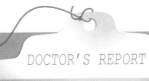

STRESS AND THE IMMUNE SYSTEM

Doctors have long linked stress with headaches, backaches, and gastrointestinal problems. More recently a connection has been made between stress and the immune system. Scientists are now seriously studying interactions between the mind and the body in the hope of better understanding human healing.

THE PHYSICAL RESPONSE TO STRESS

The body's natural response to stress is physical as well as emotional. The brain releases chemicals that trigger the immune system to start producing defensive antibodies. When stress is too great or lasts too long, however, the immune system can stall, leaving the body more vulnerable to illness.

Research shows that people under mental pressure are more likely than others to catch colds. Also, people with Graves' disease, a thyroid disorder, reported more problems and higher levels of stress prior to becoming ill than healthy individuals, suggesting that a combination of negative life events and genetic predisposition can increase the risk of developing this disease.

STRESS AND YOUR HEART

Although stress has been linked to high cholesterol levels in the blood, no firm connection has been proved. Psychological stress has also been linked to hypertension, but a major study found that, as a group, hypertensive individuals who attended a stress management program did no better than a control group of hypertensive people who had no program.

Research on the cardiovascular impact of stress on people who already have heart disease suggests that stress narrows artery walls. In a Boston test, men and women with histories of coronary disease were asked to count backward by sevens under time pressure. Diseased arteries proved more likely to constrict under stress than healthy arteries.

At a veterans' hospital in California, telling an anger-inciting story had no effect on the hearts of healthy men. In men with heart disease, however, telling the story produced a small but significant drop in the rate of the heart's pumping action.

CAN STRESS BE LETHAL?

Researchers can clearly show that stress causes physical changes in the body. But how stress contributes to the development of disease and how the mind-body health connection works remain a mystery. Some reports linking stress and disease have been misinterpreted to suggest that people make themselves sick. If that were true, what would explain the occurrence of dread—and even fatal—diseases in happy, relaxed people?

While state of mind affects your physical well-being, your physical health also affects your psychological state. And illnesses have their own progression. Some doctors now believe that the course of disease takes a wave form, an up-and-down pattern influenced by many factors. According to this theory, harnessing positive emotional energy may do wonders at one stage of an illness and have little or no effect at another stage.

HANDLING MIDLIFE PASSAGES

While midlife has always had its share of change and turmoil, the idea of a midlife crisis—until recently the explanation for any unusual or bizarre behavior—is yielding to the more orderly notion of midlife transitions, life changes most people cope with in their forties and fifties.

THE EXPANDING PERIOD OF MIDLIFE

Midlife is often a time for accepting limitations and facing signs of aging. But because it is also a period when many people decide to take stock of their lives and re-evaluate directions, midlife can also result in exploration, change, and new beginnings.

Surprisingly, midlife crises tend to be rare. Social psychologist Gilbert Brim believes that while most people in their forties expect to experience such a crisis, only one in ten actually does. Most of the significant changes you undergo during midlife—grown children leaving home, retirement, the deaths of parents, grandparenthood—are usually spread out over a period of 20 to 25 years. A midlife crisis is most likely to occur when several of these events take place close together, producing an unusual amount of stress and straining your ability to cope.

WOMEN AND THE EFFECTS OF MENOPAUSE
Contrary to many popular myths, most women go through menopause with few if any problems.

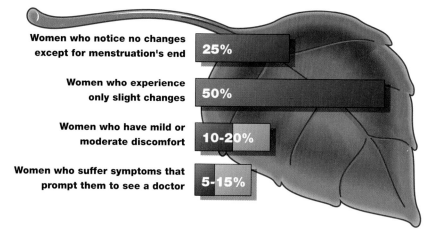

Women who notice no changes except for menstruation's end — 25%

Women who experience only slight changes — 50%

Women who have mild or moderate discomfort — 10-20%

Women who suffer symptoms that prompt them to see a doctor — 5-15%

WOMEN AND MIDLIFE

For women, menopause remains the most definitive marker of midlife. In the past, its onset was mistakenly believed to cause depression, emotional upheaval, erratic behavior, and an end to sexual activity. But while menopause does usher in major biological changes, women seldom suffer from any severe psychological repercussions. The physical symptoms also tend to be mild (see chart below).

The anthropologist Margaret Mead claimed that many women actually become more vigorous after menopause, a phenomenon she called post-menopausal zest. Research has confirmed her observation. Many women do feel healthier, more in control of their lives, and more energetic after menopause. While some women are depressed at midlife, this condition can occur for a variety of reasons: because they are getting older, are suffering from uncomfortable menopausal symptoms, or are undergoing exceptional stresses in their personal or working lives.

MEN AND MIDLIFE

Although there is no such thing as a male menopause, more men than women expect to be, and are, among the 10 percent who suffer midlife crises. Some experts believe the reason for this is the competitive career-based aspect of many men's lives, others that the cause is more complex. Men

How We Divide Our Time

In this age of computers and jet lag, when it often seems as if time itself has speeded up, many people feel they have too much to do in too little time. Those suffering the most from this time crunch are between the ages of 30 and 49 and have child care responsibilities. Sometimes, however, the need to help aging parents prolongs the demands on people's time.

Paid employment. Seventy-five percent of all men and 59 percent of all women over the age of 16 are in the work force. Men average 42 hours a week on the job; women, 36 hours. About 6 percent of all workers say they have a second job, often to help make ends meet. According to one study, workers put in 160 hours more a year (equal to a 13th month) than they did 20 years ago, and the incidence of paid work on weekends has more than doubled since 1965.

Household chores. Women average 20 hours a week on housework; men, 10 hours. Working mothers spend more than 80 hours a week on the job, on child care, and on housework. Over a 20-year period, women have decreased their housework from 6 times to 2 times the amount done by men. Men have more than doubled the time spent on domestic chores, but 70 percent of those chores are traditional male tasks such as yard work and home repairs.

Leisure time. Forty-eight percent of workers claim they don't have enough time to spend with their spouses; 57 percent say they don't have time to relax or have a hobby. Most people complain that they don't get enough sleep—an estimated 1 to 1½ hours less a night than they need to stay healthy and alert. Over the last 10 years, workers' paid time off has shrunk by 3½ days. In one study, 84 percent of workers said they would give up all or part of a raise for more time off.

Child and parent care. Thirty-nine percent of working adults say they don't have enough time with their children. Many find child care arrangements difficult, even though day care at work sites is increasing. Services to help people take care of elderly parents are also increasing, but as yet there is no data on how much time adults actually spend caring for their parents.

---

at the top may despair at having nothing left to achieve; others may realize that they have advanced as far as they are going to. Some may regret the loss of their youth or may desire a "last chance" to fulfill long-held dreams or to make major changes in careers or intimate relationships. As more women follow male career paths, they may face some of the same midlife crises.

THE NEW TRANSITIONS OF MIDLIFE

The changing nature of our society in the second half of the 20th century has produced some new midlife transitions, which often require different ways of coping. Because of the high divorce rate, one of these is being single again, with all the social and financial adjustments that such a state can entail. Another transition that many women make at midlife is returning to the work force or entering it for the first time. Yet another for both sexes is early retirement. And because of the increase in the average life span, many adults find themselves finishing up child-rearing duties only to then take on the task of helping their elderly parents.

CHANGING RELATIONSHIPS
WITH PARENTS

. . . .

After nearly a lifetime of turning to your mother and father for advice or help, you may find this situation beginning to reverse itself in your middle years as you increasingly have to tend to your elderly parents' needs.

GIVING YOUR PARENT FINANCIAL ASSISTANCE

If you are helping a parent with finances, arrange for direct deposit of his or her Social Security payments and other income and for as much automated bill paying as possible. Ask your parent for a "durable power of attorney" to manage assets in case he or she becomes unable to do so. Sit down together and make up a list of your parent's assets so that you can investigate and discuss possible new investments to make the most of them.

Make sure your parent sends in medical insurance claims and help with this job as needed. It's also a good idea to have your parent's supplemental health insurance company send you duplicate bills in case your parent forgets to mail in premiums.

LIVING WITH YOUR PARENT

If you and your elderly parent agree to live together, you should try to resolve the following issues beforehand. How are finances to be handled? Will everyone be assured of sufficient privacy? What household responsibilities, if any, will your parent assume? What are the possibilities of power struggles? And how will conflicts be resolved?

All too often, families find themselves forced to make vital decisions in moments of crisis. If possible, arrange a family discussion about household sharing before any crisis arises. Keep the lines of communication open. And, of course, any living arrangement you agree on should be subject to modification.

CHOOSING A NURSING HOME

In the event that your parent needs nursing-home care, follow these guidelines.

■ *Ask for referrals* from medical personnel; state, religious, and volunteer organizations; and relatives and friends.
■ *Read the latest annual state report* on any home you are considering.
■ *Make several visits* at different times of the day to observe daily routine, hygiene, and how staff members interact with residents.
■ *Ask to see the home's Medicare and Medicaid certifications* and the Residents' Bill of Rights. Is there a residents' or family advisory council? Can you talk freely with residents and their families?
■ *Is there a physician on call?* What is the ratio of residents to nursing staff? Is the home affiliated with a nearby accredited hospital?
■ *Check on safety precautions* such as bathroom grab bars and a fire safety program.
■ *Are there planned activities* and outside excursions?
■ *Do you have a "gut" feeling* that your parent will be happy and well cared for in the home?
■ *Are the home's location* and visiting hours convenient?

BECOMING YOUR PARENT'S CARETAKER

Role reversals can be emotionally trying for both the adult child and the aging parent. Even with the best of intentions, some adult children simply take over. Most older people cherish their independence, especially when it is limited. A parent who feels you are usurping power is likely to respond with anger. On the other hand, loneliness and disability can make your parent dependent, increasing your caregiving burden. Senior citizen centers and other support services (see box, right) can lift some of this burden.

Becoming your parent's caretaker can be rewarding too. Giving something back to the person who raised you feels good. And as you spend quiet time together, conversations may reveal things you never knew—about your parents, other family members, your own childhood. Such moments can add powerful new dimensions to your relationship.

THE SO-CALLED SANDWICH GENERATION

If children are dependent on you at the same time that your elderly parents require care, you belong to the "sandwich generation," people who are squeezed between the needs of younger and older family members. Some experts feel that the sandwich generation will expand even more in the 21st century. Others claim that this generation does not exist in any significant numbers and that the major worsening midlife crisis is serial dependency, in which people complete their child-rearing duties only to then take on parent caretaking.

CARING FOR BOTH OF YOU

If you are your parent's primary caregiver, take care of yourself too. Respite care provides help so that you can take time off. Other forms of assistance include physical therapists, visiting nurses, homemakers, home health aides, and meal-delivery programs. Adult day-care programs are another option to consider so that your parent gets a change of scene and a chance to socialize while you work. Medicare and private insurers may cover some of these services.

To find care providers, ask friends and trusted professionals for referrals. Always check references. If you or other relatives live far away, you may need a local manager to coordinate help for a parent. Children of Aging Parents (CAPS) in Levittown, Pennsylvania, and the Older Women's League (OWL) in Washington, D.C., are good general resources.

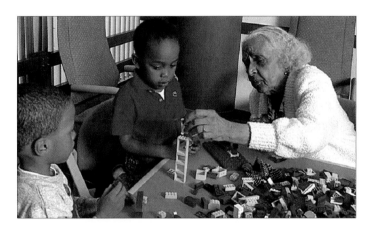

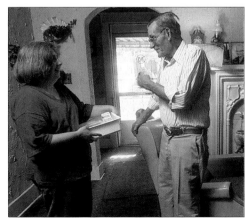

Parent care. At an intergenerational day-care center (above), old and young can socialize if they wish. The family of a senior living alone (left) has arranged for a hot meal to be delivered to him every day.

MAINTAINING YOUR MARRIAGE

As your marriage evolves over the years, keeping your relationship vital is well worth the effort it takes. Studies show that people in long-term marriages tend to be healthier and more emotionally and financially secure than other people their age.

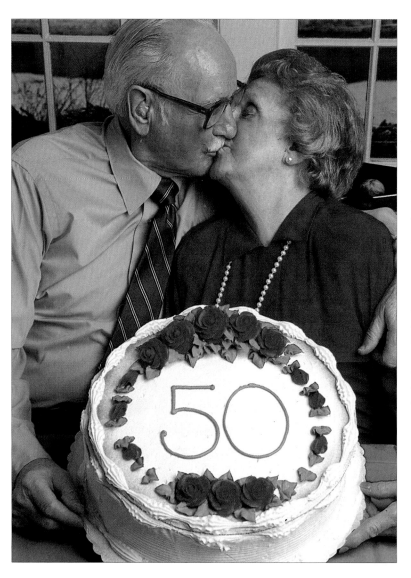

HOW MARRIAGES CHANGE

Any couple who can look back on a long marriage will recognize stages that were almost like different marriages. Ideally, the romantic early years give way to the parenting phase, then to the empty nest and the subsequent transitions to retirement and aging. In general, researchers believe that the most difficult stage in a marriage is the child-rearing one when the marital partners, focused on their children's needs, may inadvertently neglect their own relationship.

But even couples who have maintained their closeness must work at dealing with the emotional and physical changes that midlife brings and renew their relationship accordingly.

For husbands, the middle years are often a time for revising goals. Many men redirect their energies back toward the home. Enjoying the intimate satisfactions of marriage becomes more important. Wives, however, are often pursuing postponed ambitions. Some may be taking their talents seriously for the first time. In many marriages, a role reversal takes place. Husbands may resent their wives' outside activities, and wives may be frustrated by their husbands' demands on their time.

Couples also face major and sometimes difficult transitions—among them, retirement and the deaths of elderly parents. Sexual problems can develop when one or both spouses are concerned about losing their youthful vigor or are adversely affected by normal biological changes.

KEEPING YOUR MARRIAGE HEALTHY

In a healthy marriage, the partners are able to grow and change together through the years. Psychologists and marriage counselors encourage couples to foster each other's individual growth by combining independence with intimacy. You should allow time for personal interests as well as shared ones, for private moments and for together time.

Most successful marriages today involve an equitable balance of power between the partners. Decision-making is shared, as is the responsibility for making the marriage work. If fair ground rules are set up for handling disputes, the couple can communicate respectfully and effectively.

You should appreciate your differences as well as understand (and forgive) each other's weaknesses. Also important are mutual trust and respect, the willingness to be open with each other, frequent expressions of love and affection, sensitivity to each other's needs, and, last but not least, a sense of humor.

HOW TO BE A STEPPARENT

About half of all marriages in the United States are remarriages for at least one of the spouses; 40 percent of them involve stepchildren. According to one study, remarriages with stepchildren are nearly twice as likely to result in divorce. And even if the marriage succeeds, the period of adjustment can be stormy and take anywhere from 2 to 7 years, especially if the children are adolescents. If both spouses have children from a previous marriage, conflicts may also arise from differing child-rearing practices.

If you become a stepparent, don't rush in and try for a closeness that may need years to evolve—if it happens at all. Children are often resentful of the stranger who is so intimate with their parent, fiercely loyal to their other parent, and angry that their dreams of parental reconciliation didn't come true. Because girls tend to bond more closely to their mothers after a divorce, they can be especially disturbed by a new stepfather. Respect the boundaries your stepchildren set. Aim to earn their friendship and respect. Above all, don't try to replace the absent parent.

Initially, it may be better to leave discipline to the biological parent. If this is not practical, talk over the situation with your spouse and decide on basic ground rules, then present them to the children together. The more they see you acting as a couple, the sooner they may come to accept the situation.

THE EMPTY-NEST SYNDROME: MYTH AND REALITY

For many a marriage, the empty-nest stage may be one of the happiest. Child rearing leaves little private time for parents. Studies confirm that marital satisfaction is highest in the years before the children are born and after they have grown up and left home.

Traditionally, psychologists felt that women were the likeliest victims of the so-called empty-nest syndrome, a depression brought on by the last child moving out. For full-time mothers, the reasoning went, this child's departure was equivalent to losing a job or being forced into retirement. The transition was seen as easier for fathers and mothers with careers because they had social and creative outlets outside the home.

But recent studies suggest that some fathers suffer more from the syndrome than mothers. Many men who focused on their careers during the early child-rearing years may regret not having been more involved with their children. Fathers who changed diapers, supervised play groups, and led Scout troops tend to harbor fewer second thoughts.

Divorce: A Major Shift in Status

· · · · · · · · · · · · · · ·

More common today than it was just a generation ago, divorce has become easier legally and its social stigma has lessened considerably. The emotional toll on both partners, however, can still be very high.

THE STRESS OF MIDLIFE MARITAL BREAKUPS

Divorce at any age makes many people feel that they have failed. But when the breakup follows 20 or 30 years of marriage, the experience can be devastating, especially if you haven't anticipated the possibility. Wives who have spent their adult lives as homemakers may be vulnerable financially. Lifelong alimony is rare today, and finding a rewarding job at midlife is hard.

Some couples acknowledge growing apart but wait for the children to grow up or some other catalytic moment before actually separating. For them, divorce can be liberating—a chance to start over. For many people, however, midlife divorce is painful.

If you are facing such a divorce, give yourself time to work through your feelings before making big changes in your life. If you can avoid it, don't move, change jobs, or make any other major decisions during the first 6 months after the split-up. You may regret choices you make before you have started to heal.

· ·

PICKING UP THE PIECES

Emotional recovery from a divorce can take some people several years. First, sticky questions surface about money, splitting up possessions, and sharing responsibility for children. You must learn to be a single person again.

Counseling may help you sort out your feelings and come to terms with them faster. For most newly divorced people, relations with the former spouse are not the only problem. Children frequently take one parent's part. Friendships change, especially with married couples who don't want to seem to take sides.

Recovery begins when you start taking pleasure in life again. You are buoyed by old friends who come through for you and by the promise of new friendships that you are forming. Self-confidence gradually returns.

HOW TO GET APPROPRIATE LEGAL AID FOR A DIVORCE

When both partners agree to separate, they can save money by using a divorce mediator, a third-party legal expert who helps splitting spouses negotiate a fair distribution of assets; this is spelled out in a separation agreement drafted by the mediator and checked by each spouse's lawyer. To find a mediator, ask for referrals from your lawyer or friends or look in the Yellow Pages under "Mediation services." If your state allows it, you can save more legal fees by filing for a no-fault divorce based on the signed separation agreement.

When any part of a divorce is contested, however, each spouse needs a separate lawyer who specializes in divorce law. Battles over custody of children or division of assets can be lengthy, emotionally draining, and extremely costly. For families of modest means, such legal expenses can greatly diminish the financial resources of both spouses.

REMARRIAGE RATES AFTER DIVORCE

For more men than women, remarriage fulfills the needs they experience after divorce. Remarriage at midlife is complicated. Potential spouses come with former partners, aging parents, debts as well as assets, and children who see you as a threat to their inheritance. Prenuptial agreements are crucial.

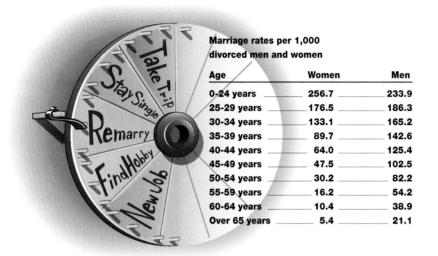

Marriage rates per 1,000 divorced men and women

Age	Women	Men
0-24 years	256.7	233.9
25-29 years	176.5	186.3
30-34 years	133.1	165.2
35-39 years	89.7	142.6
40-44 years	64.0	125.4
45-49 years	47.5	102.5
50-54 years	30.2	82.2
55-59 years	16.2	54.2
60-64 years	10.4	38.9
Over 65 years	5.4	21.1

EFFECTS OF DIVORCE ON ADULT CHILDREN

It is a myth that college-age or older children are not affected by their parents' divorce. It can be very upsetting for young people just starting out on their own to have to worry about their parents' problems as well as their own.

You can help adult children weather the changes in the family by being sensitive to their needs during this time. Don't allow yourself to become emotionally dependent on adult children.

Tempting as it may be, don't put them in the middle of your squabbles with your former spouse because you think they are old enough to grasp how badly you've been treated. And don't disparage your former spouse or discourage the children from seeing that parent.

Concentrate instead on rebuilding your own life and showing your children how self-sufficient you can be. If you sometimes are hurt by an adult child's seeming preference for the other parent, talk it out with a sympathetic friend or counselor who will understand your feelings. Don't burden your son or daughter with petty jealousies.

. . . .

MAKING A NEW LIFE

Whether or not you remarry, your best bet for re-establishing a full life after divorce is to cultivate your network of family and friends. Don't be afraid to take the initiative in suggesting outings or offering dinner invitations.

Some old friends—and family members—may have trouble acknowledging the changes in your life. Your newfound independence may make them feel uneasy. Concentrate on the activities that interest you most and let your social life develop around those affinities and the friends— old and new—who share them.

A WISE WIFE'S FINANCIAL INVENTORY

For her own protection— and her family's in an emergency—no wife should be ignorant of the family's finances. Nor should she be without resources of her own. Whether they are kept in a desk, at a lawyer's office, or some other safe place, a wife should be able to access the following personal financial papers:

▇ Deeds to property
▇ Stocks, bonds, and other investments
▇ Life insurance policies
▇ Other insurance policies (health, liability, disability, and auto)
▇ Loan agreements (mortgage and car loan, for example)
▇ Pension benefit papers, including Social Security cards for all family members and any discharge papers from the armed services
▇ Trusts
▇ Wills
▇ Income tax returns

A wife also should have independent means for taking care of herself if something should happen to her husband or if she is uncomfortable in her marriage and divorce is a possibility. Her minimum resources should include the following:

▇ A credit card in her own name to use as a convenience and to establish a credit history
▇ A bank account in her own name

DEALING WITH LOSS

*T*he death of a close relative or friend is a trauma everyone dreads. You can't really prepare for such a loss, but facing the inevitability of death and understanding the grieving process can help you through the mourning.

INITIAL REACTIONS TO THE DEATH OF SOMEONE CLOSE

Most people who lose a loved one feel the pain like a physical blow—excruciating at first and only gradually subsiding. How difficult any loss will be generally depends on several factors.

When an illness precedes a death, the process of mourning may actually begin before death occurs as relatives prepare for the end of a family member's life. When death strikes suddenly, shock and disbelief may delay mourning.

If a loved one suffers a violent death, horror and anger complicate the mourning. And when suicide is the cause of death, survivors often experience an array of emotions from rage to guilt.

A RANGE OF FEELINGS

The sudden or unexpected death of a child may be the most devastating loss because society expects the young to survive their elders. Whether it is an infant or an adult child who dies, the parents' grief is especially agonizing because the death is out of the natural order.

When a contemporary friend or colleague dies, you are not only saddened by the loss but also reminded—perhaps for the first time—of your own mortality.

At midlife, the loss of an elderly parent cannot be unexpected but may nevertheless be difficult. A parent's death often brings to the surface unresolved emotional

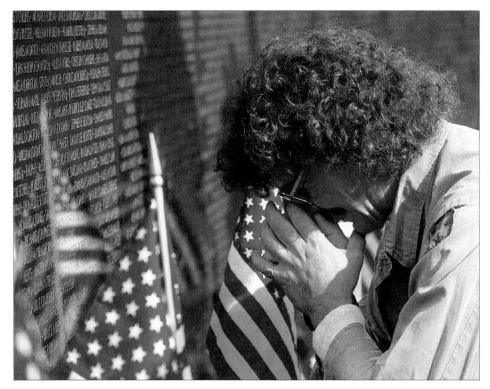

At the Vietnam memorial in Washington, D.C., a friend mourns the death of a war buddy whose name is engraved on the wall. Such rituals—religious or secular—allow the bereaved to formally pay their respects to the dead and go on with living.

issues within the family. Sibling rivalries may be rekindled during a parent's final days. Deathbed reunions ending long family estrangements are rarer in real life than in fiction, but most people do have feelings they need to communicate to a dying parent—even if the message is as simple as "thank you" or "I love you."

Losing a spouse is particularly traumatic because this death severs your primary—and often long-lived—relationship with another person and redefines your status in the community. After years of doing things in partnership, facing life alone may at first seem daunting, if not impossible.

THE STAGES OF GRIEF

The grieving process generally goes through stages. The initial shock and denial are followed by anger, depression, and sometimes guilt. In successful mourning, the loss eventually is accepted, and feelings of sadness are incorporated into fond memories of the loved one.

Until recently many psychologists felt that the process of mourning followed a predictable pattern. People who deviated from that pattern—mourning too long or not long enough—were suspected of having emotional problems. New research suggests that most people go through similar stages of grief, but not necessarily in the same order or at the same pace. Strong emotions can come in waves, and grieving people have good days and bad days.

Acute bouts of grief frequently recur for a year or two after the death of a close relative or friend. Bereaved parents and spouses may take longer to come to grips with their loss.

PRACTICAL ASPECTS

When someone close to you dies, there are logistical matters you must deal with right away. It helps if the person who died left instructions or discussed personal wishes with you. If not, enlist a trusted friend to help you keep lists of the people to notify and the kindnesses received. Also let a friend help you make arrangements with your religious adviser and the funeral home staff, asking questions and keeping notes on what is decided.

Immediate concerns
- Notify relatives and close friends.
- Make burial or cremation arrangements. A funeral home can take care of cremation as well as embalming and will help you obtain a burial plot if your family doesn't have one.
- Plan a service with your religious adviser or the family.
- Send a death notice to the newspaper that includes the date, time, and place of the service and, if you prefer, a charity to which donations can be sent in lieu of flowers. (A friend or the funeral home will do this for you if you ask.)
- Prepare the house for friends and relatives who may visit after the funeral.
- Locate and put in a safe place important papers for settling the estate (p.213) along with at least six official death certificates.
- Notify Social Security and, if appropriate, the Department of Veterans Affairs of the death (there may be burial benefits).

Later
- Acknowledge the gifts, flowers, kind gestures, and condolences.
- Start the probate proceedings.
- File estate and inheritance tax forms.
- File the income tax return for the deceased's last year's earnings.
- Make appropriate changes on insurance policies, property titles, credit cards, and other financial papers.
- Redo your own will.

RESOLUTION AND THEN RECOVERY

Healing begins when you accept the reality of the loved one's death and find some way to put the loss into perspective. If that resolution doesn't come, grief can form the basis for long-lasting psychological problems.

When you lose a spouse, learning to live alone comfortably becomes a part of the recovery process. Things you always did together may be painful when you do them by yourself; you may need to change your routine.

Holidays and anniversaries can be particularly difficult for people who are in mourning. It's natural to feel your losses more at moments that remind you of happier times. Gradually, however, the intensity of your grief will subside, and you will be able to treasure old memories while you slowly develop new rituals.

STAYING WELL

The stress of losing someone close may actually inhibit the functioning of your immune system, making you more susceptible to a variety of diseases. Many people in mourning experience appetite loss, stomach disorders, headaches, dizziness, and insomnia. Men in particular are prone to serious health problems following the death of a close family member. Most likely to get sick are those men who have a hard time expressing their feelings. Relatives and close friends should pay particular attention to such men when they are grieving.

The older you are, the more vulnerable you are to the physical stresses of bereavement. Taking care of yourself—eating properly, exercising regularly, avoiding cigarettes, and limiting your alcohol consumption—is vital to your well-being during mourning.

THE HEALING PROCESS

Don't be too surprised—or unforgiving—if some family members and friends disappoint you during your bereavement. Your loss may create anxieties for them, or they may feel clumsy and tongue-tied around you. You'll likely have a few friends and relatives who are strong enough to cope with your pain and to help you heal.

Remember that facing the world again doesn't mean forgetting the person who died. Cherish memories of the deceased as you recover, and you will be doing what that person would want you to do—getting on with your life.

Eventually most widows and widowers discover that living alone and being lonely are not the same thing at all. If you concentrate on enjoying the simple pleasures in life, contentment will gradually follow.

REACHING OUT

Paradoxically, learning to live alone also means reaching out to other people. Weekends and evenings can be especially lonely, so it's a good idea to schedule interesting activities for those times. Check your local paper for events that you might enjoy. You can ask a friend to accompany you, or you might even enjoy going alone. Don't be afraid to introduce yourself and initiate a conversation when it is appropriate.

Volunteering is another way to get outside yourself. Check with friends or a local social service agency about jobs that need your skills. You might serve at a soup kitchen, run a booth at a charity fair, or tutor a child with learning problems. Your church or synagogue may need a helping hand; so might your local hospital.

WHEN A FRIEND IS GRIEVING

Because grief is intensely personal, there are no ironclad rules about how to handle it. The guidelines below should make you feel more confident in helping a mourning friend.

Don't worry about intruding. Caring friends are what a mourner most needs. Don't stay away just because you feel awkward or don't know what to say.

Simply saying "I'm sorry" is always correct. Recalling the good nature and charm of the person who has died is appropriate too.

Listen sympathetically. Bring a meal to share or offer to accompany your friend on necessary errands

What you shouldn't say. Unless your friend seems suicidal or is drinking heavily, don't criticize his or her behavior; expressions of grief are idiosyncratic. Never tell anyone that you know exactly how they feel. You don't. If you have undergone a similar loss, it's okay to talk about the grief you have experienced if you avoid making direct comparisons. Don't try to minimize your friend's loss by imagining ways the situation could have been worse.

Outside help. Support groups and counseling services offer help to the bereaved. Some mutual-help groups specialize, giving solace to widows, widowers, or parents who have lost children. Other groups assist people who have lost loved ones to suicide, murder, or AIDS.

After the funeral. When the ceremonies end, the relatives go home, and the neighbors stop sending casseroles, your friend may need you the most. Take the initiative. Invite your friend over for dinner. Periodically drop a note or a newspaper clipping in the mail. Arrange a regular activity you can do together—perhaps a daily walk or a weekly movie.

SUICIDE AND THE ELDERLY

Older Americans have a 50 percent higher suicide rate than the general population. The elderly take their own lives because they live in constant pain, they suffer from incurable and degenerative diseases, they fear being institutionalized, or they are recently bereaved. Elderly men in particular may be inclined to suicide if they are socially isolated. Their wives may have maintained the ties with family and friends.

Elderly people who live alone have the means for suicide at their disposal. They can stop eating or refuse life-sustaining medications with no one to notice. Some older people on medications can simply take a lethal overdose of their regular drugs.

Older people who are contemplating suicide may signal their intentions. A verbal cue may be as obvious as "I want to end it all" or "My family is better off without me." Potential suicides may withdraw from social life and begin to neglect themselves. Or, on the contrary, they may suddenly rush to put their personal affairs in order, to give away their most treasured possessions, or to find other means of saying goodbye to loved ones.

Some elderly people, depressed by their isolation, pain, and poor health, may bring up the subject of "rational suicide" with members of their families. In some cases, these aging people indeed have examined the future and found it to be unbearable. Some psychologists, however, are convinced that in many instances elderly people who talk about rational suicide are desperately lonely and are really asking family members to reconfirm their love and affection.

Profile

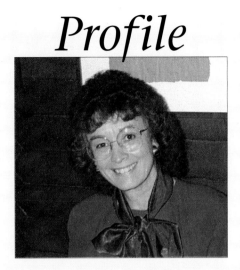

GLENYS BITTICK:
A FULL LIFE AFTER WIDOWHOOD

Glenys Bittick was 50 years old when her husband died suddenly. The shock was compounded by financial worries—her husband had left only a modest insurance policy. A part-time nurse, Bittick never expected she would have to support herself. To add to her problems, within weeks of her husband's death, Bittick was switched to the night shift on a new floor of the hospital. "My sleep pattern was a mess," she says, "and I didn't know anyone." She was too worried about paying the bills to protest.

The first year of widowhood was long and lonely. "When I went out with my married friends, I was a fifth wheel," Bittick recalls. Finally she joined a self-help group for widows and widowers called Life After Death of Spouse (LADOS). "I had gone to a counselor at the hospital, but the widowed people helped me more," she says. At LADOS, she developed a new group of understanding friends.

Today Bittick works full-time, but she also canoes, bicycles, dances, travels, plays with her four grandchildren, and works at a community theater. And she still attends LADOS meetings: "I want to help others in the same position I was in," she says.

ALCOHOL AND MIDDLE AGE

Tolerance for alcohol decreases with age. As a result, older people who continue to drink heavily increasingly risk not only addiction but also the toxic side effects of alcoholism.

DEFINING THE PROBLEM

An estimated 2.5 to 3.5 million older Americans are dependent on or abuse alcohol. The number is hard to establish because many older people hide their addiction. Retirees who live alone, for example, may drink without scrutiny. Others may fool themselves and family members (and sometimes even doctors) by seeing the symptoms of alcoholism—sudden mood changes, angry outbursts, depression, confusion, memory losses—as "normal" aspects of aging.

The majority of older alcohol abusers are early-onset alcoholics who, in midlife or later, begin to show the effects of drinking too much for too long. A smaller group begin to drink compulsively in response to specific problems—boredom in retirement, grief at a spouse's death, or chronic pain. These late-onset alcoholics are more likely to respond well to treatment.

THE NATURE OF ALCOHOL AND ITS ABUSE

Alcohol taken in large quantities is a dangerous drug. It depresses the central nervous system, slowing down brain activity and impairing alertness, judgment, physical coordination, and reaction time. Prolonged drinking not only can lead to addiction but can damage vital organs (facing page and below). Alone in sufficient quantity or when combined with other drugs such as tranquilizers, alcohol becomes lethal.

Although many experts define alcoholism as a chronic and progressive disease, some psychologists balk at calling an addiction a disease. Whether alcoholism, which often runs in families, is primarily a genetic condition or a learned behavior has long been debated. Many experts now believe that several factors—genes, family and cultural attitudes toward drinking, and life events—put some people at risk.

TESTING YOURSELF

Most people who drink do not become alcoholics, but about 10 percent—many who start as social drinkers—slip into alcoholism. If you're worried about your own drinking, try limiting yourself at the next party. Decide to have two drinks and then switch to seltzer. If you always have a cocktail before dinner, try juice instead. If you can't make these changes, you may have a drinking problem (see *Warning Signs of Alcohol Abuse* on page 199).

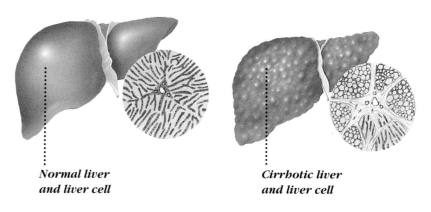

Normal liver and liver cell

Cirrhotic liver and liver cell

The liver can be destroyed by alcohol abuse. Too much alcohol can cause a normal liver (left) to enlarge and accumulate fat in its cells. Some damaged liver cells regenerate and form nodules, an aspect of cirrhosis. Other liver cells become inflamed and irritated; when they heal, scar tissue forms (right). Eventually, the scar tissue impedes the flow of blood through the liver, leading to liver failure and death.

HOW ALCOHOL CAN ABUSE THE BODY

Every system in the body is affected when you sip an alcoholic drink. The liquid irritates the tissues of the mouth and esophagus on its way to the stomach, where some of it is absorbed, but most continues into the intestines. The alcohol passes through the walls of the intestines into the bloodstream, which carries it throughout the body where it is absorbed by the cells. Finally, the alcohol is metabolized by the liver, a process that requires 3 hours for each ounce of alcohol.

Jaundice—*a sign of liver damage —causes the whites of the eyes and skin often to yellow.*

A bulbous nose *often results from alcohol damaged blood vessels.*

Ascites, *the collection of fluid (as much as several liters) in the abdomen is caused by a failing liver; it puts pressure on internal organs and makes breathing difficult.*

Enlarged veins in the esophagus, *which can rupture and cause fatal bleeding, result from blood backing up from a damaged liver.*

The heart *can develop cardiomyopathy, a disease that enlarges it and destroys its muscle. Compare the normal heart, above, with the heart of an alcoholic, below. Alcohol use is also associated with high blood pressure.*

A healthy brain *(above) loses cells at a steady rate during the adult years without impeding mental activity. Chronic drinking speeds up cell deterioration and causes the brain to shrink, or atrophy (above right), which can affect the memory. A buildup of toxins in the blood can contribute to dementia.*

Enlarged breasts *in men (and shrunken testicles) can be caused by a hormone imbalance brought on by liver failure.*

Easily bruised skin *may be a result of cirrhosis.*

Muscle loss *in the face, neck, and arms may be due to alcohol-related malnutrition.*

An enlarged spleen *is also the result of blood backing up from the liver.*

The stomach lining, *irritated by alcohol, may develop inflammation and ulcers. Alcohol can also prevent absorption of nutrients, contributing to malnutrition.*

FINDING HELP

The first step in controlling alcoholism is to stop drinking. Some people (usually late-onset drinkers) can quit by themselves, particularly if they are supported by a mutual-help group. For people with a serious alcohol dependency, however, weaning from alcohol is best accomplished in a detoxification center or hospital where the physical effects of withdrawal (shaking, dry mouth, nausea, sweating, depression, and—in extreme cases—agitation and hallucinations called delirium tremens) can be treated and psychological counseling be started. The alcohol-dependent person is then referred to a support group for help in staying sober.

Since the 1930's, many Americans have maintained their sobriety with the help of Alcoholics Anonymous (AA), a voluntary organization of former addicts who call themselves "recovering" alcoholics and never use their last names. More than 2 million people around the world attend AA meetings every day. The fellowship they find there helps them to stay sober. There is no charge for attending meetings.

Some people are uncomfortable with the AA program's emphasis on finding a "higher power." Other organizations offer similar sobriety programs without the religious overtones.

The payoff is real. No matter how they do it, alcohol-dependent people who stop drinking live longer and more rewarding lives. Most people who quit drinking take a good look at themselves, acknowledge their pain, learn to live with it, and then find ways to satisfy their compulsive tendencies with healthier interests and activities.

LIVING—AND COPING—WITH A PROBLEM DRINKER

When someone you love—a spouse, parent, or child—abuses alcohol, it is difficult to maintain a normal relationship. You never know what to expect next—affection or anger, cooperation or chaos. You must already know, for example, that it is useless to argue with someone who is drunk because that person will distort or forget the exchange. You probably don't know, however, that you may be   lovingly and with the best intentions—encouraging the abuser's addiction over and over again.

Alcoholics Anonymous describes alcoholism as a disease of denial. As long as the alcoholic can deny that he has a problem, he sees no reason to get help. Families, embarrassed by the alcohol abuser's behavior and concerned for his welfare (they often love him, after all), sometimes help perpetuate that denial.

When you clean up the mess made by an inebriated alcoholic wife, you help her deny she ever threw plates at the kitchen wall. Seeing and dealing with the results of her drinking the next day when she is sober might bring her closer to admitting that her drinking is out of hand.

If you call your husband's employer and say he has the flu instead of a hangover, you are lying to the boss, abetting your spouse's addiction, and publicly denying the real problem. Even when it is potentially embarrassing or even harmful to the family, you must allow the person who drinks too much to make his own excuses and to live with the consequences, whatever they are.

Covering up for the person who is dependent on alcohol feeds his belief that he really hasn't behaved badly at all and that his drinking is benign.

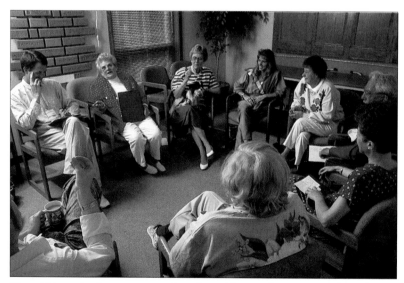

Therapists and volunteer counselors share ideas and compare notes in a staff meeting at the Older Adult Recovery Center in Ann Arbor, Michigan, one of the first and most respected rehabilitation facilities designed exclusively for drug abusers age 55 and over.

WARNING SIGNS OF ALCOHOL ABUSE

To evaluate your own dependency on alcohol or that of a family member or friend, pay attention to the following signs of alcoholism:

■ *Drinking for a reason*—to calm down, to forget about troubles, or because you're bored.
■ *Gulping drinks* or ordering doubles (needing more alcohol to feel good).
■ *Drinking before*—or continuing to drink after—social drinking occasions.
■ *Drinking alone* with increasing frequency.

■ *Getting drunk often*—more than three or four times in the past year.
■ *Being told that you are drinking too much* by people close to you.
■ *Lying* about your drinking habits.
■ *Acting irritable and uncomfortable* during nondrinking periods.
■ *Using alcohol as an excuse* to do things you wouldn't ordinarily do.
■ *Developing drink-related problems* at work, with your health, or in your social life.

HELPING YOURSELF WHEN YOU CAN'T HELP THE DRINKER

It's important to remember that you are not the cause of your loved one's alcoholism (whatever the alcoholic may imply) nor will you be the cure. The problem drinker will commit himself to treatment only when he finally confronts the price of his addiction. You can't do it for him.

Look at your situation realistically and gently separate yourself from the dangers and sorrows that the loved one's drinking can bring you. Don't let the abuser drive when he's been drinking, and tell him why when he is sober. If your loved one ruins family gatherings, go alone and explain your reasoning when she is sober.

Try to get perspective on how living with alcoholic behavior has affected you. Join Al-Anon, a support group started by husbands and wives of AA members to help families and friends. (Call the Alcoholics Anonymous number listed in the telephone book for Al-Anon information.)

Or seek help for yourself through other programs. Many chemical dependency treatment centers provide outpatient counseling for families of alcoholics. (Look in the Yellow Pages under "Alcohol Information and Treatment Centers.")

GETTING THE ALCOHOL ABUSER INTO TREATMENT

Until recently experts concluded that a problem drinker had to hit rock bottom before he would submit to a recovery program. Some professionals now suggest that there are pressures that can sometimes get an alcohol abuser to seek help much sooner.

If a problem drinker works for a company with an Employee Assistance Program (EAP), a boss concerned with the employee's deteriorating work performance can refer him for a confidential evaluation by a drug dependency expert. The evaluator may confirm the boss's suspicion of alcohol abuse and recommend that the employee enter an alcohol treatment program. Confronted with the choice of going immediately into treatment or losing his job, the problem drinker usually picks the treatment program.

Families also have an option. Working with an experienced professional, family members can try a technique called intervention to motivate the problem drinker to get help. In essence, an intervention is a carefully orchestrated surprise confrontation with the alcohol abuser in which family members and close friends calmly and lovingly tell the person about the pain she has caused them. A successful intervention, scheduled for a time when the alcohol abuser is sober, takes many hours of preparation with all the participants and the leader. A successful intervention ends with the problem drinker immediately entering a treatment facility. A botched intervention, however, may leave frustration and bad feelings all around.

No one should try an intervention without hiring a qualified professional. Seek recommendations from a reputable treatment center. You must trust the person you choose to lead an intervention completely. You have too much at stake not to feel totally confident in your choice.

STARTING A NEW CAREER

A generation ago, people at midlife seldom made major career changes. Today, in contrast, many are starting new chapters in their lives. Some seek to fulfill lifelong dreams; others, to reinvent themselves because of a job loss or financial pressures. And some retirees need to supplement their pensions.

give workshops on acquiring the interpersonal skills needed to bring about those changes as well as on marketing yourself creatively and effectively. Some will help with job placement. Check to see what programs are available in your area and how they can enhance your new career prospects.

EDUCATION FOR A CAREER CHANGE

Many men and women accomplish their career transitions by going back to school. Acquiring new skills (such as computer literacy), updating old ones (a refresher course in nursing, for instance), or earning an advanced degree (in education perhaps) all can help open the door to new employment opportunities. Besides colleges and universities, there are high schools, Y's, and technical institutes offering specialized programs and individual courses for people making midlife career changes. Many also

LOOKING FOR WORK IN YOUR NEW FIELD

When you are ready to embark on your new career, be practical and diligent. Make hunting for a job your job. Establish a daily schedule and stick to it. Let your friends and acquaintances know that you are looking for work and

---

A PROGRAM FOR GETTING STARTED

Experts say that the biggest stumbling block to making a successful career shift is a negative attitude. Most people have more options than they realize. And while many face changes, even the ones they choose themselves, with trepidation, taking action (no matter how minor at first) helps dissipate the fear and gets them moving toward their goal.

Step 1	Make a list of all your skills, talents, and interests, including those you want to develop more as well as the ones that are already developed. Don't leave out anything. Even a hobby or a volunteer activity can provide the nucleus of a new career.
Step 2	Try to match what you have to offer with what's in demand. See how your abilities and interests correlate with various career areas. Consider career counseling (see p.206). A responsible counselor will spend several hours with you assessing possibilities based on your test results, life circumstances, available opportunities, and degree of motivation.
Step 3	Do the necessary research once you have decided on your goal. In addition to reading books, magazines, and professional journals, try to interview up to 10 people in your chosen field. Ask detailed questions about how they got started, their financial problems, the skills they needed, and the risks they had to take.
Step 4	Write out a step-by-step plan for achieving your goal based on your research. Then put together a realistic timetable for accomplishing each step.

ask all of them about job opportunities. Get as many names and introductions as possible.

A well-crafted résumé is essential, but it's the interview that gets you the job. Practice with your friends or family. Have them ask you tough questions (check your library or bookstore for career books that include them). In any interview, accentuate the positive: your job qualifications and the assets that maturity brings, such as reliability, practiced skills, good judgment, and grace under pressure. If the job involves working for a younger person, tactfully emphasize your adaptability and eagerness to learn.

Seek out companies with fewer than 20 employees; they are more likely to value your experience than large corporations, many of which are downsizing anyway. Don't neglect going through the want ads either. "Cold" phone calls to firms in your field are a good idea too. If you have trained as a paralegal, for instance, go through the list of law firms in the Yellow Pages. Consider taking any available part-time or temporary work in your new career area until you can find something better. Such a job gives you an opportunity to show what you can do, make contacts, and may even lead to a full-time permanent position.

If you are starting your own venture, consider working at it part time and remaining in your current job until your new business begins to build.

With determination and some hard work, you can recharge your life at almost any age. Taking a chance may be scary at first, but in the long run, people who follow their dreams are much more satisfied than those who let them wither and die.

Profile

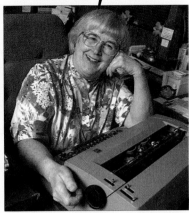

VIRGINIA SNYDER, FLORIDA'S SENIOR-CITIZEN PRIVATE EYE

*I*n 1974, Virginia Snyder, a 53-year-old investigative reporter for the Boca Raton News in Florida, went away for the weekend to accept two reporting awards and came in on Monday to find she was out of a job.

Her career options weren't encouraging. "I saw what happened to older women reporters. I knew they'd be wanting me to write recipes," she says. Her husband suggested she start a private investigative service. Snyder received her license in 1976 and soon had so many cases that both her husband and nephew became partners. The second woman in Florida to become a licensed private detective, she is the oldest and longest-licensed one in Palm Beach County.

Snyder's biggest challenges were murder cases in which innocent people were convicted. Her investigations helped get six clients off death row (two were freed), and five clients stays of execution. Now in her seventies, Snyder has written a book about her most fascinating cases. "To me, there's no difference between work and play," she says. "My work is fun, challenging, rewarding, and contributes something to society. If I were independently wealthy, I'd work for free."

YOUR RETIREMENT YEARS

*N*owadays, as more people live into their eighties and nineties, retirement is often a new beginning rather than an ending. As you reach midlife, you should ask yourself what kind of life you would like to be leading in 10 or 15 years.

SETTING GOALS

Where will you live when you retire? Will you play golf? Work part-time? Start a second career? Once you clarify your goals, you can take the steps to attain them. If you're not sure of your retirement goals, you may want to try a "retirement rehearsal" by taking a leave of absence from your job. Another option might be to settle into retirement in stages by going from full-time to part-time work.

FINANCIAL PLANNING

Besides good health, the main prerequisite of a happy retirement is an adequate financial base—one with 60 to 70 percent of your current pretax income. Social Security usually provides only a minor portion of that amount, so if you are not already saving for retire-

ment, start now. Open a tax-deferred retirement account (an IRA or a Keogh). If your firm has a 401(k) plan, enroll in it. To find out what Social Security will add to your retirement income, fill out and send in a Personal Earnings and Benefit Estimate Statement (PEBES). Get the form from your local Social Security office or by calling 1-800-772-1213.

Because inflation can reduce the purchasing power of your retirement income, learn how to manage your money. Decide how much risk you can afford, make some conservative investments (such as Treasury securities), and then make some careful choices in stocks and bonds where the potential for gain is greater.

For help with financial planning, try one of the retirement counseling programs offered by the American Associaton of Retired Persons (AARP) and the National Council on Aging (NCOA). Workshops are also given at Y's, senior centers, community colleges, and by other organizations.

ENJOYING RETIREMENT

Family and friends are your best insurance for health and happiness in retirement. Men and women with solid social networks cope better with stress and may actually live longer. Keeping a large circle of acquaintances is less important, however, than acquiring at least one close friend who is a confidante. Having several close friends is best, since no one person (not even your spouse) can fulfill all your needs.

You don't have to be wealthy to enjoy retirement. Your age and status can entitle you to many special deals and discounts. Senior citizens often pay half fare on public transportation, get discounts on movie and theater tickets, and qualify for special plane and train fares. Some banks provide free checking, and many local government programs offer a reduction in real estate taxes as well as fuel cost allowances.

ENRICHING YOUR LIFE WITH EDUCATION

Older adults are going back to school in unprecedented numbers. Hundreds of thousands of Americans over the age of 50 are enrolled in college courses. Thousands more attend lectures, belong to various study groups, and take trips that combine travel and

EARLY RETIREMENT

While some people keep on working well past retirement age, many others take early retirement. Three-fourths of American men and more than four-fifths of American women now collect Social Security checks before their 65th birthdays.

If you decide on early retirement, review all the possible consequences beforehand. Obviously, you will need a larger nest egg to cover the extra years you won't be working. You may also lose a portion of your pension. And if you begin collecting Social Security at 62 instead of 65, your benefits will be permanently reduced by about 20 percent. If you plan to supplement a fixed income by working, investigate your prospects for part-time work in your field well in advance.

Although the law bans age discrimination and mandatory retirement because of age, some firms offer bonuses and special deals to encourage older workers—many only in their fifties—to retire early. With the right conditions, this may be a golden opportunity. But proceed carefully and get good advice. In any such proposal, all pension penalties should be eliminated. Many companies offer a substantial lump-sum payment to make the package more appealing. Consider also asking for bridge payments to supplement your pension until you begin getting Social Security. You should be given a reasonable amount of time, from 1 to 3 months, to weigh the proposal. Your employer should also tell you what to expect if you don't take it. Are layoffs planned? Will you be given a heavier workload to make up for those people who do retire?

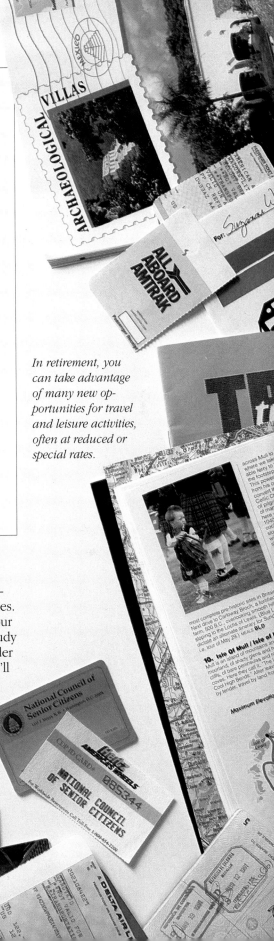

In retirement, you can take advantage of many new opportunities for travel and leisure activities, often at reduced or special rates.

learning. Most of them are studying for the sheer pleasure of it.

Keeping your mind active provides benefits that extend beyond what you learn. Research shows that it's good for your health and also improves mental ability. One study of 64- to 95-year-olds found that those individuals whose faculties had declined could recover some of their losses by challenging themselves intellectually.

Local high schools, colleges, and universities are obvious first choices for a study program. Senior centers, Y's, and special-interest groups also offer courses. Check the listings section of your newspaper for independent study groups and book clubs. Consider convenience and cost too. You'll be more inclined to follow through if getting to a class is easy. Most community programs are inexpensive or free, and many colleges offer courses to older people for free or at a nominal cost (financial aid may sometimes be available).

Another option is peer group study, known generically as Learning in Retirement. More than 160 such seminar-like programs exist, most of them under university sponsorship. In consultation with an adviser, the students design a program of study. While there are no educational requirements, grades, or exams, the courses are rigorous, the discussions spirited, and each student must take a turn preparing a lesson and leading the class.

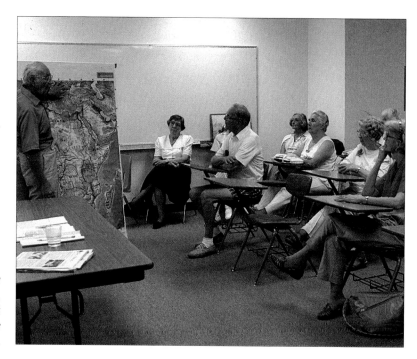

At Rio Salado Community College in Phoenix, Arizona, retirees attend a class in current affairs taught by a retired State Department official.

TRAVEL AND STUDY PROGRAMS

Travel is always a learning experience, but specific travel-study programs have been increasing in popularity. The nonprofit Elderhostel, based in Cambridge, Massachusetts, is probably the largest of many organizations (including some major museums and universities) that offer such activities.

Geared to people age 60 and over, Elderhostel provides a wide variety of courses lasting from 1 to 4 weeks at more than 1,900 colleges and educational institutions in the United States and in 49 foreign countries. Accommodations vary, but they are usually simple and inexpensive.

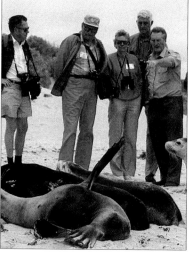

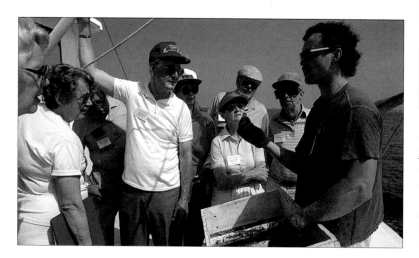

Some Elderhostel members participate in a marine biology program at Hampton University in Virginia (left), while others study sea lions in their natural habitat on a remote island beach (above).

EMPLOYMENT AFTER RETIREMENT

Increasing numbers of people are working after retirement, most of them part-time. Some just want to remain active, while others wish to supplement their retirement income. Still others find retirement unsatisfying and return to full-time work, even embarking on new careers (see pp.200-201).

Opportunities for work in retirement are there if you look for them. Some corporations offer special programs designed for older workers. These include job sharing, in which two part-time employees share one job, and flextime, which lets you choose the hours that you work. Many companies maintain job banks that draw on retirees for temporary or part-time work.

Other places to seek employment include banks, which often hire older workers as tellers or customer-service representatives; travel agencies, which value the rapport older workers have with peers who travel frequently; and temporary agencies, which allow flexibility. Home improvement chains and hardware stores have discovered that older workers have a fund of knowledge to impart to the growing do-it-yourself crowd. Although the pay is usually low, nonprofit organizations are another employment possibility. There is also a need for workers of all ages in the service industries.

But perhaps your dream has always been to go into business for yourself: to start a bed-and-breakfast, for instance, or to open a shop to sell the patchwork quilts or wood carvings you've been making for years. Prospective entrepreneurs can obtain expert business advice from SCORE, the Service Corps of Retired Executives, a volunteer-run division of the Small Business Administration. Free counseling is available at SCORE centers throughout the United States. To get the address of

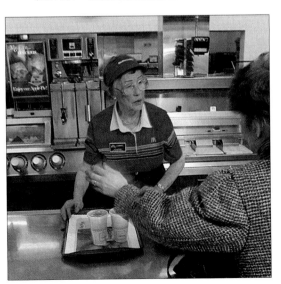

Many senior citizens find full- or part-time work in offices (right) or in fast-food restaurants (below).

FAST FACTS

■ Isolation can be hazardous to your health. People living alone have more heart attacks, perhaps because medical help is not readily available or because close human contact brings a protective mind-body response.

■ Women's death rates are highest in the week after their birthdays; men's, shortly before, a recent study shows. The reason may be that men tend to view birthdays as a time of stocktaking and focusing on goals they have not met, whereas women tend to welcome them as an opportunity to reaffirm treasured relationships.

■ A third of all workers who take early retirement regret it within 6 months, some because they miss their jobs, others because they haven't planned what to do with their free time.

■ Women with demanding jobs have a lower risk of heart attack than women who don't work. The reason may be that they have more of a sense of control over their lives, a feeling linked to a lower illness rate.

■ The happiest people, regardless of their station in life, are those who have worked hard and accomplished a goal that is meaningful to them.

the SCORE center nearest you, call the Washington headquarters.

If you want to work but aren't sure what you're best suited for, it's a good idea to take some time to assess your skills and experience (see the *Getting Started* chart, p.200). Think about the kind of working environment you'd prefer, what hours you wish to work, and how much money you want (or need) to earn. If matching your tastes and talents to a job isn't easy, consider talking with a vocational counselor. Many senior centers, religious organizations, community colleges, and professional and trade associations offer job-counseling services. Local chapters of the American Association of Retired Persons (AARP) may also be able to help you with your job search.

Keep in mind that your Social Security benefits will be reduced if you earn more than a certain amount. Your local Social Security office (or local AARP chapter) can tell you what your earnings limit is. In general, when you exceed that limit, you forfeit $1 of Social Security for every $2 you earn.

VOLUNTEERING IN RETIREMENT

If staying active and involved is important to you but money is not a consideration, try volunteering. Returning something to society isn't just doing good for other people; it's doing good for yourself too. People who give to others report a reduction in chronic pain and an increased sense of optimism.

There are as many ways to volunteer as there are volunteers. Lifelong learners can aid their school systems or community libraries. Others can help local theater or music groups. Hospitals and church or community social programs always need people, and the politically inclined can assist in local campaigns or register voters. On a wider front, the American Red Cross trains volunteers throughout the country for domestic disaster-relief work.

ACTION (American Council to Improve Our Neighborhoods), the federal agency for domestic volunteers, coordinates several programs. The largest is RSVP (Retired Senior Volunteer Program), in which participants serve on a part-time basis in one of the 750 RSVP community programs in the United States. Other ACTION programs include the Foster Grandparent Program and the Senior Companion Program. The more demanding VISTA program (Volunteers in Service to America) assigns people to serve for 1 year in poverty-stricken communities,

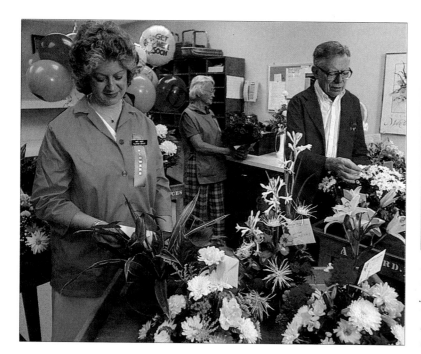

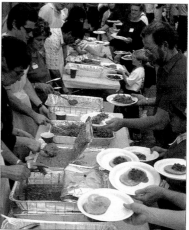

In a Raleigh, North Carolina, hospital (left), volunteers prepare flowers for delivery to patients, while volunteers in a Los Angeles shelter (above) serve Christmas dinner to the homeless.

where they work on projects with local people. Peace Corps volunteers perform VISTA-type services in other countries, usually for a 2-year term.

If you'd like to do some hard physical work, Habitat for Humanity, headquartered in Americus, Georgia, always needs volunteers to build and rehabilitate low-income housing—working side by side with the people who will live there—in the United States and abroad. Global Volunteers in St. Paul, Minnesota, sends people all over the world on similar "working vacations."

If you can't find the right spot for you, contact the AARP Talent Bank in Washington, D.C., or Volunteer: The National Center in Arlington, Virginia. Before applying, decide how much time and effort you want to put in; then help the organization place you by coming up with some concrete ideas about what you can do.

· ·

FINDING THE RIGHT PLACE TO RETIRE

Many popular retirement communities are overbuilt, congested, and expensive. But new ones are constantly being built, and other alternatives, such as small towns (especially college towns) have been gaining appeal. To get leads, browse through the travel and shelter magazines at your local library. Then talk to real estate agents—at home or when you travel—about places where housing buys and retirement prospects are good (see the checklist on page 208). Don't finalize arrangements right away. If, for instance, you've always dreamed of retiring to the rocky coast of Maine, rent for a year first to make sure that is where you really want to live.

Profile

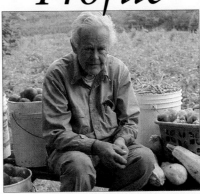

WILLIAM LIDDELL: A RETIREE WITH "A FULL-TIME JOB"

"I *never thought about what I'd do when I retired, and then this happened," says Bill Liddell. "This" is growing more than 40,000 pounds of vegetables a year on a ¾-acre plot in Hamden, Connecticut, and donating the bounty to the Connecticut Food Bank in New Haven for distribution to local soup kitchens, homeless shelters, and church pantries.*

Liddell took up gardening in the late 1940's while enrolled in the graduate history program at Yale University. He planned to teach but took a job with a seed company instead. Meanwhile he continued to tend his garden, giving away bushels of produce to friends, relatives, and a New Haven homeless shelter. When Liddell retired in 1985, he decided to make a career of his gardening. From observing vegetable farmers over the years, he had learned how to get the most from his space.

To achieve his yield, Liddell has the help of 16 regular volunteers. He produces two or three crops of at least a dozen kinds of vegetables annually. "For a retired person, it's a full-time job," he laughs. "I'm lucky to have the land, time, friends, and neighbors to help me. I plan to keep doing this for as long as I can."

MAKING THE RIGHT RETIREMENT HOUSING DECISION

Deciding on your retirement living arrangements is a highly individual matter, and the only right decision is what is right for you. The following checklists, however, may help you in making that decision. Once you have isolated the housing considerations that are the most important to you, stack them up against your assessment of what assistance you or your spouse may need. Then review the financial checklist to see what steps, if any, you may still need to take to get the living arrangements you want.

WHAT HOUSING CONSIDERATIONS ARE MOST IMPORTANT TO YOU?

	Very Important	Moderately Important	Not Very Important
1. Staying in your present home.			
2. Living near family and friends.			
3. Living near your place of worship.			
4. Keeping housing and living costs to a minimum.			
5. A large amount of living space.			
6. Access to public transportation, stores, and community services.			
7. Having outdoor and home maintenance services available.			
8. Feeling secure in your home and neighborhood.			
9. Privacy.			
10. Companionship.			
11. Keeping pets, furnishings, and other personal items.			
12. A homelike environment.			
13. Numerous recreational activities.			
14. Readily available health care services.			
15. Living in a climate you like.			

DO YOU NEED OR WILL YOU NEED ASSISTANCE WITH THE FOLLOWING?

	Now	Within a Year	Within 5 Years
1. Preparing meals.			
2. Personal care.			
3. Getting around the house.			
4. At-home medical care.			
5. Housekeeping.			
6. Outdoor maintenance.			
7. Transportation.			
8. Managing finances.			

WHAT FINANCIAL CONSIDERATIONS HAVE YOU TAKEN INTO ACCOUNT?

	Yes	No
1. Do you currently spend the recommended 30 percent or less of your gross income on housing (including utilities)?		
2. Will your anticipated budget over the next 5 years provide you with comfortable housing?		
3. Would you be willing to alter your housing arrangements to adjust to any change in income?		
4. Would the financial benefits of living with others make you want to adapt to a new living arrangement?		
5. Would the rental income from an accessory apartment or a home sharer be worth the alteration costs to your residence?		
6. Are you eligible for subsidized rent, fuel assistance, or property tax breaks?		
7. Have you talked to other older retirees about their experiences?		
8. Have you carefully reviewed all the living arrangements available to you?		
9. Have you discussed your housing options with members of your family? With friends, a housing counselor, or a financial adviser?		

STAYING PUT IN RETIREMENT

Surveys show that most older people prefer not to move. Such a decision should depend on the condition of your home, your financial situation, how well your home (and neighborhood) will meet your needs as you age, and your adaptability.

For instance, if your house is big and expensive to maintain, consider home sharing, which has both economic and social advantages. Your housemate could be a friend who shares not only expenses but also meals and leisure. Or you might choose a student or other young person who does household chores and yard work in exchange for a low rent.

If zoning laws permit it, you can add an apartment onto your home or create a self-contained unit within it that you can either rent out or let a relative or friend live in (with both of you able to maintain your privacy).

A concept that is gaining popularity is ECHO (Elder Cottage Housing Opportunity). A prefabricated cottage is set up near a single-family home (if zoning laws permit) so that people can live near relatives, usually their adult children, without having to share quarters.

Another option is co-housing, which provides private living spaces with a communal kitchen, dining room, and recreational area. Residents of all ages live as a large, extended family and make major household decisions together. When older residents become frail, co-housing communities may also provide health care services. Some older people set up their own, less formal co-housing arrangements by banding together with a few good friends to live communally.

LIVING ARRANGEMENTS THAT PROVIDE HELP

While everyone hopes for good health in the retirement years, it's wise to research alternate living arrangements in case you or a loved one ever needs physical assistance. These fall into three basic categories: Board-and-care homes provide meals and housekeeping but vary on other services. Some of their residents may be highly independent; others may need help with personal care. Congregate housing is a group living situation with communal dining, some housekeeping services, and organized social activities. Continuing-care retirement communities are for people who live independently now but want housekeeping and health care services to be available if and when they need them.

Before you sign up for any of these communities, make sure that all the services you need—or might need in the future—are provided. The best communities usually have long waiting lists, so it's a good idea to start looking far in advance.

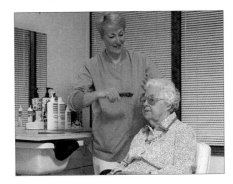

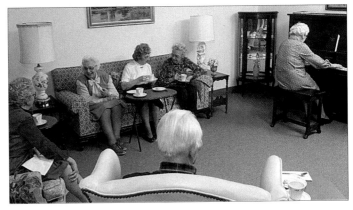

Hair care is one of the services available in this board-and-care home (left). Residents in a group home (below) enjoy a piano recital by another resident.

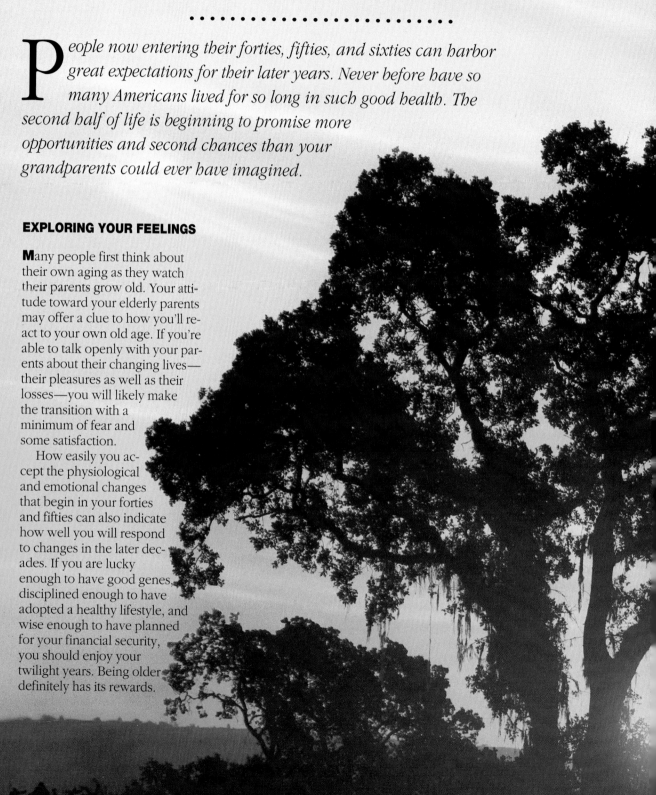

GETTING OLDER

· ·

People now entering their forties, fifties, and sixties can harbor great expectations for their later years. Never before have so many Americans lived for so long in such good health. The second half of life is beginning to promise more opportunities and second chances than your grandparents could ever have imagined.

EXPLORING YOUR FEELINGS

Many people first think about their own aging as they watch their parents grow old. Your attitude toward your elderly parents may offer a clue to how you'll react to your own old age. If you're able to talk openly with your parents about their changing lives—their pleasures as well as their losses—you will likely make the transition with a minimum of fear and some satisfaction.

How easily you accept the physiological and emotional changes that begin in your forties and fifties can also indicate how well you will respond to changes in the later decades. If you are lucky enough to have good genes, disciplined enough to have adopted a healthy lifestyle, and wise enough to have planned for your financial security, you should enjoy your twilight years. Being older definitely has its rewards.

A KEY TO HEALTH: THE RIGHT ATTITUDE

Bitterness and inflexibility are not natural results of aging; they often develop when people feel they have lost control over their lives.

Giving in to old age—becoming helpless and incompetent—may actually shorten your life; such submissiveness certainly affects the quality of your later years. Elderly people who prop themselves in front of a TV and complain about their fate can't enjoy life as much as their peers who fill each day with purposeful activity. Passivity and inactivity take a physical toll on the body. Passivity and indifference take the joy out of life.

Experts agree that the people who age most successfully maintain a positive outlook. They accept their limitations by adapting to them. If, for example, they can't live near their grandchilden, they establish a correspondence with them. If they can no longer play a sport, they help run meets for younger athletes.

> **"***One of the unanswered questions of life is: When is old age? My answer would be: When I have ceased to wonder.***"**
>
> —British diplomat and author Sir Harold Nicolson (1886–1968)

REMINISCENCE

Most people like to think back over the past. Purposeful reminiscence, sometimes called life review, is a form of therapy that contributes to self-knowledge and self-esteem.

Everyone reminisces—even preschoolers talk about when they were babies—but older people get the most benefit from looking back. Reviewing your life, you can assess your successes and failures over the long term, discern patterns in your behavior, deepen your sense of identity, and find ways to cope with personal losses.

Through reminiscing, you take responsibility for your life. You can savor the moments of triumph and forgive yourself some mistakes. You can work through conflicts that may have disturbed you for years. You may also discover tasks left undone that you can take care of now.

A good way to review your life is to tell your story to an interested listener. If you'd like to document your life history—or just enjoy an afternoon of reminiscing—ask a friend to prompt you with questions. Plan to talk about your family history—where your grandparents lived, how your parents met, your first memory of them, the impact historical events had on you and your family. Try to remember your first date, your first job, your wedding day, your best friends through the years.

You might want to write down your life story or tape-record it as a gift to your family. If you're not camera shy, let a relative videotape your reminiscences.

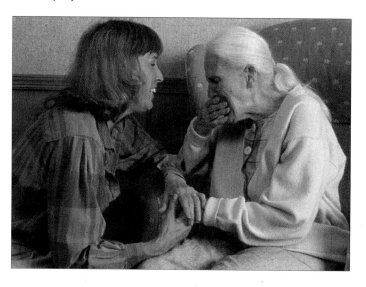

THE SECRETS OF GROWING OLD GRACEFULLY

Not everyone deals with aging in the same way. One gerontologist, to simplify the issues, divides approaches to aging into two broad categories: digging in and digging out. Those who dig in hold tightly to the familiar, even when it no longer makes sense. Those who dig out take risks. They are willing to make new friends and try new endeavors to redefine their lives and themselves.

Psychologists who work with the elderly have identified a number of lifelong habits that seem characteristic of the people who most savor their later years. Such people set themselves goals to work toward. They celebrate their own successes but also cheer on their families and friends.

People who age well never seem to lose their curiosity or sense of adventure. They balance a familiar routine with bursts of spontaneity. They keep learning. They juggle their social schedules with private moments and still save time for helping others.

LATE-LIFE TASKS

Although the subjects may be difficult for you and your family to bring up and discuss, how you feel about a mentally incapacitating illness or injury, where and how you want to be buried, and how you want your property divided after your death are vitally important issues. If you want your wishes to be carried out, you must communicate your thoughts to your family or close friends. In addition, you must put some of your wishes into a proper legal form so that doctors, hospitals, and state courts can honor them.

Drawing up a will

A will legally protects your wishes about the disposition of your property after your death. It also speeds up the settlement of your estate and saves your heirs high probate court costs.

To draw up a will, first make an inventory of what you own and decide what you want to go to each of your beneficiaries (you may want to designate a percentage of the value of your assets). Name a guardian for any dependent children and an executor (usually your spouse or an adult child) to oversee the carrying out of the will. A lawyer will see that the document conforms to your state's laws.

Don't postpone making a will. If you die without one, the court will divide your property according to state law and take out hefty fees for doing so. If your estate is large or complicated, you should consult a lawyer or an accountant who specializes in estate planning. Be sure to revise your will if you move to another state or if there's a birth, marriage, divorce, or death in your family.

Considering a living will and a health care proxy

Hospitals and nursing homes in the United States are required by federal law to inform their patients about state statutes on living wills and health care proxies, the legal means for telling doctors when to withhold care if you can't speak for yourself.

If you don't want to be kept alive by technology when you are no longer aware of what is going on, you can sign a living will, a document that spells out your views on prolonging your life artificially. You can also designate a relative or friend as your health care proxy (p.222), a person legally empowered to act on your behalf. The legal forms for a living will and a health care proxy differ from state to state. Consult your lawyer or write to Choice for Dying, 200 Varick St., New York, NY 10014.

Keeping important documents

Your will and other important papers should be kept in a secure place at home (a safe or fireproof box) or at your lawyer's office. Don't store crucial documents in a safe-deposit box; your heirs won't have quick access to them.

Immediate access to the following papers will make your family's life easier at your death:

- Living will
- Health care proxy
- Uniform donor card
- Social Security card
- Birth certificate
- Marriage certificate
- Insurance policies
- Deeds and mortgages
- Safe-deposit box key
- Tax records
- Veteran's discharge

Making arrangements

You save your heirs worry and confusion if you leave clear written instructions for the kind of burial arrangements and memorial service you would like to have. If you own a burial plot or have a membership in a memorial society, include the relevant papers. Writing your own obituary—by yourself or with someone you love—can also save your heirs a task that is difficult for people in mourning.

You may want to leave money specifically for funeral expenses. Don't prepay a funeral home, however. You may leave the area before you die, or the funeral home may go out of business.

WHY OLDER CAN BE BETTER

■ ***You become smarter.*** Although you continue to lose brain cells throughout your life, as you grow older you increase the depth and breadth of your knowledge and experience.

■ ***You are tougher.*** A physical change in the brain may be part of the reason that older people take life's ups and downs in stride more easily than younger people.

■ ***You gain power.*** By the time you are middle-aged or older, you are secure in what you know from study and from experience. You may be working at the peak of your powers.

■ ***You love better.*** If you have been able to build relationships over time, your commitment makes them deeply satisfying.

■ ***You know who you are.*** The older you are, the more relaxed you become about your identity and your opinions.

■ ***You become kinder.*** Midlife and the later years are the time for giving back to the family and the community. Older people are more altruistic than younger ones, more likely to be mentors to the aspiring or to volunteer when help is needed.

■ ***Your spirituality deepens.*** With time to reflect, your inner life develops, and you find yourself blessed with new wisdom.

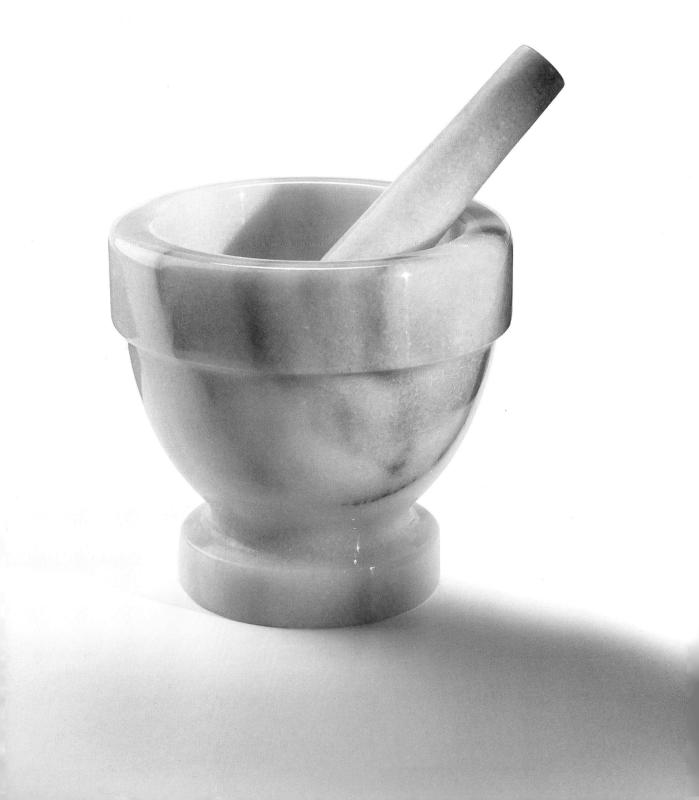

Chapter 6

MAINTAINING HEALTH

▨ TAKING RESPONSIBILITY FOR YOUR
HEALTH CARE *216*

▨ HANDLING A HOSPITAL STAY *220*

▨ PAYING FOR MEDICAL CARE *224*

▨ MAKING THE MOST OF MEDICAL TESTS *226*

▨ USING DRUGS WISELY *230*

▨ SEXUALITY ACROSS THE LIFESPAN *238*

▨ KEEPING YOUR MEMORY SHARP *240*

▨ SMOKING: HOW TO BREAK A BAD HABIT *242*

▨ MANAGING HEADACHES *246*

▨ THE SCOURGES OF WINTER:
THE COMMON COLD AND THE FLU *248*

▨ GETTING A GOOD NIGHT'S SLEEP *250*

▨ TAKING CARE OF YOUR BACK *252*

▨ NUISANCE PROBLEMS OF THE
DIGESTIVE SYSTEM *256*

▨ KEEPING YOUR FEET HEALTHY *260*

TAKING RESPONSIBILITY FOR YOUR HEALTH CARE

P reserving your health is important throughout life, but especially as you grow older. If you don't already have a primary care provider, it's crucial to find one to give you periodic check-ups, tend to your basic medical needs, and serve as a gatekeeper to the world of specialists and high-tech medicine.

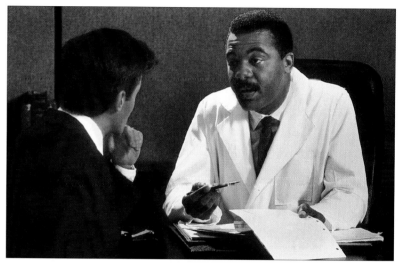

Don't hesitate to ask your doctor any questions you might have about your health. If you are anxious in a medical setting, bring a written list.

CHOOSING A PRIMARY CARE PHYSICIAN

A doctor who knows you and is familiar with your medical history can spot the early signs of disease, give you personal support in emergencies, and help you avoid unnecessary tests and treatments.

To find a suitable doctor, get names from friends, medical professionals you know, your state or local medical society, and nearby teaching hospitals. If you have a chronic ailment, ask the medical society for a list of physicians who specialize in treating that condition. Once you have gathered some doctors' names, you should check their credentials. The *American Medical Directory* or the *Directory of Medical Specialists,* which are available in most libraries, can tell you where a doctor trained and is licensed and whether he is certified by a professional specialty board.

Medical competence, though, is not enough. You want a doctor who will listen sympathetically to your complaints and explain findings clearly and candidly. You may also have preferences regarding age or sex; a younger doctor, for instance, is more likely to be around as you grow older.

To decide if a doctor is right for you, make an appointment; investing in a consultation now may prevent misunderstandings later. The medical staff can answer your questions about office hours, fees, insurance claims, and telephone consultations. In your meeting with the doctor, inquire about his hospital admitting privileges, availability in emergencies, who covers in his absence, and how he feels about your particular health concerns. A conscientious doctor will not be offended, and you will learn how well the two of you are able to interact.

GETTING THE MOST OUT OF YOUR FIRST VISIT

To ensure that your visit to a new doctor is as productive as possible, ask what you should bring with you. Usually you will need proof of insurance, a list of any

How Some Alternative Treatments Can Help

People frustrated by traditional medicine sometimes turn to unorthodox forms of treatment. While medical doctors dismiss many of these alternative therapies as quackery, they do accept some of them, especially for treating chronic, stress-related complaints. Some of the most widely used alternative treatments are described below.

Acupuncture. An ancient Chinese technique, acupuncture involves inserting thin needles at specific points on the body to treat disease. Some Western doctors now use acupuncture, or else refer patients to practitioners, to alleviate such ailments as stubborn back or joint pain or chronic headache. Many states license acupuncturists; others allow only medical doctors with training in acupuncture to use the method.

Chiropractic. The manipulation of the spinal column to treat disease, chiropractic was long condemned by the medical profession. Recent studies show, however, that it can relieve back and neck pain. Licensed in all states, chiropractors cannot perform surgery or prescribe drugs.

Herbalism. Herbalists use plants to treat and prevent many illnesses. While some remedies may contain valuable ingredients, keep in mind that many plants are toxic. Check with your doctor to make sure that an herbal medication is safe for you to take.

Homeopathy. This uses extremely diluted solutions of substances that, in large doses can cause symptoms similar to the ailment. For instance, a diluted solution of poison ivy or poison oak may be prescribed for dermatitis. Many traditional doctors attribute homeopathic cures to suggestion, but some believe they merit further study.

Naturopathy. The field of naturopathy incorporates several alternative therapies, including herbal and homeopathic remedies. Although not licensed to prescribe drugs unless they are M.D.'s, naturopaths sometimes work with traditional doctors.

Osteopathy. Once regarded with the same suspicion as chiropractic, osteopathy is now recognized as largely equivalent to traditional medicine. Practitioners emphasize a holistic approach that includes massage and manipulation, but they are also trained in conventional medicine and are licensed in all 50 states to practice medicine and surgery.

drugs you take, and all available records of any recent tests or treatments you have undergone. You should be prepared with facts too—70 percent of what a doctor learns in an office visit comes directly from the patient's history, that is, your own words.

If your visit is related to sickness, give the doctor as many specific details about your complaint as you can. You will also be asked about other symptoms, past illnesses, and your family's medical histories and lifestyles as well as your own. This information can be vital to keeping you healthy and is kept confidential.

"Cures" That Don't Work

This year, one out of four Americans will contribute to a $25-billion-plus industry for products and services that are useless, dangerous, or both. The industry is medical quackery, and its customers are people who feel that traditional medicine has let them down. Unfortunately, medical science does not offer quick, easy, and certain solutions for many problems. Quacks do. But their solutions not only don't work, but they also may keep a person from seeking treatment that could be beneficial and even lifesaving, especially in the case of cancer, which, if treated early and appropriately, may be curable.

Medical quacks often dress like medical professionals, have impressive offices, and display fake degrees. Some even have medical degrees. But what they all have in common is phony solutions to real problems.

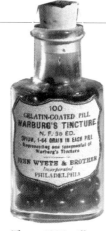

These 1890 pills contained opium.

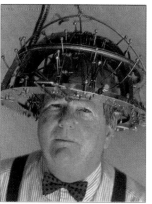

This 1930 Psycograph "diagnosed" traits dangerous to a person's health.

It's Medical Quackery If They...

Promise quick, easy cures for illnesses such as cancer and arthritis. Such cures do not exist.

Promote "secret" medicines, often sold via mail from only one distributor. Medicines that work are not secret and can be readily obtained.

Offer testimonials from satisfied users as proof that a medicine works. Prescription medicines must be tested for effectiveness and safety,

WHAT TO EXPECT IN A ROUTINE PHYSICAL EXAMINATION

During a checkup, the doctor (or her nurse) weighs you, takes your temperature and blood pressure, listens to your chest with a stethoscope, tests your reflexes with a rubber hammer, and takes blood and urine samples for analysis. You may also be given a stool test to do at home. (See *Types of Screening Tests,* pp.228–229.)

The doctor checks your general appearance, your skin, eyes, ears, nose, and throat, and feels your neck, armpits, and groin for enlarged lymph nodes. She then inspects your joints for swelling, palpates your abdomen, and probes your rectum. Examination of a man's prostate and testicles and a woman's breasts and pelvic organs (including a Pap smear) is also routine. Your medical history may suggest other exams. If you have a specific problem, ask about available treatments and any possible side effects.

THE BENEFITS OF A SECOND OPINION

Get a second—or even a third—opinion if you have a rare or life-threatening disease, if the diagnosis or treatment is in doubt, or if a suggested procedure is controversial, risky, or new. Choose a board-certified expert in the same field, but one with a different specialty from the first doctor. If a heart surgeon recommends a coronary bypass, for instance, consult a cardiologist who does not perform surgery. Have your records sent to the second doctor to avoid repeating any tests, and make sure the second opinion is sent in writing to the first doctor so that you can all discuss it before a decision is made.

IF YOU DON'T IMPROVE

Talk to your doctor if you are dissatisfied with your treatment. The problem may be bad communication, not bad medicine. You can also complain to your insurer or local medical society—or file a lawsuit. But keep in mind that doctors win most malpractice

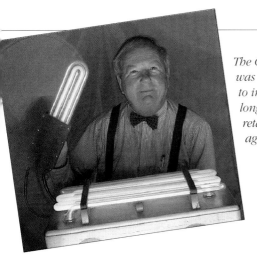

The Color-Therm was thought to increase longevity and retard the aging process.

YOU CAN CHECK...

A doctor's credentials with your local medical society.

A medicine with your local FDA office.

A health care facility or company with your local Better Business Bureau, your state's attorney general, the Federal Trade Commission in Washington, D.C., and your local postmaster or postal inspection service.

with accompanying reports in reputable scientific or medical journals, and approved for use by the Food and Drug Administration (FDA).

Sell a medicine or promote a diet to cure many conditions. Most medicines and diets are useful for one or, at best, a few conditions.

Claim their medicine is a scientific breakthrough that traditional doctors are trying to suppress. Responsible doctors quickly accept any medicine that is scientifically proven effective.

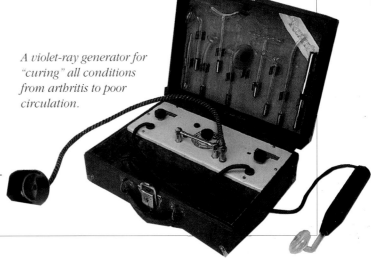

A violet-ray generator for "curing" all conditions from arthritis to poor circulation.

suits. You must prove not that the treatment failed but that it was below community standards and caused you physical or financial harm. Consult a malpractice lawyer to see if you have a valid case. Then consider whether you can handle the expense and trauma of a trial.

YOUR MEDICAL RECORDS

Your right to see your medical records is protected by law in many states. Go over them with your doctor so that you understand all the technical terms and their implications. Records may be shared with insurance companies, employers, and others; so check their accuracy.

ADULT IMMUNIZATIONS

Immunizations are important for children, but you need to keep up your immunity as an adult too.

■ ***Diphtheria and tetanus*** (usually given together). Even if you had these immunizations as a child, you need a booster every 10 years.

■ ***Influenza vaccine.*** Flu viruses change so rapidly that a new inoculation is needed each year. It is recommended for those over 65 and younger people with chronic ailments. You cannot catch the flu from the vaccine. But anyone allergic to eggs should forgo it because eggs are used in its preparation.

■ ***Pneumococcal pneumonia.*** Everyone over the age of 65 should have this vaccine, as should younger people with chronic ailments. Some experts suggest a booster after 6 years for those considered at high risk.

■ ***Other immunizations.*** Check with your doctor about other inoculations, especially those required if you travel abroad.

HANDLING A HOSPITAL STAY

No one looks forward to time in a hospital, but the experience will be more positive if you have confidence in the facility—and if you understand how much your own participation in your treatment can affect the quality of your care.

CHOOSING A HOSPITAL

Your options for picking a hospital may be limited. Doctors can treat you only in the hospitals where they have staff privileges. Also, your insurance may specify the hospital you must use.

If you want to check out a hospital before choosing a doctor or insurance plan, call its public relations department and ask if it is accredited by the Joint Commission on Accreditation of Health Organizations. A probational rating suggests a problem.

Also ask about the hospital's financial structure. Private for-profit hospitals are often comfortable but costly and may lack the staff or facilities to treat complex problems. Voluntary (nonprofit) hospitals may give more personal care for the money but may lack extensive facilities. Teaching hospitals—those affiliated with medical schools—generally have expert medical staffs and the latest technology. City or county and Veterans Affairs hospitals have the advantages of teaching hospitals at a lower cost but are likely to be overcrowded.

Check the nurse-to-patient ratio (1-to-8 is good). The local nurses' association may know the turnover rate for nurses; a stable staff suggests a well-run facility.

EASING HOSPITAL ADMISSION

Once a hospital stay is scheduled, you may be asked to fill out insurance forms a few days ahead in what is called advance admission. Some diagnostic tests may also be scheduled during the week before you are admitted.

Pack lightly for a hospital stay. You will need proof of insurance if you have not registered in advance, a list of your medications, basic toiletries, a bathrobe and nightgown or pajamas, slippers, your reading glasses and reading material, a notepad and pencil, and a few dollars for incidentals like newspapers. Leave valuables such as rings at home.

THE IMPORTANCE OF AN ADVOCATE

Having a friend or relative act as your advocate while you are sick relieves you of worry about dealing with doctors and other hospital personnel. In the absence of such an advocate, you can enlist the hospital's patient representative, or ombudsman, to resolve problems that come up.

The more responsibility you and your advocate can take for your care while you are hospitalized, the better you will fare.

You—or your advocate—should understand your treatment program and know exactly which tests, procedures, and medications your doctor has prescribed for you and why. Be sure you are given those that are listed on your chart; reject those you have not been told about. If a pill you normally take doesn't look familiar, don't take it until you have seen the bottle. Mistakes do happen.

You or your advocate should also make sure that the meals you receive conform to any special diet you require. (If the food is what the doctor ordered, eat as much as you can; poor nutrition can slow recovery.)

GETTING READY FOR SURGERY

Before you undergo surgery, you can relieve some of your anxiety by learning about the procedure. Ask your surgeon such questions as these: Exactly what will be done? How long will it take? How long is the recovery period? Who will actually perform the operation, you or an assistant? If I will need blood transfusions, can I donate my own blood in advance to avoid the possibility of contamination or incompatibility?

Ask about the pain you can expect after the operation and how it will be controlled. Also ask if you will be given a self-administered painkiller (see photos, facing page) or if you will need to call a nurse. Studies have shown that recovery is faster if analgesics are given before pain becomes severe, but in some situations,

WHO'S WHO IN THE HOSPITAL

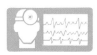 MEDICAL STAFF

Attending physician. The doctor—primary physician or surgeon—in charge of your care at the hospital.

Consulting physician. A specialist called in by your doctor for a procedure, special tests, or an opinion.

Fellow. A doctor who has finished a residency (below) and is pursuing a specialty.

Resident. A staff doctor who is taking advanced training after completing medical school. A resident gives medical help under the supervision of an attending physician or surgeon. Most residents serve 2 or 3 years.

Medical student. After the first year of medical school, students may draw blood or do other simple tasks but not more complex procedures.

 NURSING CARE

Nurse. A registered nurse (RN) has had 2 or more years of theoretical and practical training. A nurse can monitor your temperature, blood pressure, and other vital signs, give medications, set up intravenous lines, and relay questions about your illness to your doctor. A licensed practical or vocational nurse (LPN or LVN) has less technical training but has passed a state licensing examination. LPN's and LVN's are supervised by doctors or RN's. RN's who have more advanced training work as clinical specialists such as midwives or nurse anesthetists.

Nurses' aide, orderly, and attendant. Hospital employees who help with custodial tasks such as bathing, feeding, and lifting patients.

 SUPPORT STAFF

Medical social worker. An MSW helps patients work out medical financing and arranges for any post-hospital health-care services prescribed by the doctors. An MSW can also offer psychological counseling.

Medical technologist. A person trained to administer laboratory or diagnostic tests.

Patient representative. A hospital employee (or volunteer) who handles patient complaints and helps resolve patient-staff problems.

Therapist. A specialist in rehabilitative training. Physical and occupational therapists help patients regain strength and flexibility. Speech therapists teach patients to communicate again after a stroke or other injury.

---

doctors feel self-administered drugs are inappropriate.

The better drugs and safer procedures that have been developed for anesthesia in recent years make putting you to sleep less risky than it once was. Before surgery, the anesthesiologist should interview you about your medical history and any sensitivities you have to anesthetics or other medications. The doctor may also order tests before choosing the safest drug for you.

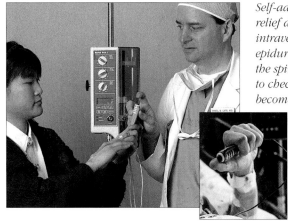

Self-administering pain-relief drugs through an intravenous line or an epidural catheter into the spine allows a patient to check pain before it becomes debilitating.

Such pain control often requires less of the analgesic than the doctor might otherwise have prescribed.

WHAT TO EXPECT BEFORE AND AFTER THE OPERATION

You will be asked not to eat or drink for 8 to 10 hours before surgery to avert the chance of your vomiting and choking. The area of the incision will be shaved and cleansed to prevent infection. An intravenous line will be inserted in a vein for administering medication and fluids and you will probably be given a sedative before going to the operating room.

A local anesthetic may be injected into skin or tissue to numb a limited area. A regional anesthetic is injected into the spine or other nerve area to block sensation in a larger part of your body. General anesthesia involves two steps—first an injection, which puts you to sleep, and then additional anesthesia is given through the IV line or pumped directly into your lungs through a tube in your throat.

After surgery, your vital signs will be monitored in the recovery room while you regain consciousness. If you had general anesthesia, you may feel nauseated and your throat may be sore from the breathing tube. Nurses will encourage you to breathe deeply (to clear out your lungs), change your position often (moving prevents bedsores), and walk (physical activity helps speed recovery).

ADVANCE DIRECTIVES FOR MEDICAL EMERGENCIES

Trauma victims and their families can be hurt as much by lack of forethought as by accidents. Without directives, doctors in a trauma center must try to save the threatened life at all costs.

Publicity about comatose patients kept alive artificially with no hope of recovery has led many people to sign living wills to protect themselves and their families from such a tragedy. These documents, however, are more often honored for terminally ill patients than for physically strong people who become severely brain-damaged.

A living will alone can be hard to interpret: The terms are vague because you can't know the exact procedures that will be involved in a future crisis. Without specific instructions, many doctors—respectful of life or fearful of lawsuits—hesitate to limit care.

Appointing a proxy to talk to the doctor through a "durable power of attorney for health care" is a solution. You legally designate a friend or relative to make health decisions for you if you are unable to do so. Doctors can then discuss choices with your surrogate as they would with you.

Talk out your feelings about what makes life meaningful with the person you choose as your proxy. Life and death issues call for serious reflection. Ponder your religious beliefs. Putting your thoughts on paper will clarify them and leave clearer evidence of your wishes if they are ever in dispute.

Some states have special forms for preparing advance directives and appointing health care proxies. Forms for each of the 50 states are also available from Choice for Dying (p.213). You may want to discuss the wording with your lawyer. Give copies of any documents you sign to your doctor and your proxy. Carry a card in your wallet that indicates that you have such documents.

A PATIENT'S BILL OF RIGHTS

First approved voluntarily by the American Hospital Association in 1973, the patient entitlements spelled out below are now legal rights in some states.

■ You are entitled to considerate and respectful care.

■ You have a right to privacy. No unidentified person should be present while you are examined. Your records are confidential.

■ You should not face discrimination because of race, color, religion, sex, national origin, or the source of your medical payments.

■ You have the right to know the names and duties of all the medical personnel who care for you.

■ You are entitled to a clear explanation of your diagnosis, the recommended treatment and any alternatives, and the likely outcome.

■ You have the right to refuse any treatment.

■ You are entitled to criticize hospital practices without fear of reprisal.

■ You may leave the hospital at will after signing a release. You can't be discharged, however, without some warning.

■ You have a right to continuing care after you leave the hospital and assistance in arranging for it as well as for medical follow-up.

■ You are entitled to see your bill and to receive an explanation of any part of it, no matter who is paying.

WHAT'S WHAT IN THE INTENSIVE CARE UNIT

During a serious illness or after a major operation, you may be placed in the intensive care unit (ICU), where your condition can be continuously monitored and emergency measures can be speedily implemented if they are needed. As intimidating as ICU machines may look, few are actually invasive, and together they can—and quite frequently do—save lives.

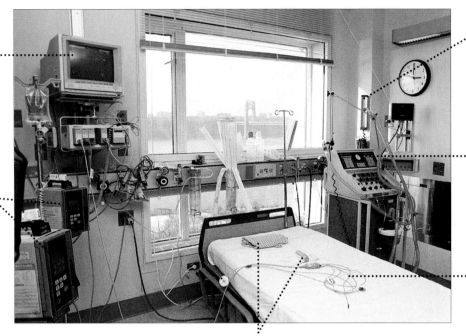

A large TV-like monitor gives a constant reading on the status of the heart.

Special equipment measures precise amounts of drugs, fluids, and painkillers to be delivered intravenously.

Blood pressure monitoring equipment

A ventilator pumps oxygen into a patient's lungs to stabilize breathing after a trauma.

Electrodes and leads, attached to appropriate parts of the body, monitor the heart, the lungs, or the brain.

Suction apparatus and irrigation solutions stand on the window shelf. An oxygen pressure gauge and a code button for alerting emergency crews are beneath the shelf.

A clean hospital gown and a bag of intravenous fluid await a patient on a hospital bed, which can be raised or lowered to facilitate the person's care.

EMERGENCY FACILITIES

Hospital emergency rooms and trauma centers deal with crises that cannot wait for a doctor's appointment—heart attacks, broken bones, head or eye injuries, and burns, for example.

If you are in a serious accident or have a potentially life-threatening symptom such as severe chest pain, you will be taken by ambulance to the closest available emergency facility. If you call a private ambulance or can provide your own transportation, you may have a choice.

Check out nearby emergency services before you have to use one. Look for an emergency room with "full basic" service, which means a doctor is on duty 24 hours a day, or a trauma center, which keeps a doctor and a surgical team on duty around the clock.

Walk-in clinics and surgical centers, often located in shopping areas, are another option for urgent care (when the problem is serious but not life-threatening). Such facilities may be independent businesses or extensions of a hospital. To check a clinic's credentials, write to the Accreditation Association for Ambulatory Health Care, 9933 Lawler Ave., Skokie, IL 60077.

Paying for Medical Care

S oaring health care costs have made a serious illness the greatest financial threat to most Americans. Everyone needs medical insurance; even people entitled to government policies may need a supplementary plan.

HEALTH INSURANCE

The entire healthcare delivery system and insurance industry are in a state of flux, with both state and federal governments looking for ways to lower costs and ensure universal coverage. In the meantime, there are myriad insurance and third-party payment programs. The federal Medicare program provides basic insurance for people over the age of 65. Medicaid covers the poor, although regulations vary from state to state. If you do not qualify for these government programs, you need one of three general types of medical coverage—a fee-for-service plan, a health maintenance organization (HMO), or a preferred provider organization (PPO). Group coverage is less costly than individual policies; you are wise to participate in a plan offered by your employer, union, or other affiliated group.

Traditional fee-for-service plans, usually the most costly, allow you to choose your doctors and hospitals. Coverage varies widely; some cover only hospital expenses, others pay all hospital expenses plus up to 80 percent of all doctors' fees, medical services, and drugs after a yearly deductible of $150 to $500 or more. Many do not cover checkups and limit reimbursement for specific procedures to a figure that is "usual, customary, and reasonable" in the area. If your doctor's fees are above the limit, you pay the difference.

HMO's offer prepaid medical services through their affiliated doctors and hospitals. Usually less expensive than fee-for-service plans, HMO's generally charge an annual fee plus $5 to $10 per doctor visit with no deductible, and cover all or most medical and surgical expenses.

Preferred provider organizations are hybrids and cost somewhat more than HMO's but usually less than fee-for-service plans. Like HMO's, PPO's offer a roster of participating doctors and hospitals who follow the PPO's rate schedule (in return for patient referrals). If you elect to go to other doctors or facilities, the PPO pays its rate and you must pay the difference.

CUTTING MEDICAL COSTS

Even with medical insurance, treatment can be financially draining. There are ways to curb expenses, however.

Discuss the cost of each procedure with your doctor ahead of time. You have a right to know the price and to negotiate. Ask your doctor to accept the Medicare or insurance company "reasonable fee" allowance.

Question the necessity of tests. Doctors and hospitals, concerned about malpractice suits, often try to cover themselves with a battery of tests that may be of questionable value in your case.

Ask about alternatives to surgery before you agree to an operation. What would happen if you waited to see if you really needed it? Can the procedure be done as an outpatient? Could drugs or lifestyle changes possibly make the operation unnecessary?

Check whether your insurance covers prescription drugs. Ask your doctor if there is an accept-

---

MEETING LONG-TERM MEDICAL COSTS

Medicare payments for nursing home stays and in-home custodial care are limited to 100 days per diagnosis and only a percentage of the cost. Medicaid covers both types of care for people with very low incomes. If you are not eligible for Medicaid, you may want to look into private insurance for long-term care. Shop carefully; these policies are not uniform and many have severe limitations. When comparing long-term care policies, be sure to ask the following questions:

- Is there a waiting period before the policy goes into effect?
- Will you be covered if you enter a nursing home directly from home rather than from a hospital?
- Will the policy cover you even if you haven't had skilled care in a nursing home?
- How much is the deductible that you must pay?
- How much will the policy pay for each day of care?
- Will your benefits go up with inflation?
- Will you receive benefits for only a limited time or for life?
- How does the policy treat pre-existing conditions?
- Is renewal of the policy guaranteed? Will the premium rise?

---

able generic version of a drug or a less expensive alternative that is equally effective. If you take the drug for a chronic condition, buy it in bulk. For costly medications that you will be taking long-term, consider buying through a reputable discount mail order vendor.

When you must be hospitalized, insist on an itemized bill and check it carefully (95 percent of all hospital bills contain errors).

GETTING GOVERNMENT HELP

Medicare is the federal health insurance plan for Americans aged 65 or older. If you are eligible for Social Security or Railroad Retirement benefits, you are eligible for Medicare. (Some younger people with disabilities or chronic kidney disease also qualify.) To sign up for Medicare, contact your local Social Security office a month or

two before your 65th birthday.

Medicare has two parts—hospital insurance (Part A) and medical insurance (Part B). Part A covers hospital stays and short-term follow-up care in a nursing facility or at home. Part A also pays for hospice care for the terminally ill at home or in an approved facility. You pay nothing for Part A insurance, but you must satisfy a yearly deductible before you receive benefits.

Part B, for which you are charged a monthly premium, pays 80 percent of "reasonable" bills for doctors, outpatient hospital and laboratory work, medical equipment, medical therapy, and some home health care. To supplement Medicare Part B insurance, which has a number of restrictions, you can buy one of 10 federally mandated private health care policies known as medigap insurance.

Making the Most of Medical Tests

Routine physicals for healthy people include screening tests, which can often spot diseases at an early, curable stage before any symptoms are noticeable. More extensive diagnostic tests and procedures are used to help identify the causes of symptoms and then monitor the course of treatment.

IS THIS TEST NECESSARY?

Medical tests can be expensive, both in time and in money. Be sure that any test your doctor prescribes is really needed and that you understand why. A screening test should help your doctor identify a treatable disease or rule out one for which you are at risk either from exposure or because of your family medical history.

Conscientious physicians consider three criteria before ordering a test: the value of the specific information it may give about you, the discomfort it will cause, and the risks it entails. The importance of the knowledge to be gained through the test should outweigh any potential harm.

In diagnosing a disease, doctors usually start with the least invasive and less costly tests. if you have occasional bouts of chest pain, for example, a doctor will do an electrocardiogram and other noninvasive studies, reserving cardiac catheterization as a more advanced test.

PREPARING FOR TESTS

Once you agree to a battery of medical tests, you can make the experience more pleasant and the results more useful if you are relaxed during the procedures. Blood pressure, for example, is often raised by anxiety about having it measured.

If you know what to expect and how long the procedure will take beforehand, you will be more at ease. You can get that information from your doctor, the assistant who sets up the appointment, or your public library.

Make appointments for lengthy procedures on a day when you have plenty of time and won't become irritated if the doctors or technicians involved run late (they often do). Bring a book or a magazine so that you won't feel waiting time is wasted.

Carefully follow the instructions for pretest preparation, such as fasting overnight or avoiding certain foods for 48 hours. If you have questions, call your doctor.

FREQUENCY

There are no hard-and-fast rules that are appropriate for everyone about how often screening tests should be repeated. Your doctor will make recommendations for you based on your health, your family medical history, and environmental factors (such as living with a smoker or working with dangerous chemicals). The American Cancer Society, the American Heart Association, and other health groups make general recommendations about some tests.

HOME MEDICAL CHECKS

Devices for home monitoring of medical conditions are a great convenience—if they are used under a doctor's supervision. Several types of machines measure blood pressure and pulse. For diabetics, an electronic meter quickly analyzes a drop of blood for glucose levels. A less expensive version uses a chemically treated strip that reacts to glucose by changing color.

Home tests to detect urinary tract infections in urine and occult (hidden) blood in the stool have been approved by the Food and Drug Administration, as has a new one to measure cholesterol levels. These tests are similar to those used by doctors, but you should consult your doctor to make sure that you are interpreting the results correctly.

TESTS YOU CAN DO YOURSELF

Tests that you perform at home can be valuable in detecting several types of cancer. More than half of all malignant breast tumors, for example, are discovered by women themselves. Doctors recommend examining your breasts once a month so that you will notice any changes in their

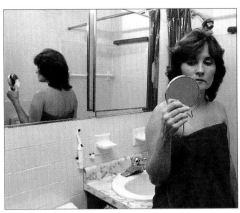

feel or appearance. Report any new lumps or other abnormalities to your doctor. Most breast lumps are benign, but early diagnosis of a cancer could save your life.

For men, self-examination of the testicles can also be life-saving and takes only 1 or 2 minutes a month. Any lumps or other irregularities you find are probably benign but should be seen by a doctor. Testicular cancer is rare after age 35 but can appear at any age. Diagnosed early, it is almost always curable.

TO EXAMINE YOUR BODY FOR SKIN CANCER

1. Using your fingers, feel for lumps, thickened skin, or scabs from your scalp down to your toes.
2. Stand in good light near a mirror and inspect directly or by reflection any suspicious spots. Use a hand mirror as shown to examine inaccessible body areas like your back.

Both men and women should thoroughly examine their entire bodies monthly for skin cancer (above). Look for changes in the color, size, or shape of moles or birthmarks; new rough, scaly areas; or sores that have oozed or bled for more than a week. Caught early enough, many skin cancers (p.265) can safely be removed in a doctor's office.

TO EXAMINE YOUR BREASTS

1. Stand facing a mirror, arms at your sides, and study both breasts for puckering, dimpling, or scaling. Raise both arms and look for changes in the shape of your breasts. Next, press your hands firmly on your hips, lean slightly forward, and tense your shoulder and arm muscles. Again, look for any changes. Check side views as well.
2. Raise your right arm (right). Use the middle fingers of your left hand to firmly feel the right breast for lumps or thickened tissue. Work in a circle from the outside inward as shown. Reverse arm positions and examine the left breast in the same fashion. (Note: This step can be done while showering. Wet, soapy breasts are easier to examine than when the skin is dry.)
3. As a final check, lie down with a pillow under your right shoulder. Raise your right arm and explore the right breast area with the fingers of the left hand. Reverse sides and check the other breast.

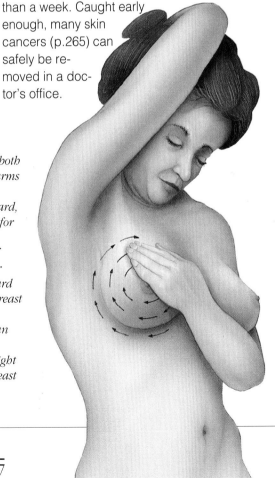

CHECKING OUT A LAB

Before undergoing any medical tests that involve laboratory work, ask about the credentials of the facility your doctor uses. Sloppy lab work can give you misleading results, causing needless worry or a false sense of security.

A good lab is accredited by the College of American Pathologists or the American Society of Cytology, licensed by a state agency, or certified by the U.S. Department of Health and Human Services. Federal legislation to improve quality standards in laboratories should eventually result in federally certified laboratories throughout the United States. Certain states, including California, Connecticut, Florida, Illinois, Maryland, New York, and Pennsylvania, already have strict licensing requirements.

Be wary of doctors who refer you to labs in which they have a financial interest; their choice may be dictated by a desire for gain. This is also prohibited by Medicare and some state laws.

FALLIBILITY OF TESTS

Doctors know that all screening tests are not equally reliable. For example, studies show that 15 to 40 percent of middle-aged men have positive exercise stress tests, but do not have heart disease. An abnormal Pap smear doesn't mean that a woman has cervical cancer—it alerts her doctor to do further testing. So-called false-positive test results—indications of disease in well people—have many causes: the testing equipment or technician may be at fault, or the patient may not have followed instructions. Always discuss test results with your doctor.

TYPES OF SCREENING TESTS

Test	Purpose
Blood chemistry tests	To analyze chemicals in the blood such as sodium, potassium, glucose, bilirubin (related to liver function), and creatinine (related to kidney function).
Blood pressure	To detect high blood pressure (hypertension) or low blood pressure, a cause of dizziness or fainting.
Chest X-rays	Once used routinely to screen for tuberculosis and lung cancer, chest X-rays are now recommended as diagnostic tools to explore symptoms of respiratory diseases (such as persistent cough or chest pain).
Cholesterol count	First, to measure the total cholesterol level in the blood and, second, to measure triglyceride, or fat, and the different kinds of cholesterol (high-density lipoproteins, or HDL's, and low-density lipoproteins, or LDL's) in the blood and their ratio to each other.
Complete blood count (CBC)	To measure the various components (red blood cells, white blood cells, and platelets) present in a given volume of blood.
Electrocardiograms (ECG's or EKG's)	A resting ECG detects abnormal heart rhythm and evaluates symptoms of heart disease. An exercise ECG, or stress test, determines whether you have coronary artery disease and indicates your safest maximum heart rate for exercise (see p.97, p.101).
Fecal occult blood test	To detect traces of occult (hidden) blood in the stool, which may signal a number of disorders, including colon cancer, which is most curable in its early stages.
Mammogram	To detect breast cancer in women. Mammograms can detect cancers of microscopic size, long before they can be felt manually, at a time when they can often be removed without disfiguring surgery.
Pap test or smear	To detect cervical cancer at an early stage when the disease is readily curable.
Purified Protein Derivative (PPD)	To test for a tuberculosis (TB) infection.
Sigmoidoscopy	To check the interior of the lower gastrointestinal tract (sigmoid colon, rectum, and anus) for tumors, polyps, inflammation, hemorrhoids, and other bowel diseases. Sigmoidoscopy is also used to remove small polyps and to take tissue samples for biopsy.
Urinalysis	To check the health of your kidneys and bladder and to screen for such conditions as diabetes, kidney disease, and urinary tract infections.

Procedure	Frequency
Blood is taken from a vein, usually in the arm, for analysis by a machine.	At your doctor's discretion.
A cuff placed around your upper arm is inflated and then released to measure the force of the blood pumped through your arteries. In a reading (such as 120/80), the first number is systolic pressure, recorded when your heart is pumping, and the second number is diastolic pressure, recorded between heartbeats when the heart is resting.	Every 2 years if your reading is normal; at your doctor's discretion if it is not.
Jewelry and clothing above the waist must be removed. Standing, you will be positioned against a film holder with your arms out of the way for one or two views. You hold a deep breath while the film is exposed.	At your doctor's discretion.
Blood is taken from a vein, usually in the arm. For a triglyceride and HDL count, you must fast (but you can drink water) for 12 hours (from dinner for an early appointment the next morning) before the blood is drawn.	Every 5 years if your cholesterol level is less than 200; otherwise, at your doctor's discretion.
Blood is taken from a vein, usually in the arm, for analysis by a machine.	At your doctor's discretion.
For a resting ECG, you usually wear a hospital gown and lie on your back on a bed or table. Electrodes are taped to your chest, arms, and legs. While you lie quietly, a recorder traces your heart's electrical activity on a screen or strip of paper.	At your doctor's discretion.
A small stool sample, taken by the doctor during a rectal exam or collected yourself, is treated with a chemical that turns blue in the presence of blood. For 2 days before the test, avoid red meat, turnips, radishes, horseradish, vitamin C and iron supplements, and aspirin, which may affect the results.	Annually after age 50; at your doctor's discretion before age 50.
A mammogram is an X-ray that requires a specially trained technician. Choose an accredited facility (facing page). You must remove all clothing above the waist for the X-ray. Each breast is then gently compressed against a plate while several pictures are taken from different angles.	The American Cancer Society suggests a baseline mammogram between ages 35 and 39, a mammogram every 2 years between ages 40 and 49, and an annual mammogram from age 50 on.
Usually done by a gynecologist or an internist as part of a woman's pelvic examination; the test involves taking a sample of cells from the cervix (the neck of the uterus) and sending it to a lab where it is examined under a microscope for the presence of cancerous or potentially cancerous cells.	The American Cancer Society urges a Pap test every 2 or 3 years for all adult women (and more often for those with high risk of cancer).
A small quantity of purified protein from tuberculosis bacteria is injected into the skin. If you have active or dormant TB, or have been exposed to the bacterium in the past, redness and swelling will develop in the next 48 hours.	At your doctor's discretion.
A thin flexible tube containing light-carrying fiber-optic bundles is inserted into the rectum and 10–12 inches up the lower part of the colon. Light beamed through the tube illuminates the area and allows images to be transmitted back to a lens, which can focus and magnify them. The procedure, which is done in a doctor's office, may be uncomfortable but is not usually painful.	The American Cancer Society recommends that you have a first and second sigmoidoscopy at ages 50 and 51. If both are negative, you should have subsequent tests every 3–5 years.
A urine specimen is tested with chemically treated dipsticks in the doctor's office. The doctor can also send a urine specimen to a laboratory for additional and more–complex analysis.	At your doctor's discretion.

USING DRUGS WISELY

rugs can halt the spread of infections, eliminate pain, and help you to live a healthier life. By learning to use medications wisely, you can enjoy their benefits while minimizing their potential problems.

TYPES OF DRUGS AND WHAT THEY DO

Drugs are divided into groups according to how they work.

Drugs for infections

■ *Antibiotics* either kill bacteria or inhibit their growth so that the body's defenses destroy them.
■ *Vaccines, antiserums, and immune globulins* prevent infectious diseases. Vaccines cause the body to produce antibodies against diseases like polio and measles, thus making it immune to them. Antiserums and globulins contain the antibodies themselves; an unvaccinated person exposed to tetanus or rabies would be treated with them.

Cardiovascular drugs

■ *Antianginals* relieve the chest pain (angina) caused when the heart muscle does not get enough oxygen. Some work by opening (dilating) small blood vessels; others cause the heart to beat slower or less forcefully.
■ *Antiarrhythmics* regulate an irregular or too fast heartbeat.
■ *Antihypertensives* treat hypertension (high blood pressure). Diuretics lower blood volume by helping eliminate water and salt. Other drugs block nerve impulses that constrict small arteries; still other antihypertensives work through the brain, kidneys, or muscles, or act on the heart.
■ *Digitalis* drugs strengthen and slow down the heartbeat.

Drugs that affect the nervous system

■ *Analgesics* relieve pain. Non-narcotic ones such as aspirin are effective for mild pain, and some also reduce inflammation. They do not affect consciousness, as the narcotic analgesics used for severe pain can. Narcotics also are addictive.
■ *Anesthetics* eliminate sensation. A general anesthetic causes unconsciousness; a local deadens feeling only in the part of the body to which it is applied.
■ *Anti-anxiety drugs,* or tranquilizers, have a calming effect by slowing brain activity.
■ *Antidepressant drugs* increase the levels of mood-elevating brain chemicals.
■ *Hallucinogens,* or psychedelic drugs, distort the senses.
■ *Stimulants* increase nervous system activity, thereby increasing alertness. Some, such as amphetamines, can be addicting.

HOW A DRUG PASSES THROUGH YOUR BODY

To produce its benefits, a drug must be absorbed into the bloodstream. Medications taken orally are processed by the stomach and intestines, which may reduce their assimilation. Some drugs are injected directly into the bloodstream; others are inhaled. With skin patches, the drug passes slowly into the bloodstream through the skin. Other methods for delivering drugs over time include surgically implanted pellets, mini-pumps, and slow-release tablets and capsules. Suppositories are given to people who can't take drugs orally. They are also used for drugs that might irritate the stomach or that might be destroyed by the stomach's acids or enzymes.

Once the drug is in the bloodstream, it is distributed throughout the body. Drug metabolism —the drug's breakdown into other chemicals—usually occurs in the liver. Some drugs become active only after being metabolized by the liver. Although metabolized drugs are eliminated mostly in the urine, they are also excreted in tears, sweat, saliva, solid waste, and exhaled breath.

PROBLEMS WITH DRUGS AS YOU GROW OLDER

The percentage of fat in your body typically increases as you grow older, while that of muscle and water decreases. Drugs stored in fat tissues can accumulate to levels higher than may be safe. These drugs also may stay in your body longer than is desirable because the liver and kidneys take more time to break down and eliminate them. For these reasons, it's a good idea to

> **"*Almost everyone takes them.... It is an age of pills.*"**
>
> *British humorist*
> *Malcolm Muggeridge*
> *(1903-1990)*

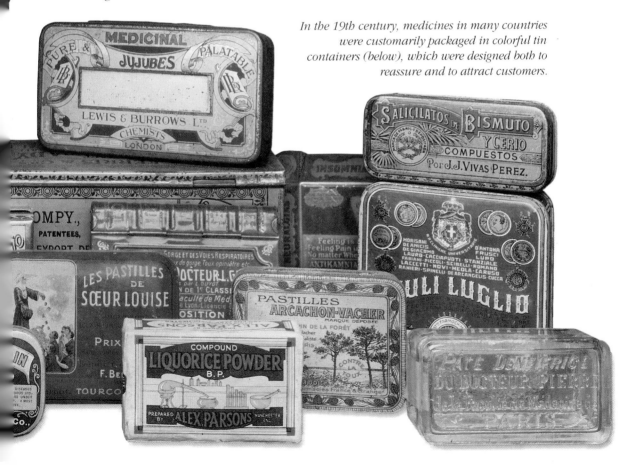

In the 19th century, medicines in many countries were customarily packaged in colorful tin containers (below), which were designed both to reassure and to attract customers.

ask your doctor if your medication should be adjusted.

Because older people are likely to have multiple ailments, they are also likely to be taking more than one drug. This sets up the possibility of a dangerous drug interaction, especially if more than one doctor is prescribing medication. Prevent this by showing your doctor a log of all the drugs you are taking (including any over-the-counter drugs and vitamins), indicating how long you've been taking them and why, before he prescribes any new drug.

Finally, because most drugs have been tested only on younger people, a "normal" adult dose can often turn out to be too high a dose for an older person— although sometimes it is too little. Occasionally older people have the opposite reaction to a drug that a younger person has. To remedy this problem, the Food and Drug Administration (FDA) now requires all drugs to be tested on the population group that will be using them.

Regardless of your age, you may be able to eliminate some drugs or reduce dosages through lifestyle changes. An evening walk and a glass of warm milk, for example, may take the place of sleeping pills. If you think that this could work for you, continue to take your medication, but talk to your doctor about possible alternatives.

DRUG ALLERGIES

Almost any drug can cause an allergic reaction in sensitive people. Usually this is not serious, but occasionally individuals may experience more dangerous reactions: severe asthma, swelling of the throat, or anaphylaxis. The symptoms of anaphylaxis can range from widespread hives and intense itching to difficulty in breathing and shock. The condition requires immediate medical treatment. If you are allergic to a drug, make sure that you always wear an alert necklace or bracelet.

When you tell your doctor about any drug allergies, also mention substances to which you are allergic, since drugs often contain colorings, preservatives, binders, or alcohol in addition to the medicine.

ADVERSE DRUG INTERACTIONS

Whenever your doctor prescribes a new medication, ask what drugs or foods, if any, you should avoid during the time you are taking it.

Medications can sometimes produce adverse reactions when they are combined with other prescription or nonprescription drugs. Tranquilizers taken with nonprescription antihistamines, for example, can cause extreme drowsiness. Taking a nonprescription indigestion remedy can make iron pills being taken for anemia ineffective.

Some foods can also have adverse interactions with drugs. The therapeutic effect of anticoagulant drugs (blood thinners), for example, can be partially neutralized if you eat foods that contain large amounts of vitamin K, such as broccoli and liver. When taken with alcoholic beverages, some drugs that are used to treat heartburn can greatly exaggerate the effects of the alcohol. Even something as benign as natural licorice can cause problems if you are taking a medication for high blood pressure.

YOUR ANNUAL BROWN BAG REVIEW

At least once a year when you visit your primary care doctor, or whenever you visit a new doctor, bring with you all the prescription and nonprescription medications you are taking or have taken in the last month. This is a good way to check for such problems as the following:

■ *Duplication.* People seeing several doctors sometimes inadvertently take the same drug under more than one name.
■ *Side effects,* allergies, and adverse drug interactions.
■ *Improper use.*
■ *Medications that have expired* or that you no longer need to take.

PROBLEMS WITH SIDE EFFECTS

Prescription drugs often come with a daunting list of possible side effects, but most of them rarely occur, and if they do, they are usually mild and short-lived. Common ones include drowsiness, diarrhea, nausea, headache, and skin rash. If you experience any of these or anything else unusual, ask your doctor if your dose should be lowered or if another drug should be substituted.

ABUSE OF LEGAL DRUGS

Drug abuse involves not just illegal drugs but also the misuse of legal prescription and nonprescription drugs.

If taken for too long, some drugs can cause dependence or addiction. With dependence, the person needs larger and larger doses to achieve the desired effect; with addiction, the user becomes both physically and psychologically reliant on the drug and cannot stop taking it without unpleasant and sometimes dangerous withdrawal symptoms.

Treatment usually involves a slow, safe withdrawal under medical supervision. This is especially important with tranquilizer abuse, since withdrawal symptoms can include anxiety, nausea, appetite loss, sleeping difficulty, blurred vision, trembling, twitching, muscle pain, and, in severe cases, delirium or convulsion. The symptoms of tranquilizer abuse itself include drowsiness, slurred speech, lack of coordination, impaired memory, confusion, trembling, agitation, and paranoia.

For chronic pain sufferers, alternatives to potentially addictive narcotics include relaxation techniques, acupuncture, psychotherapy, and biofeedback.

If you think that you are addicted, your doctor can recommend a specialist in addiction problems, or you can call a local mental health clinic. Support groups can aid in preventing a relapse. If you think someone you know is misusing a drug, talk to him about it. Offer to sit down with him and make a list of all his medications, then go to the doctor with him to discuss the problem. Find out about available local help and tell him about it.

FAST FACTS

■ The urge to sleep in the middle of the day appears to be natural. Experiments have shown that people's alertness and ability to perform tasks drop during the midafternoon whether or not lunch has been eaten.

■ Some legal substances can give false-positive results in drug tests—cough syrups can read as opiates, herbal teas as cocaine, diet pills and decongestants as amphetamines.

■ To stop persistent hiccups, try rubbing the roof of your mouth with a cotton swab in the area where the palate changes from hard to soft.

■ The thermometer doesn't have to read 98.6° F for you to have a normal temperature. A recent study shows that a "normal" temperature can range from 96° to 99.9°, with a mean of 98.2°.

■ Nicotine news: Wearing a nicotine patch and smoking can put you at risk of a heart attack. Drinking coffee when you chew nicotine gum will block absorption of the nicotine.

■ Many drugs can cause a dry mouth, among them antihistamines, decongestants, antidepressants, and antihypertensives.

HOW TO READ A PRESCRIPTION

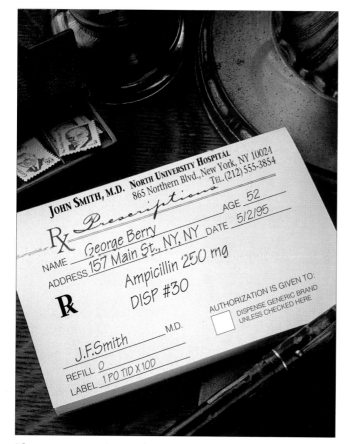

The following are some of the abbreviations that doctors use when writing prescriptions.

ABBREVIATION	MEANING
AA	OF EACH
AC	BEFORE MEALS
AM	MORNING
BID	TWICE A DAY
C	WITH
CAP	CAPSULE
CC	CUBIC CENTIMETER
D	DAYS
DISP	DISPENSE
GT	DROP
GTT	DROPS
H	HOUR
HS	AT BEDTIME
ML	MILLILITER
OD	RIGHT EYE
OS	LEFT EYE
PC	AFTER MEALS
PM	EVENING
PO	BY MOUTH
PRN	AS NEEDED
Q	EVERY
QD	ONCE A DAY, EVERY DAY
QID	FOUR TIMES A DAY
S̄	WITHOUT
SIG	LABEL AS FOLLOWS
STAT	AT ONCE; FIRST DOSE
TAB	TABLET
TID	THREE TIMES A DAY
X	TIMES

The prescription above is for 30 pills of ampicillin in a strength of 250 mg (ampicillin 250 mg DISP # 30). One pill is to be taken by mouth three times a day for 10 days (1 PO TID X 10D). Ampicillin is an antibiotic prescribed for such ailments as earaches, sinus infections, and other bacterial infections.

BRAND-NAME DRUGS VERSUS GENERIC DRUGS

A company that creates a new drug has a patent on it; after the patent expires, anyone can make the drug as long as the "copy" has the same amount of the active ingredient as the patented drug. Such copies are called generics, and they cost less, often much less, than their brand-name counterparts. The basic difference is cosmetic: generics are not permitted to look like the brand-name drug. Although it is unusual, problems can develop because the coloring agents and fillers used in the generic drug may differ from the patented drug, and these may alter the drug's metabolizing time or cause side effects. For example, a lactose-intolerant person may be adversely affected by changing from a patented drug with little or no lactose filler to a generic with a lot. Always consult your doctor about the right drug for you, whether it is a brand name or a generic.

THE BENEFITS OF A GOOD PHARMACIST

A good pharmacist acts as a check on physicians, to make sure they have prescribed the correct drug at the proper dosage. He can also help you select nonprescription drugs that are the most appropriate for you.

Your pharmacist should keep a record of all your prescription and nonprescription drugs, as well as any food and drug allergies you may suffer from. Have all your prescriptions filled at the same pharmacy so that your pharmacist will be able to advise you of any potential problems with drug interactions.

It's a good idea to shop around for a pharmacist, especially if you take medication regularly. You can compare prices by telephone; also be sure to ask about home delivery, charge accounts, and senior citizens' discounts.

. . . .

BUYING DRUGS BY MAIL

Mail order drug suppliers often offer big discounts as well as convenience for people who need to keep taking medication over a long period of time. After you enroll in a program, you can call in your prescription on a toll-free number. Your order is confirmed by phone with your doctor, then mailed to you.

If you are interested in trying this service, remember to add the handling and shipping charges to your drug costs to see how big your savings really are.

One disadvantage of mail order drugs is that several days elapse before your prescription arrives. Another is that the suppliers cannot offer the personal service that a good pharmacist can.

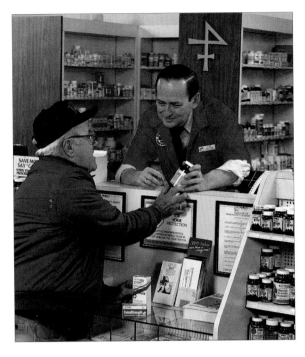

Your pharmacist can help you with a variety of problems, from advising you of your prescription's side effects to making sure your medicine has an easy-to-open cap.

USING OVER-THE-COUNTER DRUGS SAFELY

While most nonprescription drugs are safe to use and effective in relieving symptoms, all have potential side effects, and all of them can have serious consequences if misused.

Read the label carefully even if you've used the drug before; manufacturers occasionally change the strength of their products. If you are confused, ask your pharmacist to advise you. The following are some common warnings:

▪ ***Who should avoid this drug.*** Use may not be advisable for people over or under a certain age or for those with heart disease, high blood pressure, diabetes, asthma, or glaucoma.

▪ ***Do not drive or operate heavy machinery.*** Antihistamines can cause drowsiness and slow reaction time.

▪ ***Do not drink alcohol.*** When mixed with alcohol, some medications for allergies, colds, and insomnia cause extreme sleepiness or even difficulty breathing. Sometimes alcohol can neutralize the beneficial effect of a drug.

▪ ***Side effects and drug interactions.*** While few people suffer the side effects listed, if you are one of them, stop taking the drug at once and call your doctor.

▪ ***Foods or other drugs that should be avoided.*** Aspirin, for example, should not be taken with acidic foods, vitamin C, or alcohol. Check with your doctor or pharmacist if you are already taking a medication.

▪ ***If symptoms persist, consult your doctor.*** Your problem may require a doctor's care, or you may have used the medicine for too long. The labels on nasal decongestants, for example, advise against using them longer than 3 days because after that they can actually cause congestion.

USING DRUGS SAFELY AND EFFECTIVELY

 Store your medications in a dry place at room temperature and away from sunlight so that they won't deteriorate and become ineffective or toxic. The bathroom medicine cabinet, because it is humid, may be the worst place to store drugs. Some drugs need refrigeration, but be careful never to freeze them.

 Keep medicines in the original containers with their original labels. Don't put two different drugs in one container for the sake of convenience; you may confuse them, and some drugs can even lose their potency. To preserve freshness, always keep the container lids tightly closed.

 Discard unused medicine unless your doctor tells you to keep it for future use. You should also discard any medication that is past its expiration date; it may deliver a weaker or stronger dose than you need.

 Never take your medicine in the dark and never keep it by your bed. When you are not able to see something clearly or are still half-asleep, it is very easy to take an overdose or the wrong drug.

 For easier pill swallowing, stand or sit up straight and put the pill far back on your tongue; then swallow it as you take a drink of water. Drink some more water and stay upright for a few more minutes. If the pill is stuck, eat part of a banana and drink more water. You can also try burying the pill in a piece of banana and swallowing that.

 Ask your doctor for samples of a newly prescribed medication—this way you can determine whether you will experience any side effects and try out the drug before going to the expense of having the prescription filled.

 Keep a bottle of ipecac syrup in your bathroom in case you need to induce vomiting because of an accidental overdose. Usually an extra dose won't do you any harm, but with some drugs, such as anticonvulsants, it can be dangerous. Call your doctor, a poison control center, or an emergency room at once.

 To avoid mixups or overdoses, ask your doctor if she can prescribe a drug that you need to take only once or twice a day. If you have to take several medications, see if you can get pills that look different from one another.

 If you use syringes, ask your doctor or pharmacist how to dispose of them safely, or follow the instructions on the package they come in. You should not discard them with your everyday garbage because they are considered to be dangerous medical waste.

 Never take someone else's medication (and don't share yours!), even if you appear to be suffering from the identical symptoms. Doing this can have dangerous and sometimes even fatal consequences. Prescription drugs are available only on a doctor's order precisely because of their potential for harm if they are used improperly.

THE SYMPTOMS OF ILLEGAL DRUG USE

If a friend or a relative begins to exhibit one or more of the following behavioral changes it may indicate the use of illegal drugs or abuse of legal ones.

■ Sudden changes in mood
■ Unusual displays of temper
■ Consistent absences from school or work or sudden poor performance
■ Abrupt resistance to rules at home or school
■ Borrowing of money from relatives or friends
■ Stealing from parents, friends, or employers
■ Secrecy about activities and companions
■ New friends, especially if they use drugs

For information on dealing with illegal drug abuse, write or call the Center for Substance Abuse Treatment, 11426 Rockville Pike, Suite 410, Rockville, MD 20852, 1-800-662-4357.

Common illegal drugs and controlled substances

■ *Amphetamines* make users feel intensely awake, energetic, self-confident, and clear-headed.
■ *Cocaine* gives users a spurt of energy and an intense feeling of well-being and confidence. Sometimes it can also make them irritable and violent.
■ *Hallucinogens* distort the senses.
■ *Heroin* produces intense euphoria.
■ *Inhalants* (such as cleaning fluids, airplane glue, and hairspray) cause a mild "high," dizziness, hallucinations, and sometimes unconsciousness.
■ *Marijuana* makes people feel relaxed, self-absorbed, and mildly euphoric.
■ *Opiates* have a tranquilizing and painkilling effect.
■ *Sedatives* reduce stress and anxiety, and induce sleep.

Name of Drug/Directions	Sun	Mon	Tue	Wed	Thu	Fri	Sat

A DRUG USE CALENDAR

If you have been prescribed more than one medication, it's a good idea to keep a drug use calendar (left) on which you list each of your prescriptions, the dose, and the times you are supposed to take it. Check off each dose as it is taken.

To make doubly sure that you remember the times and the dosages of your medications, consider placing the day's individual doses in paper cups or envelopes that you then put in a very visible spot. Another possibility is to buy special containers with small compartments that can be labeled.

Name of Drug/Directions	Sun	Mon	Tue	Wed	Thu	Fri	Sat
DRUG A – 3 times a day	8 12 5	8 12 5	8 12 5	8 12 5	8 12 5	8 12 5	8 12 5
DRUG B – once a day in A.M.	8	8	8	8	8	8	8
DRUG C – 3 times a day	8 12 5	8 12 5	8 12 5	8 12 5	8 12 5	8 12 5	8 12 5

SEXUALITY ACROSS THE LIFESPAN

Hormonal and other changes throughout life affect everyone's sexual relationships. But while the frequency of sex may decrease somewhat as you grow older, people in good health can usually stay sexually active and satisfied for as long as they live.

WOMEN AND MENOPAUSE

Menopause, the major physical midlife change for women, usually occurs between 45 and 55. The process leading up to it lasts for several years, during which estrogen levels drop and menstrual flow gradually stops. Most women have few if any problems, but some 5 to 15 percent of them develop symptoms severe enough to seek medical help—the most common being hot flashes and vaginal atrophy. If either problem continues, estrogen replacement therapy may be suggested (see facing page).

MEN AT MIDLIFE

Although men don't undergo as dramatic a change as menopause, production of the male hormone testosterone does gradually slow down—30 to 40 percent between the ages of 50 and 70.

Most men at midlife need more sustained sexual stimulation to get an erection but sometimes can maintain it longer than when they were younger. Men prone to premature ejaculation in their youth find that the problem often corrects itself in the later years.

The likelihood of impotence can increase, however, usually for health reasons. After a heart attack, a man may fear that sex is dangerous for him. (Usually, it is not.) Prostate surgery and diabetes can result in impotence. A new treatment entails injecting into the penis a medication increasing blood flow, resulting in an erection. Many patients have good results with vacuum devices. As a last resort, a penile prosthesis can be surgically implanted.

OTHER FACTORS AFFECTING SEXUAL PERFORMANCE

Many drugs can impair sexual functioning. Talk to your doctor if you are having problems; they can often be solved by halting or changing your medication.

Arthritis can make sex uncomfortable, but taking pain medication and using positions that put the least stress on affected joints can help. Stress incontinence can be inhibiting, but this problem can usually be remedied (see p.316). Depression, stress, anxiety, and fatigue can adversely affect anyone's sex life; but counseling can help, as can relaxation exercises (see pp.180–181).

AVOIDING SEXUALLY TRANSMITTED DISEASES

The only sure way to prevent AIDS and other sexually transmitted diseases is to abstain from sex. The second best way is a long-term monogamous relationship. If you are beginning a new relationship, you should know your partner's sexual history, and only have sex with someone you trust. Using latex condoms and foams, jellies, and lubricants with non-oxynol-9 can provide some, but not total, protection.

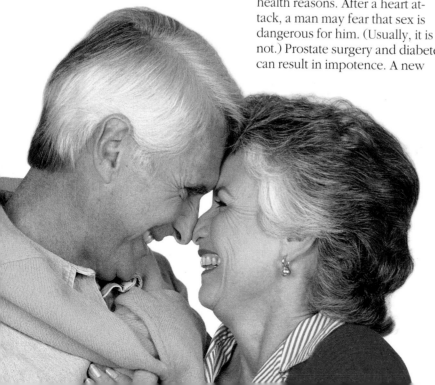

CONSIDERING ESTROGEN REPLACEMENT THERAPY

Fewer than 25 percent of menopausal women undergo estrogen replacement therapy (ERT); most do so to alleviate hot flashes and often halt treatment once the symptoms abate. Although ERT is still controversial, a growing body of medical research suggests that for the great majority of women its health benefits may outweigh the risks. ERT clearly helps prevent osteoporosis, a bone disease that mainly affects postmenopausal women and women who have had a hysterectomy. Estrogen will not rebuild lost bone, but it can help sustain bone that remains. In addition, some studies show that estrogen replacement can help prevent heart disease, the major killer of American women over the age of 50.

If a woman still has her uterus, however, the recommendation is that progesterone be given along with estrogen to decrease the risk of uterine cancer. The long-term benefits are unclear, but studies to date indicate that the combination is safer than estrogen alone. Many doctors now prescribe combination hormone replacement therapy (HRT), with much lower doses of estrogen than were used 20 years ago when ERT was found to increase the risk of uterine cancer. Combined HRT appears to eliminate this risk.

Some studies indicate that estrogen may slightly increase the risk of breast cancer, but this has not been proved; still, women with a personal or family history of breast cancer probably should avoid hormone therapy. Also, women who have phlebitis and other clotting disorders should not take estrogen.

Whether or not you opt for ERT, there are two other ways to help reduce health risks. The first is regular exercise (see Chapter 3), which can condition the heart, improve circulation, and help maintain strong bones. The second is a healthful diet (see Chapter 2) that is low in fat and high in fiber and calcium.

Some women have found that vitamin E in daily doses of 400 to 800 IU's provides relief from menopausal symptoms; research suggests that it may also help to reduce women's risk of heart disease and cancer. In addition, several nonhormonal prescription drugs may help relieve hot flashes. Check with your doctor to find out if any of these medications may be suitable for you.

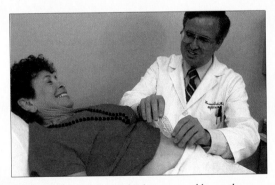

An estrogen patch, applied twice weekly on the stomach or buttocks, allows the hormone to pass directly into the bloodstream instead of going through the liver first, as oral estrogen does. Some doctors believe that this method may be safer for certain patients.

KEEPING YOUR MEMORY SHARP

Fading memory may be the phenomenon people fear most about aging. Worry that a memory lapse indicates early dementia makes older people lose their perspective. When you are in your sixties, retrieving a name from your memory may take longer than it did when you were 40. But then, after 20 years, you have many more names to remember.

HOW AGE AFFECTS THE PROCESS

Aging does bring change. As you grow older, your brain may need more time to learn new facts and to store them. Retrieving memories may take slightly longer too. Beginning in middle age, you are increasingly likely to have the frustrating experience of remembering that funny anecdote *after* you get home from the party. Very little information in your vast storehouse of memories is actually ever lost, however. With the right cues and enough time, your brain can generally retrieve whatever data you need.

THE BRAIN'S FILING SYSTEM

As you make memories, your brain sorts and stores the new impressions in its neurons, or nerve cells. The strongest neuron connections are generally made for long-term memories (important events like your wedding, a major accident, or your first child's birth). These are indelibly printed into your neural records like files kept on a computer's hard disk. Very short-term memories (a telephone number that you need to remember only long enough to dial) have always passed through your brain fairly quickly.

THE TRICKIEST MEMORY

Information you need to remember for a few minutes, a few hours, or even a few days is the most vulnerable to age-associated memory deterioration. The location of your car at the mall, the whereabouts of the book you were reading last night, and the paper pickup day in your town's new recycling program are the kinds of memories you are most likely to forget.

You don't have to accept such lapses in memory, however. Like muscles, the brain benefits from exercise. If you want to keep your memory agile, maintain your brain's powers by using them. Practice some of the memory tricks on the facing page, pursue new interests, read, and play word games. To help your concentration while you exercise your mind, avoid such distractions as the radio or television.

TEST YOUR MEMORY: NAME/FACE ASSOCIATION

Study the names and faces below for 30 seconds. Then cover this page and recall the names that go with the faces on the facing page.

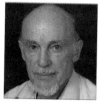
CHARLES

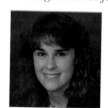
PATRICIA

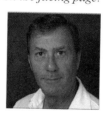
JAMES

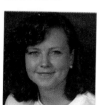
NANCY

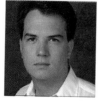
ROBERT

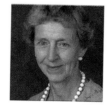
MARY

YOUR HEALTH AND YOUR MEMORY

A failing memory can be a symptom of a health problem, so if you are experiencing memory lapses, see your doctor. Infections, liver and kidney problems, anemia, heart disease, lung disease, diabetes, and dehydration can all produce memory loss. Memory lapses can also be caused by vitamin deficiencies, thyroid problems, poor blood circulation, or low blood sugar. Some older people suffer small, often imperceptible strokes that reduce memory function (p.276).

Drug reactions are a leading cause of memory loss in older people, but the condition can usually be reversed with a change in dose or medication. Alcohol, too, can impair your mental acuity. Long-term alcohol abuse can significantly—and permanently—blunt your memory.

Depression not only makes people feel sad and helpless but can also cloud the memory. Some doctors believe that the disease short-circuits your ability to focus your mind. Once recognized, however, depression can be successfully treated with drugs and psychotherapy (p.278).

MEMORY AND DEMENTIA

At the first sign of forgetfulness, some people fear that they're in the early stages of Alzheimer's disease, a frustrating kind of dementia that affects only a small percentage of the population (see p.277). Memory lapses are usually due to causes far less daunting—even a cold can make you temporarily forgetful. People who worry about their memory problems probably are not suffering from senility. Dementia patients are usually unaware of their mental losses.

MEMORY TEST RESULTS

If you are under age 50, three or four correct answers is an average score; for those 50 or older, one or two correct answers is the norm.

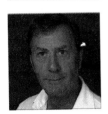
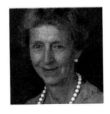
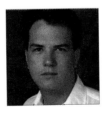

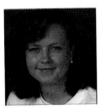
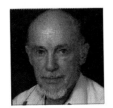
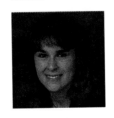

STRATEGIES FOR IMPROVING YOUR MEMORY

■ Pay attention and repeat. When you meet someone new, listen carefully to the name and say it aloud immediately. Use it several times in the course of your conversation.

■ Use mnemonic (memory-enhancing) devices. Rhyme words—"I had pizza with Lisa" for your daughter's new friend. Or draw mental pictures to associate a face with a name. A man named Mark has a mustache. You can remember that the mustache makes a "mark" across his face.

■ Make up an acronym to remember a list: TIPTOE could help you remember a grocery list of Tomatoes, Ice cream, Pepper, Tuna, Onions, and Eggplant.

■ Write things down. Leave notes for yourself in visible places such as on the refrigerator door or the bathroom mirror. Enter appointments on a single calendar and check it regularly.

■ Keep necessities in convenient places and always put them back where they belong—your keys on a hook by the door, your address book in the desk drawer, your umbrella in the stand by the front door.

■ Put "to-do" items in unavoidable places. Keep medicines you have to take beside your toothbrush. Place letters to be mailed by the door so that you can't leave without seeing them.

SMOKING: HOW TO
BREAK A BAD HABIT

· ·

The principal preventable cause of death in the United States is smoking. Since the first surgeon general's report on smoking documented the habit's deadly potential in 1964, more than 45 million Americans have quit. New research continues to confirm the hazards of smoking.

THE RISKS

Smokers are three times more likely to die of cancer than nonsmokers. Smokers are more likely to develop not only lung cancer but also cancer of the throat, larynx, mouth, esophagus, kidney, bladder, pancreas, or cervix. They are also at increased risk for heart disease, emphysema, and chronic bronchitis. People who smoke a pack a day are more than twice as likely to suffer a heart attack as people who don't smoke. (They are also more likely to die from it.)

Nonsmokers who are exposed to smokers are also at risk of developing smoking-related diseases. An Environmental Protection Agency review of smoking studies released in 1992 confirms, for example, that the nonsmoking spouses of smokers face a 30 percent higher risk of dying of lung cancer than those who have non smoking partners.

KICKING THE HABIT

It's never too late to give up cigarettes. No matter what your age, not smoking for 15 years makes your health risks comparable to those of people who never smoked (see p.244). Quitting smoking after the age of 50 cuts your risk of heart disease in half, leads to a better outcome if you already have a smoking-related disease, and reduces your num-

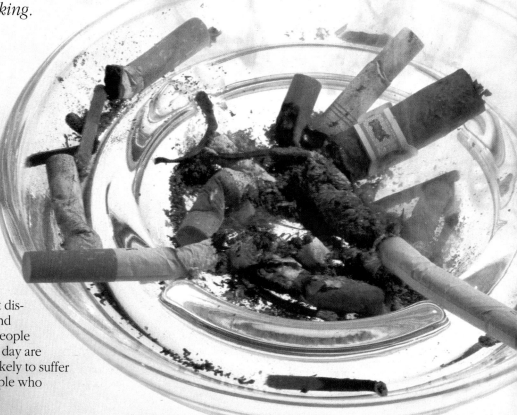

ber of headaches, stomachaches, and respiratory infections.

Quitting isn't easy. Most smokers try and fail several times before they succeed. Nicotine is an addictive drug, and you can expect withdrawal symptoms (irritability, lethargy, headaches, coughing) for several weeks. The hardest part is over for most people after about 3 months. After that, the urge to smoke when you're especially tense or when you see someone else smoking gradually fades.

Nine out of 10 smokers quit without professional help. And most do it cold turkey. There is no reason, however, not to ask your doctor to prescribe nicotine gum or nicotine patches, which can minimize the effects of nicotine

More than a smelly, messy habit, smoking affects the health of those around the smoker. The hazards increase with the amount of exposure. Research shows, for example, that children subject to secondhand smoke at home are at increased risk for ear infections, asthma, bronchitis, and pneumonia.

THREE STEPS TO QUITTING

Whether you are giving up smoking by yourself or through a group, you may benefit from this three-step program used by many people who have quit successfully.

■ *Set a quit date.* A date 2 to 4 weeks away is close enough to take seriously but also allows you time to get prepared. Some people stop smoking on vacation when they are away from their everyday routine. Others find that maintaining a regular schedule is more supportive. Don't try to quit when a stressful situation is looming. After you pick a date to quit, let friends and family members know so that they can help you. Remove all the smoking paraphernalia from the house on your quit day.

■ *Study your habit before you stop.* Keeping a diary of when and where you smoke helps you recognize situations and activities that trigger smoking and need to be changed. If, for example, you always have a cigarette with your coffee after dinner, plan to skip the coffee and go for a walk instead. If you smoke in the car when traffic slows to a halt, substitute chewing gum as a tension reliever; keep several packs in the glove compartment and remove the lighter from the car.

■ *Alter your routine to cut down on smoking as you prepare to stop.* Switch brands to reduce the nicotine content (and your enjoyment) of the cigarettes you smoke. Buy cigarettes by the pack instead of the carton to make smoking more expensive and less convenient. Confine smoking to one room in your house. Hold your cigarette in the hand that you don't normally use for smoking. Try a glass of juice instead of a cigarette for a pick-me-up. Substitute exercise for a favorite daily cigarette (it will keep you from smoking and help to boost your metabolism when you no longer have nicotine to do it). When you are down to seven or fewer low-nicotine cigarettes a day, you are ready to stop smoking for good.

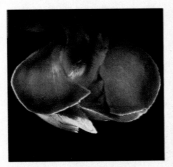

A baby's pristine lungs

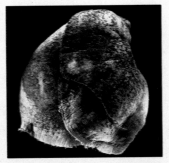

An adult smoker's lungs

DAMAGE FROM SMOKING
Compare the unblemished lungs of a newborn, left, with those of a longtime heavy smoker, right. The black patches on the smoker's lungs are tar deposits.

withdrawal. Some people find learning a relaxation technique (pp.180–181), undergoing hypnosis, or taking acupuncture treatments to be helpful.

Or you may find joining a support group beneficial. The American Cancer Society, the American Lung Association, and the Seventh Day Adventist Church run low-cost stop-smoking programs in most areas of the United States (check your local telephone directory). Many hospitals also offer programs for minimal fees. Commercial clinics, which may be more expensive, often provide intensive individual counseling.

HANDLING RELAPSES

If you relapse after quitting, don't be too hard on yourself. It takes most smokers three or four unsuccessful attempts before they give up cigarettes for good.

Most relapses occur in the first week when withdrawal symptoms are at their peak and the body is craving nicotine. You may feel sick and want comfort, or you may feel lethargic and want a shot of energy to get you going and to help your concentration. These early weeks will be your most difficult time, and you should arrange to stay busy at ac-

tivities (sports, movies, handicrafts) in which smoking doesn't fit. Ask your family and friends to help keep you away from potential smoking situations during this critical time.

More subtle relapses come during the first 3 months after quitting when events trigger an automatic response of reaching for a cigarette almost before you realize what you are doing. You may be feeling tense, and your natural association of a cigarette with relaxing will make you accept an offered cigarette without

HEALTH REWARDS WHEN YOU QUIT SMOKING

Although you may feel rotten while you go through withdrawal, the health benefits from giving up smoking begin within 20 minutes of your last cigarette. How these rewards continue to accrue after you stop smoking is shown on the chart below. A bonus is the psychological satisfaction you experience from taking control of a part of your life that was under the power of a bad habit and a bad drug.

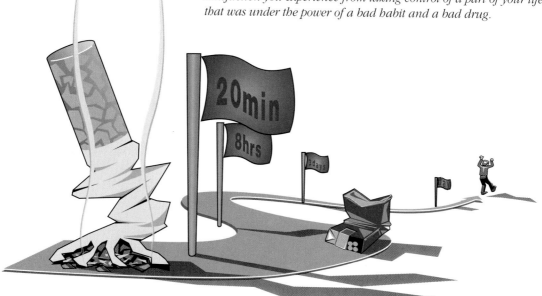

Within 20 minutes	Within 8 hours	After 72 hours	Within 3-5 years	Within 10 years
Your blood pressure and pulse rate drop to the levels they were before you smoked.	Your blood levels of carbon monoxide and oxygen return to normal.	Your lung capacity is already increasing.	Your risk of a heart attack drops to that of a nonsmoker.	Your risk of dying of lung cancer drops to the level of a nonsmoker.

Note: If you smoke just one cigarette a day, you lose all these benefits.

thinking. Such lapses are not hard to recover from if you catch yourself right away.

Many former smokers, after months—or even years—of not smoking, relapse under severe stress. Situations such as divorce, a death in the family, or the loss of a job can make them turn to the solace of cigarettes and trap them into the habit again.

The only way to avoid this type of relapse is to tell yourself that smoking is not an option, even in an emergency. Remind yourself of all the things you hate about smoking—the smell, the mess, the threat to your health, the expense. Smoking won't solve your new problems; it can only re-create an old one.

Luckily, as more people stop smoking, and smoking is banned in more offices and public spaces, the opportunities for former smokers to relapse are shrinking.

DEALING WITH ADDED POUNDS

Weight gain is another reason some individuals start smoking again. (Most people who stop smoking put on 6 to 8 pounds.) Smoking curbs your appetite and nicotine speeds up your metabolism, so that you burn off calories more quickly when you smoke. Those few extra pounds are not, however, nearly the danger to your health that smoking is. And there is another, healthier way to speed up your metabolism again—aerobic exercise.

With a healthful, low-fat diet (snacking on fruits and vegetables instead of candy, chips, and nuts) and a regular exercise program (see Chapter 3), you can keep your weight down while you quit smoking.

Profile

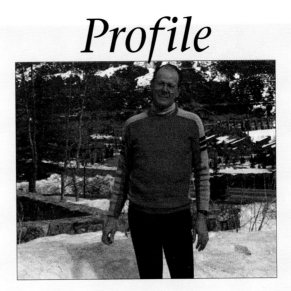

BILL BOYD: A HAPPY EX-SMOKER

Bill Boyd was 46 years old and taking practice runs down a difficult ski slope in his adopted home of Aspen, Colorado, when he was joined by another skier who was 72 years old. Feeling challenged, Boyd skied a little harder and a little faster on each run, but his companion stayed right with him. After several times down the slope, Boyd was more winded than the older man, who looked at him and said, "Why don't you quit smoking?"

Boyd, inspired by the stamina and prowess of the older man, decided on the spot to do it. "I quit cold turkey, but it took a year to get over the craving. There were nights I wanted to smoke the couch!"

During his first smoke-free year, situations in which he'd see other people smoking were agonizing for Boyd. An electrician, he had bosses who would taunt him by blowing smoke in his face. Boyd is sure that having a single cigarette during that time would have ruined his resolve. Today he avoids smoky rooms for a different reason. "I can't stand the smell anymore." Smokers ask Boyd if he's ever tempted to smoke again. He says no; he feels too good now.

245

MANAGING HEADACHES

*M*ost *headaches clear up with rest or the help of an aspirin or other analgesic. More specialized treatment may be needed, however, if you get headaches regularly. Some of them may signal a more serious underlying medical disorder.*

THE MOST COMMON HEADACHE

A tension, or muscle contraction, headache—generally experienced as a band of dull pain tightening around the head—is the kind that most people suffer. Stress, exhaustion, depression, or anxiety can bring one on, as can habitual poor posture. Aspirin, acetaminophen, or ibuprofen will usually provide relief. Sometimes, however, a tension headache can last for weeks or months and persist around the clock. In such a case, the remedy may lie in using relaxation techniques (pp. 180–181), taking antidepressants or tranquilizers, getting more sleep, or even going on a vacation.

THE INFAMOUS MIGRAINE

The often severe vascular headaches known as migraines can last from several hours to several days. They produce a throbbing or pounding pain, generally on only one side of the head. Other symptoms may include icy hands, nausea or vomiting, and extreme sensitivity to light and sound.

Some people know an attack is beginning because they develop an "aura"—they may hear sounds and see flashing lights, jagged lines, and patches of darkness; they may also have tingling or numbness in their limbs, and their speech may be impaired.

While it is not yet totally clear what causes migraine headaches, heredity may play a part. Two-thirds of migraine victims have parents who also had migraines.

Preventive measures involve avoiding stress and maintaining a regular sleeping schedule to ensure you get enough rest. In some people, migraines may be precipitated by certain foods and beverages (see facing page). Weather, changes in elevation, and menstruation may also act as triggers.

If taken at the first sign of a migraine, aspirin with coffee or other source of caffeine may stop it. Drugs used to abort a migraine include sumatriptan, ergotamine, naproxen sodium, and isometheptene. These work best for people who have an aura. Simply resting in a dark room with an ice pack on your head may help.

For people who are immobilized by an attack or who suffer more than three attacks a month, a daily dose of the beta blocker propranolol can act as a preventive, as can antidepressants and calcium channel blockers. A recent study shows that a daily aspirin dose may be beneficial too.

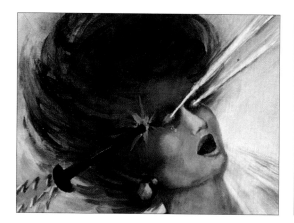

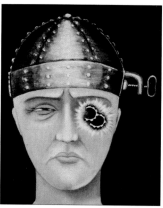

Headaches as depicted by their victims. One person (far left) experienced her headache as a screw being driven into the side of her head, causing shafts of pain to shoot from her eyes. Another (near left) felt as if a steel helmet were being tightened on his head, making his left eye radiate with double centers of pain.

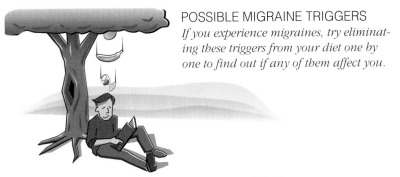

POSSIBLE MIGRAINE TRIGGERS

If you experience migraines, try eliminating these triggers from your diet one by one to find out if any of them affect you.

Additives Artificial sweeteners; monosodium glutamate in foods.

Beverages Alcohol, especially red wine, scotch, and bourbon; caffeine in tea, coffee, or colas in excessive amounts.

Chocolate

Dairy Aged and ripened cheeses such as Brie, Camembert, Cheddar, Emmanthaler, and Stilton; sour cream; yogurt.

Fruits and vegetables Avocados, bananas, citrus fruits, figs (canned), lima beans, navy beans, nuts, onions, peas.

Grains Yeast-leavened wheat products such as bread, coffee cakes, and doughnuts.

Meats Chicken livers; fermented sausages and processed meats such as bacon, bologna, hot dogs, pepperoni, and salami; herring; pâté; pork.

Preserved foods Fermented, pickled, or marinated foods; vinegar (except white vinegar).

CLUSTER HEADACHES

Occurring in groups over periods of time as short as several days or as long as several months, cluster headaches are a type of vascular headache. A person may experience one to four piercing headaches in a single cluster daily for several weeks. The headaches are usually nocturnal and strike mostly in the spring and fall. Cluster headache victims seem to be especially sensitive to nicotine and alcohol, both of which can serve as triggers. For some people, they are seasonal, coming at the same time each year.

Cluster headache pain is usually one-sided and localized as a burning sensation around or in a single eye. Other possible symptoms are nasal congestion, sweating, tearing, a drooping eyelid, and facial flushing on the afflicted side. The eye may be swollen, and its pupil may be contracted.

Drugs used to prevent or interrupt cluster headaches include lithium, ergotamine, cyproheptadine, methysergide, and steroids. During an attack, some may benefit from oxygen therapy.

ORGANICALLY CAUSED HEADACHES

Although sometimes they may indicate medical conditions of varying seriousness (see box at right), many organically caused headaches require only minor medical care or none at all. A caffeine withdrawal headache, for example, is "cured" with a caffeinated drink. A sinus headache caused by an allergy or a sinus infection is usually cleared up with the appropriate antihistamines, nasal decongestants, or antibiotics.

Since the same nerves serve both the head and the neck, peo-

WHEN TO CALL A DOCTOR

Seek medical help immediately if your headache

▨ Is very severe, sudden, incapacitating, or the worst headache you've ever had.
▨ Comes with a fever and a stiff neck that you can't move in any direction.
▨ Is accompanied by difficulty in talking or thinking clearly, nausea or vomiting, paralysis, vertigo, visual disturbances, faintness, or sensitivity to light and sound.
▨ Occurs with severe pain around the ear, temple, and one side of the jaw when you chew; and there are vision problems and a low fever—particularly if you are more than 60 years old.
▨ Produces pain around one or both of your eyes.
▨ Is very painful when you awaken and slowly worsens, especially if it does so in one area; is exacerbated by exertion, coughing, and sneezing; and is accompanied by nausea and vomiting.
▨ Fits the descriptions of cluster or migraine headaches (see left), especially if others in your family have similar headaches.

ple with osteoarthritis of the neck and spine get headaches as a result of pain in these joints. Arthritic headaches respond well to treatment with aspirin or an equivalent. Bed rest, applied heat, and special exercises and massage can also help.

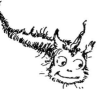

THE SCOURGES OF WINTER:
THE COMMON COLD AND THE FLU

The common cold gets less common as you grow older. By the time you are 60, you are likely to average less than one cold a year. Influenza, unfortunately, becomes more dangerous as you age.

FIGHTING OFF THE VIRUSES THAT CAUSE COLDS

More than 200 different viruses cause colds. It takes the human body many years to develop antibodies to so many viruses, which is why small children are most susceptible to colds and mature adults enjoy some immunity.

When you have a cold, you expel millions of viruses when you sneeze or cough. Others become infected by inhaling the viruses or transmitting them to their mouth or nose via the hands. Your best defense is to wash your hands regularly to get rid of viruses picked up when you touch a doorknob or other object touched by someone with a cold. When you have a cold, wash your hands frequently and use disposable tissues rather than a handkerchief. Also, try not to touch your eyes and nose, the viruses' main entryways into your body.

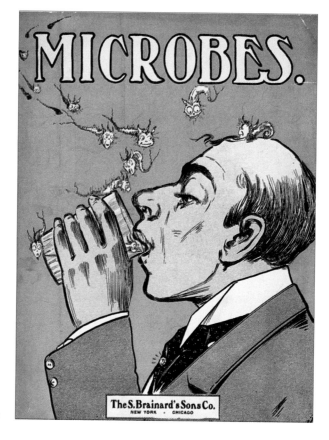

The S. Brainard's Sons Co.
NEW YORK · CHICAGO

A ditty called "Microbes," written in 1905, addressed the subject of the invisible creatures that spread colds and the flu. The sheet music cover shows an unsuspecting water drinker besieged by imaginatively depicted microbes.

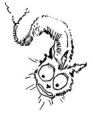

WARDING OFF THE DIFFERENT STRAINS OF FLU

There are two major flu viruses—influenza A and influenza B. Although new strains of each are continually forming, scientists have been able to compound a reliable new flu vaccine each year. Unless you are allergic to eggs (the medium in which the vaccine is grown), a flu shot in the fall or early winter should protect you through winter. If you are allergic to eggs, there is an antiviral drug, amantadine, that is effective against the influenza A virus.

Although the flu, like a cold, clears up by itself, it can lead to serious complications for vulnerable people. Doctors recommend annual flu shots for everyone over 65 and for anyone who has a circulatory, respiratory, kidney, metabolic, or immune disorder.

Flu viruses are spread through the air or by touching contaminated surfaces and people. As with colds, washing your hands often is your best defense.

THE BEST TREATMENT

Antibiotics can't fight a cold or the flu. These illnesses must run their course. Get adequate rest, use a steam vaporizer to ease breathing, and drink lots of nonalcoholic fluids to counter the dehydration caused by a fever and to loosen the mucus in your throat.

Colds creep up on you with a variety of symptoms and last a week or so, whether or not you stay in bed. Flu symptoms come on fast and hit you hard, requiring several days or more in bed.

USING COLD AND FLU MEDICINES

Drugs can't cure a cold or the flu, but they can make you more comfortable. Aspirin, ibuprofen, or acetaminophen will ease body aches and bring down fever. A decongestant will make breathing easier. A warm saltwater gargle or hard candies (cough drops may upset your stomach) will soothe a sore throat. An expectorant cough medicine will loosen mucus in your lungs. All-purpose cold or flu drugs contain more ingredients than you need. Some have both cough suppressants and expectorants, which work at cross-purposes. The antihistamines in many formulas don't affect cold symptoms and can cause drowsiness.

COMPLICATIONS

Colds and flu can leave you susceptible to bacterial infections or other complications that may require a doctor's attention (see box, right). A sore throat, for example, may indicate strep throat or mononucleosis. Hoarseness can be a sign of laryngitis, an infection of the larynx, or voice box. It usually clears up by itself, but you can speed the recovery by resting your voice (don't even whisper) and drinking plenty of liquids. If laryngitis lasts longer than a few days, call your doctor. You may have a bacterial infection that requires an antibiotic.

WHEN TO CALL A DOCTOR

Sometimes a cold or the flu leads to a complication that needs professional evaluation. Call your doctor if:
- You run a persistent fever above 100°F for several days or a low fever gets worse.
- You suffer severe pain in your chest, stomach, head, throat, or ear.
- The glands in your neck become swollen.
- You lose your voice or it becomes hoarse.
- You experience difficulty breathing.
- You cough up yellow or green phlegm or blood.
- You have a sore throat, runny nose, or other cold or flu symptom that persists for more than 10 days.

COLD-MIMICKING ALLERGIES

Many people who suffer from respiratory allergies to pollen or animal dander may not recognize their sensitivity to dust mites or molds. These household allergens are often spawned by improperly maintained humidifiers, heating systems, or air conditioners. Allergies can be relieved with antihistamines, but it's better to avoid the allergens. Control dust mites by covering mattresses and pillows with plastic, washing bed linens in hot water, and keeping humidity in the house below 35 percent (higher humidity promotes dust mite and mold growth). Frequent vacuuming of rugs and upholstery—preferably by a nonallergic person—also helps keep the allergens in check.

IS IT A COLD, THE FLU, OR AN ALLERGY?
Check your symptoms on the chart below; identifying your ailment is the first step to proper treatment.

	Cold	Flu	Allergy
Body aches	Mild	Severe	Rare
Congestion	Common	Occasional	Common
Cough	Rare	Common	Common
Fatigue	Mild	Severe	Rare
Fever	Rare	Up to 103°F	None
Headache	Common	Severe	Rare
Runny nose	Common	Rare	Common
Sneezing	Common	Rare	Common
Sore throat	Occasional	Common	Occasional

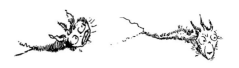

Getting a
Good Night's Sleep

As you grow older, your sleep becomes briefer, lighter, and more easily disrupted. Such changes are normal; insomnia and other sleep disorders, however, are not.

THE NATURE OF INSOMNIA

True insomnia makes you drowsy during the day and can interfere with your work or lead to accidents. The short-term insomnia caused by temporary crises can often be eased with prescription drugs, but these quickly lose their efficacy and can disrupt sleep or result in addiction when used for too long. Most over-the-counter sleeping pills are antihistamines, which tend both to be too mild to be useful and to have side effects. Insomnia is usually relieved by behavioral changes (see box at right). If these fail, your doctor may refer you to a sleep clinic.

SLEEP APNEA

A tendency to stop breathing for several seconds while asleep, sleep apnea may cause dozens of such stoppages a night. In some cases, the temporary lack of oxygen can trigger arrhythmias or heart attacks. Overweight, obstructions in the breathing passages, and the use of tranquilizers, alcohol, antihistamines, or sleeping pills are among the causes of sleep apnea.

If you are very sleepy during the day for no apparent reason and are told that you snore or gasp while asleep, see your doctor. If apnea is suspected, he may urge that you lose weight and refer you to a sleep clinic for a definitive diagnosis. If apnea is diagnosed, you may be taught to use a device that blows air into the nostrils to keep your breathing passages open. If all this fails, your doctor may recommend surgery to make an opening in the windpipe, or trachea, and insertion of a breathing tube at night.

SNORING

Only a small number of those who snore have sleep apnea. The snoring of the others usually troubles only their sleeping partners. Weight loss may help, as may sewing a marble into the back of the snorer's pajamas to wake him whenever he lies on his back (a position that fosters snoring). A new procedure using laser surgery may cure the problem.

HOW TO PREVENT INSOMNIA

■ Make every effort to get up at the same time each morning, even on weekends.
■ Try not to nap, especially in the late afternoon or evening.
■ Don't exercise vigorously just before bedtime.
■ Don't eat a heavy meal just before you plan to go to bed, and avoid caffeine, alcohol, and nicotine in the evening.
■ Wind down for an hour or two before bedtime by taking a warm bath, reading, or listening to music.
■ Sleep on a comfortable bed in a dark and quiet bedroom.
■ Use the bed only for sleeping and sexual activity.
■ Set aside "worry time" during the day so you won't bring any problems to bed with you.
■ Once you get into bed, calm your mind with meditation or by slowly relaxing each set of your muscles in turn (see pp.180–181).
■ Don't lie awake in bed for more than 20 minutes. Get up and do something until you are sleepy again.

NOCTURNAL LEG CRAMPS

Painful but not dangerous, nocturnal leg cramps strike the calf, thigh, or toes, jolting you awake. (If you suffer from more generalized cramps, see your doctor.) To alleviate the cramping, try gently massaging and stretching the muscles; a hot bath, heating pad, or cold pack may help too.

The cause of these leg cramps may involve dietary deficiencies, and potassium or magnesium supplements may help prevent them. So may doing some leg stretches before bed. A good exercise is to brace yourself against a wall or chair and lean forward until you feel your calf muscles lengthening (see p.104).

To avoid getting leg cramps in bed, wear socks to keep your feet warm, lie on your side with your legs bent, and use a pillow to raise the blankets so that they don't weigh down your legs. If nothing works, ask your doctor about the possibility of taking a muscle relaxant before bed—or even quinine pills, provided you are not sensitive to the drug.

RESTLESS LEGS SYNDROME

A sudden, irresistible urge to move the legs that generally occurs shortly after going to bed, restless legs syndrome is often relieved by just getting up and walking around. Since the condition can be related to diabetes, kidney disease, or other disorders, it should be checked out by a doctor. Alcohol, nicotine, and stress are known to aggravate the syndrome; walking and massaging your legs before bed may help prevent it. Some people find cool-water soaks to be useful; others prefer a heating pad.

Profile

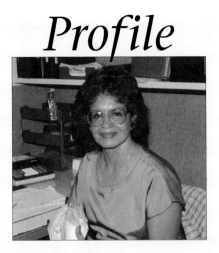

LUPE CONWAY DOESN'T "THINK ABOUT SLEEP AT ALL" ANYMORE

A good night's sleep was Lupe Conway's fondest dream. The Albuquerque resident had been suffering from insomnia for several years: "I always went to bed so tired I thought I would fall asleep as soon as my head hit the pillow. Instead, I would toss and turn for hours." Sometimes Conway took an over-the-counter sleeping medication. "It made me fall asleep faster, but it wasn't good-quality sleep, so I was still tired the next day."

Conway signed up for a sleep study at the hospital where she works as an accountant. After a doctor and nurse team questioned her extensively about her sleep habits, they determined that her problem was that she didn't need as much sleep as she used to. Over a period of several months, they pushed back her usual 8:30 to 9:00 bedtime 15 minutes at a time until she was going to bed between 11:00 and 11:30. "In the beginning, even staying up for an extra 15 minutes was hard because I was so tired."

Conway turned in a log of her sleep patterns every few weeks. After about 6 months, it showed she was falling asleep more quickly; 6 months after that, she "graduated." "The sleep I get now is restful," she says happily. "Now I don't think about sleep at all."

TAKING CARE OF YOUR BACK

Four out of five people suffer from back pain at some time in their lives. In most cases, the ache clears up in a few weeks regardless of treatment. Some kinds of back pain, however, may require more sustained therapy.

THE CAUSES OF BACK PAIN

Because your back is constantly engaged in a balancing act with gravity, just supporting the weight of the head and upper body puts a stress on the vertebrae, the cushioning discs between them, and the muscles and ligaments that hold them in place. A sudden or unusual exertion may throw off the spine's alignment, strain muscles, or tear ligaments and cause pain. The neck and lower back are the most vulnerable.

Another source of back pain is a "slipped," or herniated, disc: gelatinous material bulges out between two vertebrae, often pressing against nerve roots. This can result in severe pain that radiates into the legs (sciatica) or, if it occurs in the neck, into the arms.

Emotional stress is blamed for much lower-back pain. Although this theory is controversial, stress can certainly lead to muscle tension, thus intensifying any back discomfort.

DIAGNOSING THE PROBLEM

In most cases of back pain, elaborate diagnostic tests may not be necessary. Check the box on page 255 for those symptoms that should prompt you to seek medical help. In these cases, the doctor will test your reflexes, feel your spine to pinpoint the painful area, and perhaps do blood tests to rule out an infection, tumor, or other disorder. Additional tests may include X-rays and a CT scan (computerized tomography) or an MRI (magnetic resonance imaging). Test findings do not always match the severity of the pain—your spine may appear normal when you are in agony, while visible abnormalities may produce no symptoms.

TREATING BACK PAIN

The basic treatment for acute back pain is to lie flat on your back for at least 2 days. Experts advise against remaining in bed for more than a week, however, because the resulting muscle weakness can make your condition worse. To relieve the pain, take aspirin, ibuprofen, or muscle relaxants, and avoid making any movements that hurt. Applying ice packs for 10 to 20 minutes every 2 hours for the first 48 hours may numb the pain; after that, heating pads or hot baths may be soothing.

When the pain subsides, you should do gentle exercises prescribed specifically for your condition by your doctor or physical therapist. Recent studies suggest that spinal manipulation by a chiropractor may also help alleviate lower-back pain.

NECK PAIN

While it is much like pain in the lower spine, neck pain can signal a medical emergency when associated with certain symptoms (see pp.247 and 255). A stiff neck may also be a symptom of the flu; if all of your muscles are stiff and aching, home remedies may suffice.

A morning "crick" in the neck is usually a muscle spasm caused by an awkward sleeping position. Rest and aspirin along with applications of ice or heat will often ease the pain (some people find that ice helps; others, that heat is effective). If the spasm doesn't clear up, call a doctor. One way to prevent getting neck pain is to avoid working for long periods with your head tilted up or down.

MUSCLE ACHES AND STIFFNESS

As you grow older, muscle aches and stiffness become more common. To minimize them, experts advise a regimen of regular exercise and adequate rest. While joint stiffness may signal arthritis, the likelier culprits are strained muscles due to unusual activity. Your muscles will need about 2 days to recover; during this time, to restore your flexibility, try gently repeating the movements that led to your trouble.

PREVENTING BACK PAIN IN YOUR DAILY LIFE

You can often avoid occurrences of back pain by being careful to perform simple everyday activities correctly. Doing them the right way generally requires less effort too. Other measures that can help to prevent back pain include checking your posture (see p.103), taking off excess weight, and following a regular exercise program. Women with back pain who wear high heels should change to low-heeled shoes with good support.

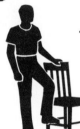

Sleeping. *Use a firm mattress or one with a bedboard underneath it. Lie on your side with your legs bent. If you sleep on your back, place small pillows or folded towels under your neck, the middle of your back, and your knees.*

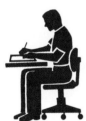

Getting out of bed. *Roll to the edge of the bed, then swing your legs over, sitting up as you do so.*

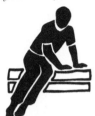

Standing. *Shift your weight from one foot to the other at frequent intervals. Resting a foot on a low rail or a chair rung also helps.*

Sitting. *Use a chair that is the right height for you and has good back support. When your feet are flat on the floor, your thighs should be parallel to the floor and the small of your back should be wedged against a back rest or cushion. Don't cross your legs. If you must sit for long periods of time, get up at regular intervals to stretch, making sure to include a backward stretch.*

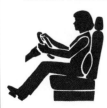

Driving. *Support your lower back with a back rest (usually available in car accessory stores). Make sure that your knees are higher than your hips and that your feet can easily reach the pedals.*

Picking up something from the floor. *Never lean over from the waist. Instead, keep your back straight and go down to the floor by bending your knees. Hold the object close to your body, and, still keeping your back straight and your head up, let your leg muscles bear the weight as you rise up smoothly and evenly. If the object is heavy, push, don't lift, it.*

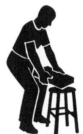

Picking up something part of the way down. *Placing one foot slightly ahead of the other, bend your front knee or both knees and, keeping your back straight, lean forward from your hips to pick up the object. Then come up by leaning back and straightening your knees.*

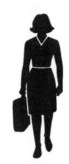

Regularly carrying a briefcase or heavy purse. *Alternate the side on which you carry a purse or briefcase. And always keep your shoulders in a straight line: don't let the weight make you tilt to one side. Consider using a backpack—many fashionable business models are now available.*

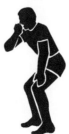

Coughing or sneezing. *Support your back by keeping it straight and by placing a hand on your thigh or on a nearby table. If you are standing, also bend your knees slightly.*

EXERCISES TO KEEP YOUR BACK HEALTHY

Back schools run by many hospitals and Y's teach simple exercises to help prevent back pain. Here are a few such exercises you can do three to five times a week. Be sure to warm up before you begin and cool down afterward (see p.109). If you have a back problem, check with your doctor before beginning any exercise program.

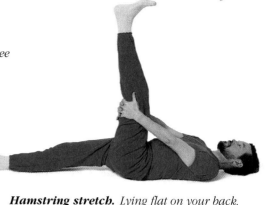

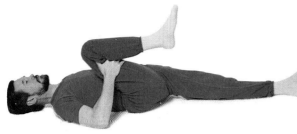

Lower-back stretch. *Lie flat on your back with one leg bent, the other straight. Put both hands behind the knee of the bent leg and pull the knee as close to your chest as you can; hold for 10 seconds. Repeat, alternating legs, 10 times on each side.*

If this exercise is easy for you, try the advanced version: bend both legs, put a hand under each knee, and pull both knees toward your chest. Repeat 20 times.

Hamstring stretch. *Lying flat on your back, bend one leg and clasp it behind the knee with both hands. Pull the leg gently up and toward you, straightening the knee until you feel a gentle stretch in the back of the thigh; your foot should be arched, with the toes pointed at your face; hold for 10 seconds, then release. Repeat 10 times with each leg.*

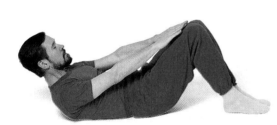

Stomach curl. *Lie on your back with your knees bent and your arms at your sides. Keeping your back flat against the floor, slowly raise your head and chest while reaching toward and touching your knees; hold for 5 seconds, then resume your original position. Repeat 10 to 15 times.*

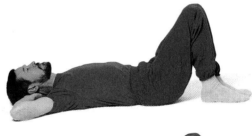

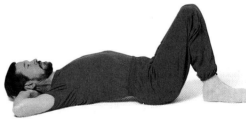

Pelvic tilt. *Lie on your back with your knees bent at a 90-degree angle, arms folded under your head or straight by your side. Then tighten your stomach muscles and push your pelvis down until you can feel that your lower back is completely flattened against the floor. Hold for 10 seconds, then release. Repeat 15 times.*

Bridge. *Lie on your back with your knees bent, arms spread out on either side. Tuck in your stomach so that your back is flat against the floor and slowly raise your hips up off the ground; hold the position for 10 seconds, then release. Repeat 20 times.*

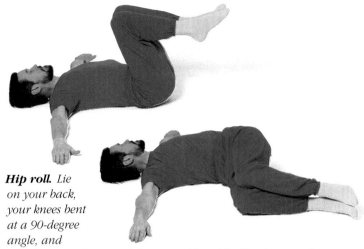

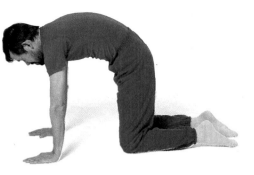

Hip roll. *Lie on your back, your knees bent at a 90-degree angle, and your arms reaching straight out to either side. Keeping your legs together, raise them up toward your chest, then slowly let them fall to the right, with your left leg on top of your right leg (your hips and lower torso will rotate when you do this); hold for 10 seconds. Then bring your legs back to your chest and let them fall to the left. Repeat 10 times on each side.*

Cat stretch. *Get down on your hands and knees and slowly dip the middle of your back downward; hold for 5 seconds. Then slowly reverse the process, rounding your back so that your torso forms an arch; hold for 5 seconds. Repeat 5 to 10 times.*

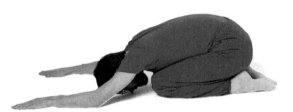

Fold-up stretch. *Sit on the floor with your legs folded beneath you. Then slowly stretch your arms forward until your forehead and arms are resting on the floor; hold, breathing deeply, for a minute or two. Repeat 5 times.*

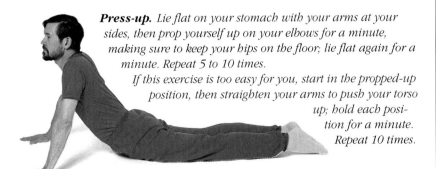

Press-up. *Lie flat on your stomach with your arms at your sides, then prop yourself up on your elbows for a minute, making sure to keep your hips on the floor; lie flat again for a minute. Repeat 5 to 10 times.*
If this exercise is too easy for you, start in the propped-up position, then straighten your arms to push your torso up; hold each position for a minute. Repeat 10 times.

WHEN TO CALL A DOCTOR

Contact your doctor if you have any of the following:

■ Severe neck pain accompanied by fever, nausea, or vomiting.
■ Severe back pain that is not relieved by shifting position or that continues or becomes worse despite 2 days of complete bed rest.
■ Back pain, numbness, or tingling that extends into the legs or arms.
■ Back or neck pain resulting from a fall or an automobile accident.
■ Back pain occurring with a change in bowel or bladder habits.
■ Back pain occurring with fever, stomach pain (including nausea or vomiting), urinary discomfort, weakness, or sweating.
■ Back pain accompanied by weakness in the arms or legs.

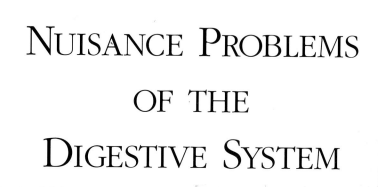

NUISANCE PROBLEMS OF THE DIGESTIVE SYSTEM

S eldom life-threatening, digestive upsets can still be debilitating. You can't avoid an occasional bug, but you can cultivate a smooth-running digestive system.

INDIGESTION AND HEARTBURN

At some time or another, nearly everyone suffers indigestion. Its symptoms include abdominal pain, bloating, and nausea. Eating too much, drinking too much alcohol, consuming foods that don't agree with you, and stress can all trigger indigestion.

Heartburn, or acid indigestion, is caused by a backup of stomach acid into the esophagus. Certain foods can provoke this reflux reaction in some people, but it is also caused by overeating, obesity, stress, and anxiety.

Although heartburn is not deadly, its main symptom—a sudden burning sensation behind the breastbone, which sometimes spreads to the throat or jaw—can easily be mistaken for a heart attack (see *The Warning Signs of a Heart Attack,* p.299). If you are not sure about the cause of chest pains, call for help immediately.

A healthy low-fat diet with a minimum of acidic foods such as citrus fruits or tomatoes will usually keep heartburn at bay. Other preventive measures include eating slowly, avoiding alcohol and cigarettes, staying erect for several hours after a meal, and remaining relaxed when under pressure (see pp.180-181). If you suffer heartburn at night, raise the head of your bed several inches.

For occasional indigestion and heartburn, an over-the-counter antacid may provide temporary relief. If you take other medications, however, ask your doctor which kind of antacid to use (some interfere with the effectiveness of certain drugs). Prolonged use of any antacid can lead to unpleasant and sometimes serious side effects. If you suffer from chronic indigestion or heartburn, discuss it with your doctor.

Type	Onset After Eating
Campylobacter	2–10 days
Clostridium perfringens	9–15 hours
Hepatitis A	15–50 days
Norwalk virus	1–2 days.
Salmonella	6–48 hours.
Scombroid poisoning	5–60 minutes.
Staphylococcus	30 minutes –8 hours

EXCESS AIR

Intestinal gas is usually caused by swallowing too much air while you eat or drink. It can also be created by the fermentation of incompletely digested carbohydrates, such as the unabsorbed sugars from milk and some high-fiber foods. (The health benefits of a high-fiber diet, however, far outweigh an occasional bout of gas.) You can cut down on gas by eating slowly, avoiding carbonated drinks, and giving up smoking. Over-the-counter products to reduce gas may provide some relief, but if you are on medication, check with your doctor to make sure that they don't interfere with the absorption of your drugs.

If you experience a sudden onset of excess gas and bloating—particularly when you haven't been eating foods associated with gas—call your doctor.

A 24-HOUR STOMACH UPSET

Intestinal (or stomach) flu, called gastroenteritis by your doctor, is a nasty but usually short-lived infection brought on by either viruses or bacteria. The disease usually involves nausea, vomiting, diarrhea, muscle aches, headache, and fever. Because dehydration can result from the excessive loss of fluids, it is very important, as soon as the vomiting has stopped, to take sips of

FOOD-POISONING FACTS

Food poisoning, or bacterial contamination, is often mistaken for stomach flu because the symptoms can be similar. Unfortunately, there is often no way of knowing if food is contaminated until it is eaten. You can, however, learn to choose foods more carefully and to handle food more safely—keeping hot foods hot (140°F or above) and cold foods cold (40°F or below) and minimizing the time that any food is left at the temperatures in between, which encourage bacterial growth. Most food-poisoning symptoms last only a few days and can be treated with rest and replacement liquids. If your symptoms are severe, however, or you have a chronic disease or an impaired immune system, you should call a doctor immediately. Some forms of food poisoning can be fatal if you don't get help right away.

Symptoms	Foods Found In	Preventive Measures
Muscle pain, nausea, vomiting, fever, and cramps; occasionally bloody diarrhea.	Meat, poultry, eggs, unpasteurized dairy products, fish, shellfish, and untreated water.	Cook meat, poultry, and eggs thoroughly; wash hands and work surfaces before and after contact with raw animal products; don't drink unpasteurized milk or untreated water.
Diarrhea and cramps.	Meat and poultry.	Keep cooked foods above 140°F while serving; store at 40°F or lower; reheat leftovers thoroughly.
Fever, nausea, abdominal pain, and loss of appetite; after 3–10 days, dark urine and jaundice.	Raw shellfish, untreated water, and any food handled by contaminated people.	Wash hands thoroughly and frequently; avoid raw shellfish.
Nausea, vomiting, diarrhea, and headache.	Raw shellfish and any food handled by contaminated people.	Wash hands thoroughly and frequently; avoid raw shellfish.
Nausea, vomiting, diarrhea, cramps, fever, and headache.	Meat, poultry, eggs, and unpasteurized dairy products.	Cook meat, poultry, and eggs thoroughly; wash hands and work surfaces before and after contact with raw animal products; don't let foods sit at room temperature for more than 2 hours; don't drink unpasteurized milk.
Facial flushing, headache, dizziness, burning sensation in the throat, hives, nausea, vomiting, and abdominal pain.	Mackerel, tuna, and bonito.	Make sure fish is fresh; if it has a peppery taste, stop eating it.
Vomiting and diarrhea; occasionally weakness and dizziness.	Cooked meat and poultry; meat, poultry, potato, and egg salads; cream-filled pastries.	Cooking does *not* inactivate the staph toxin; wash hands and utensils before preparing food; don't let food sit at room temperature for more than 2 hours.

water, flat ginger ale, or weak tea at 15-minute intervals. Acute gastroenteritis usually runs its course within 24 hours. Vomiting that lasts longer than 6 hours requires medical attention.

Gastroenteritis is easily confused with food poisoning (see chart, pp.256–257).

DIARRHEA

Watery stools, or diarrhea, may be caused by a change in diet, a different drinking water, or new medications (antibiotics or high blood pressure drugs, for example). Diarrhea may also result from a viral or bacterial infection.

Mild cases usually clear up in a day or two. To treat diarrhea, you need to replenish the fluids your body has lost and soothe your irritated intestinal tract. Drink water, clear broth, flat soda pop, or apple juice (no citrus juices, coffee, tea, or alcohol). Try eating dry crackers, rice, or half of a plain baked potato.

If you have diarrhea longer than 48 hours or if it is accompanied by a fever of 101°F or higher, severe cramping, blood in your stools, lightheadedness, or dizziness (a sign of dehydration), call your doctor immediately. Also, if you are on a medication when you experience an attack of diarrhea, check with your doctor. The drug may be flushed out of your system too quickly to take effect.

CONSTIPATION

The difficult passage of hard, dry stools—not infrequent bowel movements—defines the condition called constipation. Healthy people vary widely in how often they regularly move their bowels;

> **❝***If your stomach disputes you, lie down and pacify it with cool thoughts.***❞**
>
> —*Baseball Hall of Famer Satchel Paige in his book,* How to Stay Young

for one person, three times a day may be normal, while for another, once every 3 days is standard.

Constipation in older people often results from a poor diet and lack of exercise. Sometimes a new medication (such as a codeine painkiller or an antidepressant) will cause it. Travel and stress can trigger constipation in many people.

The best way to avoid—and to treat—constipation is to eat a balanced diet that contains plenty of fiber (whole-grain cereals and breads, fruits, vegetables, and legumes), to drink six or more glasses of fluid a day (coffee and tea don't count because they are diuretics and drain liquid from your system), and to exercise regularly (see Chapter 3). Also, don't put off going to the bathroom when you feel the urge and don't rush yourself once you are there. Use a laxative only as a last resort or on the advice of your doctor.

Overuse of laxatives can make the problem worse because your system becomes dependent on them. Discuss persistent constipation with your doctor, who may prescribe stool-softening pills or suppositories.

HEMORRHOIDS

Swollen and distended veins inside the rectum or around the anal opening, medically known as hemorrhoids, are very common in both men and women over 50. Some people are genetically prone to hemorrhoids, which are similar to varicose veins on the legs.

Hemorrhoids are aggravated by the straining associated with constipation. To make stools softer and easier to pass—thereby helping to prevent hemorrhoids—stick to a high-fiber diet and drink plenty of nonalcoholic liquids. Regular exercise will also help make your digestive system run smoother.

Despite precautions, however, you may still develop hemorrhoids. If they are not too bothersome, you can let them heal on their own. To help reduce the swelling in the meantime, you can put an ice pack on the affected area or soak in a few inches of warm water (a sitz bath) two or three times a day. To soothe irritation, apply zinc oxide ointment or petroleum jelly. (Despite all the advertising claims, no over-the-counter drug actually shrinks hemorrhoids.) If you get no relief, see your doctor.

Internal hemorrhoids can be especially painful and may require removal in a doctor's office by one of several methods—rubber band ligation, freezing, burning, or laser treatment.

STAYING WELL WHILE TRAVELING

Nothing spoils a vacation more than an unexpected bout of even a minor sickness. Although you can't travel in a sterile glass bubble, there are some measures you can take to keep yourself comfortable and able to cope when things go temporarily sour on a trip. For ways to stay in shape while traveling, see *Keeping Fit on the Road,* p.110.

On an airplane, drink plenty of water and avoid alcoholic drinks to prevent dehydration of your body and your skin (the cabin air is very dry). If you have a cold and have to fly, take a decongestant 30 minutes before takeoff and 30 minutes before landing. Swallowing or yawning opens your nose and ear passages, equalizing pressure and preventing pain.

In a car or on a boat, prevent motion sickness by taking an over-the-counter drug; if you are highly susceptible, ask your doctor for a prescription of scopolamine, a drug that is administered through a patch behind the ear. The patch slowly releases a regulated dose of medication.

Minimize jet lag by using the sun to reset your internal clock. Arriving at an eastern destination, bask in the morning sunlight (it will help you wake up earlier the next day). In the west, stay outdoors in the afternoon sun to push back your bedtime.

Avoid insects and insect-borne diseases where they are a potential problem by wearing protective clothing outdoors, using an insect repellant on your clothes, and avoiding perfumes or scented after-shave lotions, which attract insects. Stay indoors, protected behind screens or mosquito netting, from dusk until dawn.

Pack enough of your regular medications so that they last for the duration of your trip—and a few extra days to cover unexpected delays. Stow these drugs in your carry-on luggage in case the bags you've checked get lost. Also, take a copy of all prescriptions, which can be filled if your drugs get lost. For convenience, pack a medicine kit with your favorite analgesic, antacid, decongestant, diarrhea medicine, mild laxative, sunscreen, anti-itch ointment, antiseptic, and adhesive bandages. Take an extra pair of eyeglasses and a copy of the prescription.

If you travel to high altitudes (above 5,000 feet), give your body, several days to adjust to the thinner air before you try any strenuous outings. Avoid alcohol; its effects may be exaggerated at high altitudes.

When traveling abroad, consult the Centers for Disease Control in Atlanta well ahead of your trip to find out if you will need any vaccinations to visit the stops on your itinerary. If you need immunizations, get them early enough to be over any ill effects before you leave. To prevent traveler's diarrhea in underdeveloped countries, avoid drinking local tap water (including ice); use bottled water even to brush your teeth. Eat only fruits and vegetables that you peel yourself. Don't eat raw shellfish, rare-cooked meats, or dairy products (there's no way to tell if they've been pasteurized).

KEEPING YOUR FEET HEALTHY

*F*eet bear the brunt of all your weight-bearing activities, the walking and jogging that keep your heart fit and your bones strong. A little preventive care (pp.166–167) goes a long way in maintaining feet, but sometimes problems do develop.

ATHLETE'S FOOT

A fungal infection that flourishes in warm and moist places, athlete's foot attacks the skin of the toes, soles, or sides of your feet and causes itchy blisters and scaling. It can usually be cleared up with an over-the-counter antifungal medication that contains either miconazole or tolnaftate. If the condition persists longer than 2 weeks, however, see your doctor for a prescription drug.

To prevent athlete's foot, keep your feet clean and dry. Use an antifungal powder regularly (p. 166). Wear shoes made of materials that breathe, such as leather and canvas, and socks that wick away moisture (an acrylic and cotton mix, for example). Always let your shoes—especially sneakers or running shoes—dry out completely between wearings. Rotate your shoes daily, allowing a day or so between wearings.

BLISTERS

Caused by continuous friction against the skin, liquid-filled blisters should be covered with a sterile gauze pad and allowed to heal on their own. You can protect the area from further irritation with a moleskin or cotton circle designed for that purpose and available from most drugstores.

If a blister is very large, you may want to puncture it. Sterilize a needle with antiseptic (not a match flame) and prick the edge of the blister. Blot up the liquid with gauze, clean the area with antiseptic, and cover it with a sterile gauze pad.

THE STRUCTURE OF THE FOOT
The human foot is an ingenious design of 26 bones held together with muscles, tendons, and ligaments. A sturdy base for standing, the foot is also pliant and mobile. The metatarsal bones that stretch from heel to toe give it amazing flexibility. The sole of the foot has a thick skin underlaid with a cushion of fat and fibrous tissue to absorb the weight of the entire body.

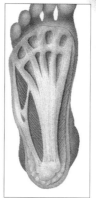

BUNIONS

The bony protrusion that some people develop at the base of the big toe is called a bunion. It may be hereditary or, in women, caused by wearing high-heeled shoes with pointed toes. Bunion sufferers should wear comfortable shoes that will not press on the affected bone. Soft pads or cushioned socks will give additional relief. Most bunions can simply be accommodated in this way. If osteoarthritis or bursitis makes a bunion chronically painful, however, your doctor may recommend surgery to realign the distorted bones.

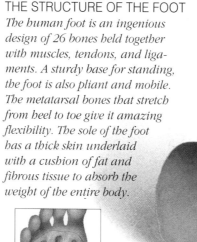

Painful heel syndrome. *A tear or swelling in the padding around your heel bone (circular area at bottom of drawing at left), this soreness is seldom caused by a bone spur, as doctors once believed.*

CORNS

Like calluses (p.166), corns are caused by rubbing and friction on cramped toes. Hard corns develop on top of toes, soft corns between toes. Both can be prevented by wearing comfortable shoes that fit properly.

You can remove some corns yourself. Soak your feet in warm water every day and gently rub the built-up skin with a towel or a pumice stone—the surface will gradually peel away. Never slice a corn with a razor blade; if the growth is stubborn or painful, see a podiatrist. In the interim, use lambswool or moleskin pads to protect the tender spots.

HAMMERTOES

A deformity that develops in the joint of the second, third, or fourth toe, a hammertoe is more common in women than in men and probably results from wearing high heels with pointed toes. Protective pads can bring relief, or your podiatrist may suggest wearing an orthotic brace to maneuver the bent toe into a more comfortable position. In severe cases, surgery may be required.

SMART SHOE BUYING

The most common cause of foot problems is uncomfortable shoes that don't fit. Some tips for shopping:
■ Always have your feet measured (sizes vary among manufacturers) and go with the size of the larger foot (no two feet are exactly alike). Try on both shoes and walk around.
■ Shop in the afternoon, when your feet tend to be swollen.
■ Be sure that a new shoe is long enough—that there is ½ inch from your toe tip to the end of the shoe—and that the width is adequate through the broadest part of your foot.
■ Don't buy uncomfortable shoes assuming that they will stretch. Buy shoes that feel good when you purchase them.
■ As the padding under your feet thins with age, look for a shoe style with a thicker, more shock-absorbing sole.

INGROWN TOENAILS

An ingrown toenail usually develops when either corner of a big toenail grows into the flesh of the toe, causing redness, swelling, pain, and sometimes infection.

A doctor or podiatrist can cut away the ingrown nail and treat the infection with antibiotics. To prevent further trouble, make sure that your shoes don't put undue pressure on the nails of your big toes. Cut your toenails straight across at the end of the toe.

If, after several treatments, an ingrown toenail keeps recurring, ask your podiatrist about surgical options for preventing it.

PAINFUL HEEL SYNDROME

As you grow older, the heel's fatty tissue thins out. Pressure on the heel causes inflammation of the connective tissue and muscle. The pain is greatest in the morning when you first stand up.

For acute discomfort, take an analgesic and apply an ice pack to the heel for 15 minutes. Gently massage and stretch the foot and elevate it whenever you can. Ask your doctor for shock-absorbing heel inserts. During an attack, which can last several months, limit your exercise to non-weight-bearing activities such as swimming and bicycling.

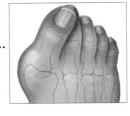

Bunion. *A minor deformity, a bunion occurs when the big toe overlaps the next toe, pushing the big toe's joint out beyond the foot's normal profile.*

INGROWN TOENAILS

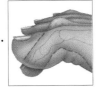

Hammertoe. *Usually a second toe problem, hammertoe may affect both toe joints, locking the bones into a clawlike curve.*

HARD CORNS

SOFT CORNS

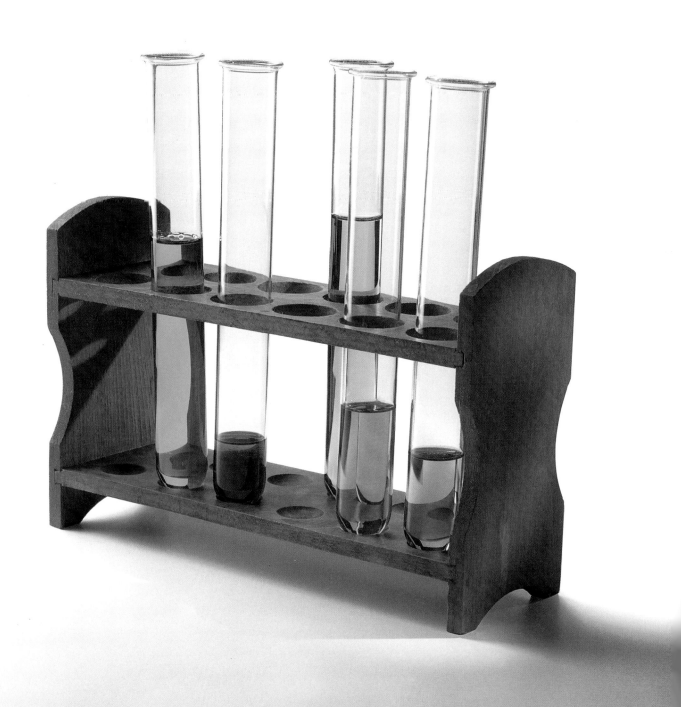

Chapter 7

LIVING WITH CHRONIC CONDITIONS AND SERIOUS ILLNESS

. . . .

PROTECTING VULNERABLE SKIN *264*

COPING WITH YOUR ACHES AND PAINS *266*

BREAKDOWNS IN THE BRAIN AND NERVOUS SYSTEM *272*

TROUBLES WITH THE ENDOCRINE SYSTEM *280*

PRESERVING YOUR EYESIGHT *284*

DIFFICULTIES WITH HEARING *290*

PROBLEMS THAT CAN AFFECT YOUR LUNGS *292*

CIRCULATORY SYSTEM DISORDERS *296*

DYSFUNCTION IN THE DIGESTIVE SYSTEM *308*

MALFUNCTIONS IN THE URINARY SYSTEM *316*

POSSIBLE PROBLEMS FOR MATURE MEN *318*

POSSIBLE PROBLEMS FOR MATURE WOMEN *320*

Protecting Vulnerable Skin

The largest multisensory organ of your body, your skin serves as a biological shield that protects you from the environment. With time, however, your skin becomes thinner, less resilient, and more susceptible to chronic diseases and injury.

INCREASED BRUISING

Older skin bruises more easily. The tissues that hold tiny blood vessels near the surface of the skin tend to shrink as you grow older, making the blood vessels more apt to rupture when the body takes a blow (or you take a fall). If the vessels break, blood leaks into the surrounding area, creating a bruise.

Dramatic as bruises may look, they usually clear up on their own within a week or two. You can reduce the pain and swelling of a large bruise by applying a cold compress with some pressure as soon as possible after the injury. Leaving the compress in place for at least 10 minutes helps to constrict the blood vessels and stop further bleeding.

Clusters of irregularly shaped, dusky purple patches on the forearms, hands, waist, or legs are characteristic of a type of bruise called senile purpura, which is particularly common in people over the age of 60. These bruises tend to fade within a week or two, and no treatment is needed.

See your doctor if a bruise persists for longer than 2 weeks, develops for no apparent reason, or appears more severe than the injury warrants. Such bruising can signal other problems.

SHINGLES

More common in older people than in younger adults, shingles is a condition caused by the re-emergence of the varicella zoster, or chicken pox, virus. In about 10 to 20 percent of adults who had chicken pox as children, the virus

BEDSORES

Bedridden people of all ages are at risk for bedsores, or pressure sores, but the older you are and the thinner your skin, the greater the danger. Bedsores start out as tender red spots; if pressure continues, they develop into open sores, which can easily become infected and destroy underlying tissue.

Although they can materialize on any weight-bearing part of the body, bedsores are most likely to develop where the bones are near the surface of the skin (see right). The constant pressure of skin against bone constricts the blood vessels and deprives the skin of its normal supply of nutrients.

Bedsores are easier to prevent than to treat. Change body position at least once every 2 hours and use egg-crate-shaped foam mattress pads, noncompressible pillows, or sheepskin pads to cushion potential pressure points.

If you (or someone you are caring for) develop a bedsore, call the doctor immediately. Bedsore infections, especially in the elderly, can be life-threatening.

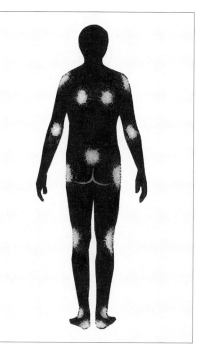

lies dormant in nerve tissue and resurfaces as a painful rash up to 50 or more years later.

The earliest symptoms of shingles are pain and a heightened sensitivity in an isolated area of skin, almost always on one side of the face or one side of the body. You may also feel a general fatigue and have a low-grade fever. Within a few days, an inflammatory rash appears, accompanied by tiny, clear blisters. The blisters eventually turn brown, dry out, and form crusts, which drop off. During the blister stage, the virus is contagious and can cause chicken pox in people who are not immune.

In the early stages of a shingles attack, mild pain can be reduced with an analgesic such as aspirin or acetaminophen and cool compresses soaked in Burow's solution applied to the affected skin.

For more severe cases, administration of the antiviral drug acyclovir within 48 hours of the onset of shingles may offer relief and shorten the course of the attack. Some doctors have also had success in controlling cases of shingles with cortisone medications. If a secondary bacterial infection of the blisters develops, it is treated with antibiotics.

SKIN CANCER

A lifetime of sunbathing takes more than a cosmetic toll—doctors find that more than 90 percent of all skin cancers are caused by overexposure to the sun during youth. The three types of skin cancer are pictured below.

■ *Basal cell carcinoma,* which usually starts as a fleshy bump on the face, ears, or hands, is the most common.

■ *Squamous cell carcinoma,* which grows more rapidly and can spread to other parts of the body, most often begins as a red scaly patch on sun-exposed skin, such as the face, rims of the ears, forearms, or tops of the hands. Both basal cell and squamous cell cancers, when brought to a doctor's attention early, are easily cured by surgical removal.

■ *Malignant melanoma,* a less common and sometimes deadly skin cancer, may develop around a molelike growth or appear spontaneously anywhere on the skin. Malignant melanomas are considered dangerous because they can quickly metastasize, invading deep into the skin and spreading cancer cells to other parts of the body.

Check your skin regularly (p.227). If you spot anything unusual—a change in the size, shape, or color of a familiar blemish or new scaling, oozing, crusting, or bleeding—see your dermatologist. Check with your doctor if a skin growth suddenly feels itchy, tender, or painful.

To recognize a malignant melanoma, the American Cancer Society suggests remembering ABCDE: Asymmetry, that is, the two sides of the sore don't match. Border irregularity, meaning the edges of the growth are ragged and uneven. Color variation from one part of the growth to another. Diameter greater than 6 millimeters or about the size of a pencil eraser (many dermatologists, however, suggest that you have a growth checked before it reaches this relatively large size). Elevation, that is, the growth sticks up from the skin.

The type, size, and location of the tumor determines how it is removed. The options include conventional surgery, electrodesiccation (removal of the tumor with electric current), cryosurgery (freezing), and radiation therapy. The earlier a melanoma is detected, the safer its removal can be.

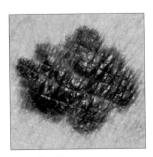

Basal cell carcinoma

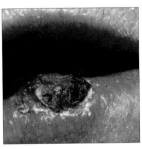

Squamous cell carcinoma

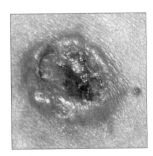

Malignant melanoma

DANGEROUS LESIONS
The sample skin cancer eruptions shown at left give you a general idea of what to look for when you make a monthly check of your body. Not all skin cancers look exactly like these, however; have a doctor check any suspicious growths.

COPING WITH
YOUR ACHES AND PAINS

Years of repetitive use can't help but have an effect on the joints. About 80 percent of all people over the age of 65 have some degenerative joint changes, and in about 60 percent, the changes have progressed enough to cause pain.

OSTEOARTHRITIS

Arthritis is the general term for a group of disorders caused by the inflammation of the joints and their surrounding tissues. One type, osteoarthritis, is common in older people, and develops when the cartilage that acts as a shock absorber between the joints gradually deteriorates. In time, the ends of the bones may be damaged from rubbing together.

Symptoms include joint pain, swelling, and loss of flexibility. People often experience stiffness in the morning; later, the accumulation of the day's stresses and activities may result in pain that continues into the night.

Treatment

There is no cure for osteoarthritis, but there are several approaches to treating it. Exercises worked out by a doctor or a physical therapist can help, as can range-of-motion and muscle-strengthening exercises. Heat—baths, hot-water bottles, and heating pads—may offer relief too. So may cold treatments. Ask your doctor which method is best for you. Aspirin and other anti-inflammatory agents can reduce pain. For severe attacks, your doctor may inject a corticosteroid drug. Arthroscopic surgery may help joint mobility by excising damaged tissue.

RHEUMATOID ARTHRITIS

Another major type of arthritis, rheumatoid arthritis, appears to be an autoimmune disease, a condition in which the body develops antibodies against its own tissues. Unlike osteoarthritis, rheumatoid arthritis affects more than one joint at a time and does so in a symmetrical fashion—that is, on both sides of the body (both knees, for instance, not just one). This rheumatic disease can also involve the eyes, heart, lungs, and other organs.

The disease's main target is the synovial membrane lining the joints, which becomes inflamed. The chronic inflammation slowly wears away the surrounding ligaments, muscles, and bones and ultimately damages the joints.

The symptoms of rheumatoid arthritis include redness, swelling, and warmth in a joint, as well as overall achiness and stiffness and loss of muscle strength. Some victims may develop deformed

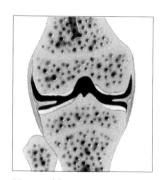

Normal knee joint

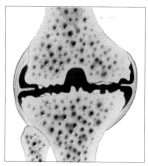

Knee joint with osteoarthritis

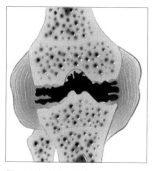

Knee joint with rheumatoid arthritis

In the osteoarthritic knee, the cartilage that covers the ends of the bones in the normal knee is eroded. In the rheumatoid knee, the synovial membrane is excessively swollen and the cartilage is being eaten away.

PROBLEMS IN YOUR BONES AND JOINTS

Over time, your bones begin to show signs of wear as well as the effects of hormonal and other physiological changes.

Osteoarthritis, *the "wear and tear" arthritis, usually strikes the finger, knee, and hip joints and the bones of the spine. Sometimes bony lumps grow on the middle or end joints of the fingers; such bone spurs do not ordinarily interfere with the use of the hands.*

Rheumatoid arthritis *may initially make its presence known by causing pain and swelling in the small joints of the hands and feet. The disease can also attack joints in the wrists, elbows, shoulders, neck, hips, knees, and ankles.*

Osteoporosis *can weaken bone to such an extent that fractures, especially of the hip and wrist, can occur spontaneously or with very little pressure. Compression fractures of the spine are also common; over time, these can result in some loss of height and the stooped-over posture known as dowager's hump.*

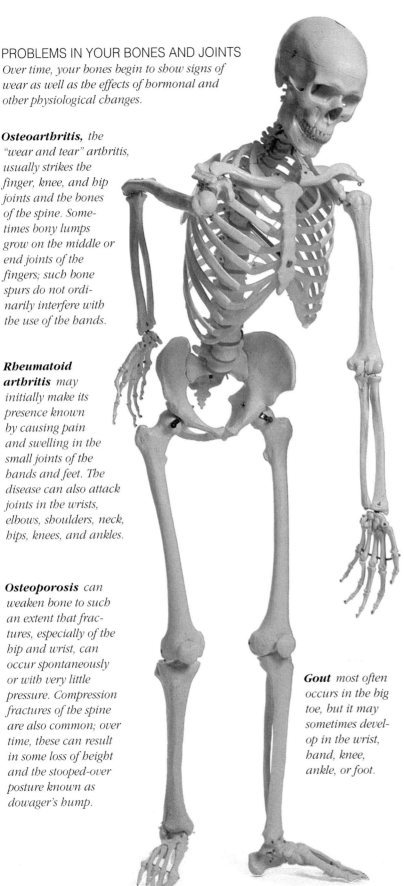

Gout *most often occurs in the big toe, but it may sometimes develop in the wrist, hand, knee, ankle, or foot.*

limbs, although the joints themselves may remain flexible.

Treatment

In addition to aspirin, several other drugs may help. They include nonsteroidal anti-inflammatory drugs (NSAID's), corticosteroids, penicillamine, methotrexate, antimalarial agents, and gold salt pills or injections.

Adequate rest and exercise are important in managing the condition. Hot treatments—a bath or shower, heating pads, hot packs, and heat lamps—can also help. Cold treatments—cold compresses or ice cubes wrapped in towels—will numb the affected area and help reduce swelling. Your doctor or therapist can advise you about which type of treatment is preferable in your case.

Sometimes surgery can prevent or correct joint deformity as well as relieve pain. Arthroscopic surgery to remove damaged tissue can enable the joint to move more easily.

. . . .

GOUT

Commonly affecting the base of the big toe, gout is the third major kind of arthritis. It may be caused by a hereditary malfunction that leads to excess uric acid in the blood. The uric acid tends to crystallize in the spaces between the joints, which results in pain and inflammation.

Attacks of gout can strike without warning, but they are often linked to specific triggers, including alcohol, organ meats, stress, and such trauma as surgery or a heart attack. Fortunately, gout can almost always be controlled. Ask your doctor about changing your diet to avoid foods rich in purine, a substance that fosters the devel-

LIVING WITH ARTHRITIS

JOINT REPLACEMENT

A person who is crippled or severely limited by arthritis can regain a good deal of mobility as well as relieve pain with a joint replacement.

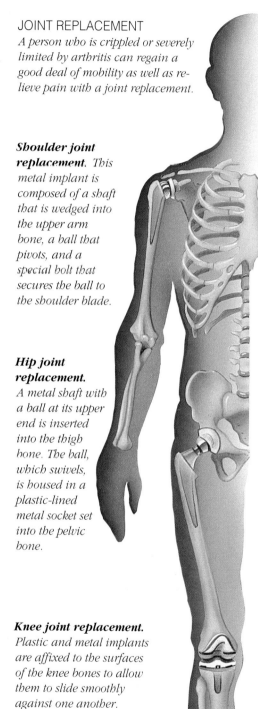

Shoulder joint replacement. *This metal implant is composed of a shaft that is wedged into the upper arm bone, a ball that pivots, and a special bolt that secures the ball to the shoulder blade.*

Hip joint replacement. *A metal shaft with a ball at its upper end is inserted into the thigh bone. The ball, which swivels, is housed in a plastic-lined metal socket set into the pelvic bone.*

Knee joint replacement. *Plastic and metal implants are affixed to the surfaces of the knee bones to allow them to slide smoothly against one another.*

There are many ways to make your life easier when you have arthritis. Going about your daily activities more efficiently (see p.253) can help reduce the stress placed on your joints. So can making some simple changes in how you handle ordinary tasks. For instance, use your larger joints whenever possible: push open a door with your hip instead of your hand, or twist open a jar with your palm instead of your fingers. Lift an object with both arms rather than with one. And be careful not to bend your joints in an awkward or unnatural fashion.

Many household aids designed for people with arthritis are sold through surgical supply houses and mail order catalogs (see right). In some cases, an occupational therapist may need to show you how best to utilize these tools.

Other helping devices available with the guidance of your doctor or therapist include splints, canes, walkers, and crutches. Used during the day or at night, splints give joints and muscles a chance to rest by taking over the task of holding your joints in place. Walkers, canes, and crutches help you to walk by relieving your lower body joints of some of your body weight. If you have rheumatoid arthritis, consult your doctor or therapist about footwear. Shoes that don't fit properly can result in foot deformity and disability.

Exercise plays a key role in controlling arthritis because increasing muscle strength can help to stabilize your affected joints. Check with your doctor about the right program for you.

As a last resort after all other treatments have failed, people with very advanced arthritis can get new joints made of synthetic materials (see left). Hips and knees are the joints most often replaced. The procedure is expensive, however, and the artificial joints themselves may need replacing in about 15 years. But newly developed materials may extend this time span to 30 years.

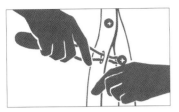

A button book enables you to fasten clothes with less trouble.

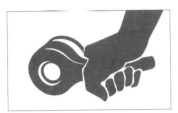

This turner attaches to the knob to help you open the door.

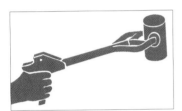

With this reacher, you don't have to strain to grasp items.

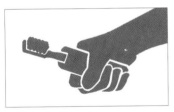

A foam holder gives you a more secure grip on your toothbrush.

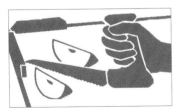

This special board and knife make cutting up food easier.

opment of uric acid. For individual attacks, the prescription drug colchicine is often effective, as are NSAID's. Between flare-ups, the drugs probenecid, sulfinpyrazone, or allopurinol may be prescribed as a preventive.

OSTEOPOROSIS

Although worn-out bone is constantly being replenished, after about the age of 35, a little more bone is lost than is restored. This loss does not affect men to any great extent because their bones are generally much denser than those of women. For women, however, the situation is more serious because bone loss speeds up after menopause.

White and Asian women with small frames are most at risk, especially those with a family history of the disease or those who had their ovaries removed at an early age. In their later years, men can also develop the condition.

Because there are usually no symptoms, osteoporosis may go untreated until the bones become so thin that they break. X-rays can detect osteoporosis only when it is in an advanced stage. It may be discovered earlier by other diagnostic techniques such as dual photon densitometry, which measures bone density by exposing the bone to a tiny dose of radioactivity and recording the amount of radiation absorbed.

Prevention

It's never too early for a woman to start protecting herself against osteoporosis. Eating calcium-rich foods will help increase and maintain bone protein and calcium. The best calcium sources are milk, yogurt, and cheese. Second best are sardines and salmon canned with bones, oysters, tofu, and green vegetables such as kale and broccoli. Experts recommend that women include at least 1,000 milligrams of calcium in their daily diet. After menopause, those women not undergoing estrogen-replacement therapy should add another 500 milligrams a day. Although it's best to try to get this mostly from food, supplements such as calcium carbonate can also be taken.

Treatment

There are three major drug treatments for osteoporosis. Estrogen decreases bone loss and helps maintain bone mass, but it increases the risk of other conditions (see p.239). The hormone calcitonin helps regulate calcium metabolism and inhibits bone loss. Another drug, etidronate, blocks bone loss and adds bone mass. Studies show that it may also reduce the risk of fractures.

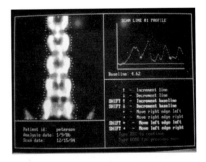

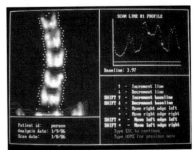

Above, a spinal column with healthy dense bone; below, a spinal column affected by osteoporosis.

Profile

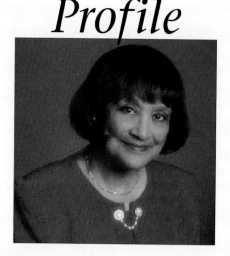

JUANITA WATSON: "WITHOUT PAIN FOR THE FIRST TIME IN YEARS"

During the late 1970's, Chicago resident Juanita Watson began to suffer from the swelling and inflammation of degenerative osteoarthritis in her hips and knees. She had aquatic therapy and took cortisone, but her condition steadily worsened until she had no more cartilage in her right hip. "My doctor said that if I didn't have hip replacement surgery, I would become crippled," says Watson.

Following surgery in 1987, Watson embarked on a rigorous course of rehabilitation. "After the first day, I was so exhausted I nearly cried myself to sleep," she says. Gradually she progressed from walking with crutches to walking with canes to jubilantly walking on her own. "I was without pain for the first time in years," she reports. She has since had her left knee and left hip replaced.

"If you learn how to cope with arthritis, you can lead a pretty normal life," says Watson, who does volunteer work with a community council at a local university and also campaigned door to door to win election to her neighborhood school council. "My major goal was to be able to get down on the floor with my grandchildren, and I made it!"

PREVENTING FALLS AND FRACTURES

Osteoporosis is one reason why older people are at risk of falls and fractures. Another is that as people age, they become less co-ordinated because of natural changes in muscle strength, re-flexes, eyesight, hearing, and bal-ance. Chronic conditions such as diabetes and heart disease also af-fect balance, and some prescrip-tion drugs may cause dizziness.

Many of the bone-breaking falls older Americans suffer each year could be prevented by fol-lowing these safety guidelines:

■ Have your vision and hearing tested regularly.

■ Don't sit up suddenly when you awaken or stand abruptly af-ter eating or sitting. The resulting sudden drop in your blood pres-sure can cause dizziness.

■ Avoid sitting in low chairs—they are difficult to get out of.

■ Set your home's thermostat above 65°F; low body tempera-tures can lead to dizziness.

■ Wear supportive, low-heeled, rubber-soled shoes rather than socks or slippers that can slip on stairs or waxed floors.

■ Keep stairways and hallways well lit and clutter free.

■ Place wires and cords out of the way; secure carpets firmly in place; arrange the furniture so that you don't bump into it.

■ Put a night light in your bed-room, hallway, bathroom, and any other places you tend to go during the night.

■ Make sure that bathtubs and showers have nonskid mats and grab bars; a grab bar should also be next to the toilet.

■ When you're away from home, plan your path to the bathroom before you go to sleep. Make sure it is clear of obstructions.

CHRONIC PAIN: A COMMON PROBLEM

Pain that lasts longer than 6 months, has no obvious cause, and does not respond to treatment is considered chronic. It affects an estimated 60 million Americans. Fortunately, in recent years there have been new developments in its diagnosis and therapy. Chronic pain is now recognized to be entirely different from acute pain and to require a totally opposite approach. Acute pain is a symptom of an injury or a disease; it is alleviated by treating the underlying cause. With chronic pain, the pain itself is the disease. Today in pain clinics throughout the country, teams of specialists work to relieve all types of chronic pain, including headache, neck and back pain, arthritis pain, muscle pain, facial pain, pain caused by the injury or compression of a nerve, postherpetic neuralgia due to shingles, pain in "phantom" amputated limbs, and pain of unknown origin.

TREATMENT

The first step in handling chronic pain is usually to ease patients off narcotic pain relievers (if they are on them). Then a comprehensive rehabilitation program is worked out to deal with the pain and to improve the patient's quality of life. Medication is one option: Aspirin, acetaminophen, and ibuprofen may help some types of pain. For people with chronic headaches, diabetic neuropathy, arthritis, facial pain, or back pain, tricyclic antidepressants may be effective.

Physical therapy can also prove useful since chronic pain is often exacerbated by lack of exercise, poor posture, overprotectiveness of the injured area, and a heightened sensitivity in the body's pain-sensing mechanisms. A regular exercise program can help make the muscles that surround and support the joints stronger, improve the body's mobility and flexibility, and provide an overall feeling of well-being. Occu-

pational therapy assists patients in managing their daily lives with graded programs in which their activity levels are slowly increased. Other treatment options for chronic pain include meditation, progressive relaxation techniques, biofeedback, guided imagery, hypnosis, acupuncture, transcutaneous electrical nerve stimulation (TENS), and psychological counseling.

DEALING WITH BACK PAIN

The most common form of chronic pain is persistent or recurring back pain. In some cases, the pain may be a symptom of a disorder of the lungs, heart, blood vessels, or kidneys. Most often, however, the pain is the result of arthritis or some other spinal disease such as disc prolapse, sciatica, lumbar stenosis, spinal arthritis (ankylosing spondylitis), or a bone disease such as osteoporosis or bone cancer. In addition to medical treatment, back pain may be temporarily relieved by applications of heat or cold (see p.252). Performing your everyday activities correctly can also help (see p. 253).

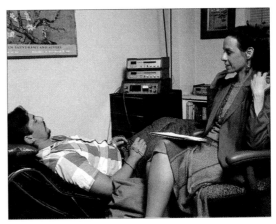

Through a series of biofeedback training sessions at a pain clinic, this patient will learn how to reduce the muscle tension that contributes to the severity of his pain.

BREAKDOWNS IN THE BRAIN AND NERVOUS SYSTEM

The complexities of the brain and nervous system are, with the use of sophisticated scanners, beginning to be more clearly understood. Although many perplexing questions remain unanswered, progress has been made in the prevention and treatment of such diseases as stroke, parkinsonism, dementia, and depression.

STROKE

Contrary to what many people think, strokes are both preventable and treatable. Although stroke remains the third most lethal disease in the United States, after heart disease and cancer, improved care and the control of such risk factors as high blood pressure and diabetes have cut the death rate for stroke to less than half of what it was in 1950.

Stroke, a form of cardiovascular disease, is localized damage to the brain caused by an inadequate blood supply. The blood can't get through because an

TYPES OF STROKES

Most strokes are caused by a blood clot that forms in a plaque-narrowed artery (cerebral thrombosis) or by a blood clot that has traveled from somewhere else (cerebral embolism). Strokes also occur when an artery bursts and blood hemorrhages either inside the brain (cerebral hemorrhage) or in the subarachnoid space between the brain and the skull.

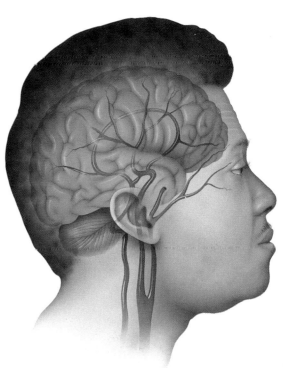

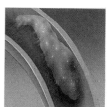

Thrombosis

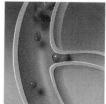

Embolism

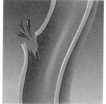

Hemorrhage

artery is blocked by a blood clot or the artery has burst. The medical term for a stroke is a cerebrovascular accident (CVA).

Brain cells can survive for only a few minutes without oxygen. They do not rejuvenate themselves. And when they die, the part of the body they controlled loses function. Depending on the specific area of the brain involved, this may affect speech, vision, use of the limbs, walking, balance, swallowing, sensation, thought, memory, consciousness, or behavior.

THE BRAIN IN CROSS SECTION

The major organ of the central nervous system, the brain controls all the body's activities, voluntary and involuntary. The largest part of the brain, the cerebrum is the source of consciousness and intelligence.

The cerebral cortex, *a thin shell of gray matter that covers the cerebrum, is where the brain performs cognitive functions such as thought and memory.*

The cerebrum *consists of left and right hemispheres joined by the corpus callosum.*

The corpus callosum, *a major communications exchange, contains more than 200 million nerve fibers.*

The occipital lobe *is the brain's vision center.*

The cerebellum *coordinates body movements and maintains posture.*

The brain stem *controls such vital functions as breathing and heart rate.*

The substantia nigra *houses the nerve cells that dispense the neurotransmitter dopamine.*

The thalamus *filters impulses from the sensory organs and relays them to the cortex.*

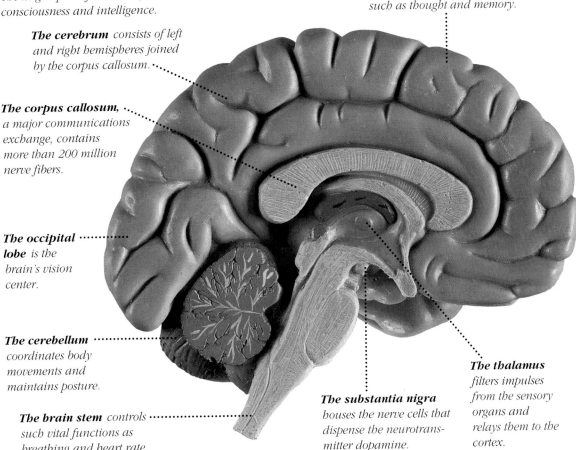

The Risk Factors

Middle-aged men are more likely to have a stroke than middle-aged women, but later the risks level out. After 65, the incidence of stroke rises sharply for both sexes. People of any age who have already had a full stroke or a short-lived ministroke called a transient ischemic attack, or TIA (p.275), are more at risk than others. People who have a family history of strokes are also more likely to have one.

The risk factors for stroke that you can do something about are diabetes, heart disease, and high

---

WARNING SIGNS OF A STROKE

Although a stroke may strike suddenly, there are often warning signs. Immediate care at a hospital or by an emergency medical team can save your life and minimize any permanent damage. Act quickly if you—or a companion—experience any of the symptoms listed below:

■ Sudden weakness or numbness on one side of the face or in an arm or a leg
■ Sudden dimness or double vision, particularly in only one eye or in one area of the visual field
■ Difficulty in speaking or understanding speech
■ Sudden severe headache
■ Unexplained dizziness or loss of balance

SURVIVING A STROKE

Anyone who has a major stroke belongs in a hospital where an emergency team can monitor and maintain breathing and circulation. Once the patient's condition has stabilized, doctors must determine what caused the stroke and try to prevent another one from occurring. They may order a brain scan or other tests, and depending on the results, the patient may be given an anticoagulant to prevent blood clots or a diuretic to eliminate water and reduce brain swelling. Or surgery may be recommended to open blocked arteries, such as the carotid arteries in the neck.

In order to prevent bedsores, lung problems, muscle atrophy, and blood clots, passive physical therapy—manipulating joints and muscles—is started immediately.

REHABILITATION REGIMEN

The site of the stroke determines the impairments the patient is likely to suffer. In general, damage to the right side of the brain causes paralysis on the left side of the body, a loss of spatial perception, and forgetfulness. Damage to the left side of the brain causes paralysis on the right side of the body, speech impairment, and difficulties with understanding language.

Rehabilitation with the help of special therapists begins as soon as the patient is able and may continue at a rehabilitation hospital. The goal is to help patients become independent. They may need to develop new motor skills to do familiar tasks in a different way. Depending on the disability, the program typically includes one or more of the following: speech therapy; special exercises to regain movement and retrain uninjured nerves to take over some of the functions from damaged nerves; and whirlpool baths to ease muscle pain.

There are many devices—from canes and other walking aids to large-button phones and clothes with Velcro closures—you can order from catalogs to make daily life easier in the aftermath of a stroke.

HOW TO HELP

Because their new physical limitations frustrate them, stroke patients need encouragement and moral support from family and friends during rehabilitation. Everyone involved must recognize that recovery will take time, effort, and patience.

Some patients make a spontaneous recovery from a stroke within the first 30 days; others experience an almost complete recovery after months of working with therapists. Most stroke patients, however, suffer permanent disabilities and must learn to live with their limitations.

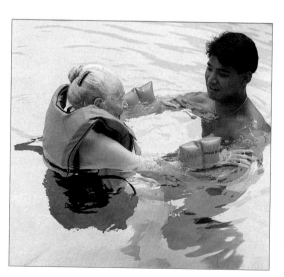

A stroke patient is helped through a water workout by her physical therapist. Water's buoyancy protects patients from impact injuries, while its resistance helps them build muscles.

blood pressure. A healthy lifestyle—eating a low-fat diet with limited intake of alcohol, exercising regularly, and giving up smoking—can keep these diseases in check. In addition, your doctor may recommend drugs or surgery to reduce your chances of having a stroke.

In some cases, small doses of aspirin or some other anticoagulant drug such as warfarin may be prescribed to help prevent blood clots. But don't take aspirin without first consulting with your doctor; for some people, aspirin increases the danger of cerebral hemorrhage.

If you are at risk for stroke, your doctor may order a test called a Doppler study, which uses sound waves to measure blood flow in the carotid arteries of the neck. If an obstruction is found, the doctor may recommend a surgical procedure called a carotid endarterectomy. In the hands of an experienced surgeon, this technique, which carries risks of its own, can help prevent strokes by removing the blockages in the carotid arteries.

TIA's

About 10 percent of full strokes are preceded by temporary interruptions in the blood supply to the brain called transient ischemic attacks (TIA's). These ministrokes, caused by a small clot that stops the flow of blood for a limited time, typically occur a few days or a few months before a full stroke and produce similar but milder symptoms that last from a few minutes to several hours.

TIA's, which have the same warning signs as full strokes (p. 273), are important alarms that shouldn't be ignored. Prompt medical attention can reduce the risk of a major stroke later.

PARKINSON'S DISEASE

James Parkinson, a British doctor, first described the disease that bears his name as "shaking palsy." A brain disorder that affects muscle control and movement, Parkinson's disease is caused by the progressive degeneration of cells in a part of the brain called the substantia nigra, which controls muscle coordination. The cells normally produce the chemical dopamine, a neurotransmitter.

When dopamine production diminishes, the symptoms of Parkinson's disease begin to appear: tremors in a resting hand, arm, or leg; stiff muscles and difficulty in initiating movement; a stooped posture and shuffling gait; a frozen facial expression; drooling; difficulty swallowing; and slow, hesitant speech.

Causes

Affecting mostly people in their sixties and older and more men than women, Parkinson's disease seems to be neither contagious nor hereditary. In fact, no one knows why the nerve cells that produce dopamine suddenly

> **❝ I looked around in surprise. There was no pain. You expect, when your life alters, a thunderclap. Nothing. ❞**
>
> *Choreographer Agnes de Mille, describing the stroke that immobilized her right side at age 69; at 82, still partially paralyzed, she presented a new ballet.*

LIVING WITH PARKINSON'S DISEASE

People with Parkinson's disease can help control their symptoms with a healthful diet and a regular exercise routine that stresses walking in a steady, relaxed rhythm. A physical therapist can suggest other helpful exercises.

A therapist may also suggest aids and adjustments that will make life easier and safer for the patient. For example, cups with spouts limit spills, and cutlery with thick handles is easier to grasp. Also, an electric stove is safer and simpler to operate than a gas stove; ramps are easier to master than stairs. In restaurants, waiters can be asked to cut up meat before serving it to the patient.

begin to die. Because exposure to certain chemicals has brought on parkinsonian symptoms in some people, environmental toxins are suspected.

Therapy

A combination of physical therapy and drugs is usually prescribed to alleviate the symptoms of Parkinson's disease, but there is no cure. Physical therapy improves muscle tone and helps the patient learn to compensate for lost motor skills. Some antiparkinsonian drugs (L-dopa and L-dopa with carbidopa) are converted into dopamine in the brain; others like amantadine stimulate the production of dopamine. All of the parkinsonism drugs require careful monitoring. Their effectiveness declines, and each can produce serious side effects ranging from high blood pressure to psychosis. A new slow-release L-dopa and carbidopa combination may stabilize the medication needs for some patients.

Research continues. A new drug called selegiline slows the decay of dopamine-producing cells. Some doctors are encouraged by the early but inconsistent results of surgical transplants of dopamine-producing cells from human fetuses into the brains of Parkinson's disease patients. Biogenetic researchers may yet create such cells in a lab.

TREMORS

Involuntary hand tremors are fairly common in middle-aged and older people. They usually occur during an activity that involves the hands, such as sewing or woodworking. The tremors generally get worse with age. Usually no treatment is necessary, but if the shaking interferes with daily activities, several medications are effective. Some people find that a glass of wine steadies the hands for an evening of close work.

TIC DOULOUREUX

Also called trigeminal neuralgia, tic douloureux is characterized by sharp flashes of extreme pain in the lips, gums, cheek, and jaw, which mimic some dental problems. The pain may be precipitated by something as simple as touching the face. Although the pain can be excruciating, tic douloureux is not life-threatening. Drugs such as carbmazepine and phenytoin may control the pain, but some patients may need surgery to relieve pressure on or destroy the nerve involved.

SENILE DEMENTIA

Losing your mental powers is not a normal part of aging. When older people suffer such a loss, something is wrong, and a doctor should be consulted. Many so-called dementias can be success-

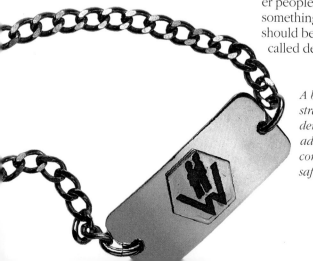

A bracelet alerts strangers to a patient's dementia and gives an address so that the confused person can be safely helped home.

SWALLOWING PROBLEMS

Older people often have difficulty swallowing, an affliction called dysphagia. The feeling may be that food is getting stuck in the throat or taking too long to go down.

Having problems with swallowing is not normal; discuss it with your doctor. Treatment will depend on the cause, and there are a number of possibilities—a neurological problem such as a stroke or Parkinson's disease, a structural abnormality, an infection, throat cancer, an obstruction (a tumor or scar tissue, for example) in the pharynx or esophagus, or a breakdown in muscle control (including spasms) in the esophagus.

If an underlying disease is at fault, treating the disease may make swallowing easier. Obstructions and abnormalities may require surgery. Spasms and other muscle problems are usually treated with drugs.

fully reversed because they are the result of drug side effects, alcohol abuse, an underactive thyroid gland, or some other treatable medical condition.

True dementia affects only a small percentage of the population. More than half of the cases are caused by Alzheimer's disease (facing page). The second most common form of mental deterioration is multi-infarct dementia, in which a series of tiny strokes destroys more and more brain tissue. The progression of multi-infarct dementia can be slowed by controlling the underlying

A prompt board reminds an elderly man with Alzheimer's disease what day it is, where he is, and what the weather is like. Such memory aids help keep dementia patients oriented within their surroundings

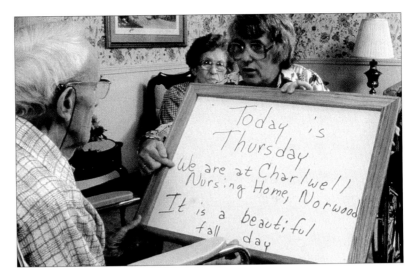

condition—usually diabetes or high blood pressure—that brings on the strokes. Other types of dementia are caused by abscesses and infections, AIDS, and brain tumors, both benign and cancerous, that crowd the brain.

Symptoms of Alzheimer's disease

Because there is no identifying marker, Alzheimer's disease is difficult to diagnose. A new X-ray procedure called PET scanning shows promise in diagnosing Alzheimer's. Otherwise, the disease can really only be confirmed by a biopsy or in an autopsy. Typical early signs include memory lapses, particularly in recent or short-term memory, and slight personality changes, such as a normally gregarious person beginning to withdraw from social interactions. As the disease progresses, thought processes and daily activities become increasingly difficult. The person may also become increasingly irritable.

In the later stages of the disease, the patient may become more disoriented and eventually may not be able to care for himself. The average course of the disease is 10 to 15 years.

Speculation on the cause

The cause of Alzheimer's disease remains unknown. In recent years, there has been speculation about a possible connection to aluminum, but this has since been discounted. Some researchers believe a virus may play a role.

About 25 percent of patients have a relative who also had the illness. But there has been no identification of an inherited defect or a pattern of inheritance.

Patient care

Most people with Alzheimer's disease can function well enough to remain at home far into the course of the disease. Only in its advanced stages do patients lose the capacity to feel and express love, pleasure, and friendship. Those close to someone with the disease can find many opportunities for positive interaction.

How much the patient is told about the disease depends on how far it has progressed. It may be cruel to tell someone that he has a progressive, incurable, and fatal disease. But he has a right to make decisions about his will and future plans for his treatment while he is still able to do so.

In the early stages of Alzheimer's, simplified routines can help reduce the patient's anxiety about performing the tasks of daily life. For some patients, nights are difficult; they wake up disori-ented and scared. A bedtime routine, a night light, and a large illuminated clock may be reassuring.

As the disease progresses, caregivers have to make difficult choices about the patient's freedoms. A person with Alzheimer's disease driving a car, for example, is a danger to himself and to others. In the house, the patient's decreased manual dexterity poses hazards. Caregivers must make the house safe for the patient.

Family concerns

Caring for an Alzheimer's patient late in the disease can exhaust a family. At some point, a day-care program for the patient may be necessary. Your doctor or a social service agency can help you find one. Later you may need to find a nursing home (p.186).

The family of someone with Alzheimer's disease needs emotional support. Regular family meetings to discuss problems may help. In addition, a support group may offer not only comfort but useful information as well; call your local Alzheimer's Association for information about such groups in your community.

DEPRESSION

At any given time, more than 17 million Americans are suffering from depression, a serious but treatable psychiatric illness. Depression is more than just having the blues for a few days. It lasts longer and can severely affect your health and your ability to function normally.

Recognizing the signs

The symptoms of moderate to severe depression include withdrawal from normal activities, disturbed sleep patterns, changes in eating habits (loss of appetite or compulsive eating), decrease in sexual desire, inability to concentrate or make decisions, loss of energy, feelings of worthlessness and guilt, and thoughts of suicide and death.

In older people, depression is often overlooked because many of the symptoms are mistakenly thought to be a normal part of aging. Or family and friends assume that an older person's sadness is a reasonable response to an advanced stage of life or a proper attitude for a widow or widower.

Causes

Depression is thought to be caused by psychological factors (childhood trauma, for example), biochemical imbalances in the brain, or both. Some forms of depression are known to run in families, but no genetic marker has been found.

Episodes of depression can be triggered by an event (a death in the family or a financial crisis), by brain trauma (a stroke or a head injury), thyroid problems, or medications. Depression also can be set off by a change in seasons; seasonal affective disorder, or SAD, is a type of depression asso-

THE ANTIDEPRESSANTS

Several types of antidepressant drugs are currently in use. The tricyclics and the monoamine oxidase (MAO) inhibitors may have nasty side effects—dry mouth, blurred vision, dizziness, and constipation. The MAO inhibitors require a restricted diet because interaction with certain beverages or foods can cause dangerously high blood pressure.

Fluoxetine, sertoline, and paroxetine, a new generation of antidepressant drugs, have fewer side effects than the older drugs. They are the most widely prescribed antidepressants in the United States.

Doctors prescribe lithium carbonate to control the mood swings characteristic of bipolar disorder, or manic depression. Like the antidepressants, lithium must be carefully monitored. Overdoses can cause tremors, vomiting, blurred vision, and diarrhea.

ciated with a lack of sunlight during the winter, which is thought to alter the body's biological clock.

Therapy

Treatment for depression, which is designed to help the patient function normally again, usually involves both drug therapy to restore chemical balance in the brain and talk therapy to help the patient perceive the world more positively and prevent relapses. Studies show that antidepressant

drugs help 80 percent of patients.

If you think you are suffering from depression, see your doctor to rule out any physical causes for the condition. Your doctor may treat you with an antidepressant drug and suggest you see a therapist or refer you to a psychiatrist who can prescribe drugs as well as provide talk therapy. You will know if drug therapy is working within a matter of months. It takes 6 months to a year to judge if psychotherapy is beneficial.

Electroconvulsive therapy (ECT), or electric shock, is also an effective treatment for severe depression. Although a minimum amount of electricity is used in modern practice, patients may experience temporary confusion and memory loss.

SAD is treated by exposure to bright light for 2 or 3 hours a day (p.349). In some cases, drugs also are used.

The role of psychotherapy

For many patients, some form of talk therapy is essential for dealing with depression. Cognitive behavior therapy (p.179) emphasizes the power of the individual to change the thinking habits that encourage depression. Interpersonal therapy concentrates on resolving problems in personal relationships that may trigger depression. Long-term Freudian therapy looks for unresolved conflicts in the patient's unconscious and analyzes the present in relation to the patient's past.

Therapy is an important adjunct to drug treatment. During the acute phases of depression, therapy provides emotional support until the drug begins to take effect. During the later stages, patients learn to understand the psychological factors that may have contributed to the depression.

WHERE TO TURN FOR HELP

There are many professionals in the fields of psychiatry, psychology, and counseling who can help people with mental health problems. Fees will vary depending on the therapist's training and on whether you choose individual sessions or group therapy (appropriate for solving family problems or working on a problem common to other people). Community health clinics may charge on a sliding scale pegged to a patient's income level.

Pastoral counselor. A member of the clergy who has taken an advanced degree in counseling, a pastoral counselor works within a religious context. Such counseling may be free or charges calculated on a sliding scale related to the patient's ability to pay. Insurance may not cover the fees.

Psychiatric nurse. A registered nurse with an advanced degree in counseling, a psychiatric nurse may work in a hospital or take private patients. Insurance may not cover sessions with a psychiatric nurse.

Psychiatric social worker. The most numerous group of professionals in the mental health field, psychiatric social workers usually have a master's degree and a minimum number of hours of counseling under supervision. Licensing requirements differ from state to state, and not all health insurance covers private treatment from psychiatric social workers.

Psychiatrist. A medical doctor with several years of advanced training in diagnosing and treating mental disorders, a psychiatrist is licensed to prescribe drugs and hospitalize patients. Psychiatrists may specialize in particular disorders or in treating particular age groups.

Psychologist. Certification requirements differ from state to state, but a clinical psychologist usually has a doctorate in psychology, supervised experience in working with clients, and postdoctoral training in counseling.

Psychoanalyst. Most often a medical doctor but sometimes a Ph.D. in psychology, a psychoanalyst who is a member of the American Psychoanalytic Association usually has 6 to 10 years of postgraduate training in psychoanalysis at an approved institution. Anyone can legally call himself a psychoanalyst, however, so check carefully the credentials, training, and affiliations of anyone you are considering.

Psychotherapist. Although the term psychotherapy legitimately refers to psychiatric or psychological counseling, the title psychotherapist denotes no specific degree or training in mental health circles. A person who identifies himself by this term alone should be asked about his training and credentials.

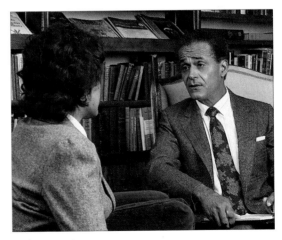

A therapist in a one-on-one relationship helps a client to explore and come to terms with her feelings.

TROUBLES WITH THE ENDOCRINE SYSTEM

. . . .

The hormones produced by the endocrine glands are chemical messengers that regulate virtually every bodily function—everything from digestion to reproduction. When hormone levels increase or decrease beyond a normal range, disorders such as diabetes or Graves' disease can develop.

THYROID DISEASES

The thyroid gland, a butterfly-shaped organ that wraps around the windpipe just under the Adam's apple, acts as the body's conductor, setting the rate of your body's metabolism. Not completely autonomous, the thyroid gland depends on the pituitary gland for a signal to release the thyroid hormones into the bloodstream. If the correct amount of hormone is secreted, the body's activities run at a normal healthy rate. Too much or too little, however, can send your metabolism into overdrive or slow it into lethargy. Both situations are usually easy to treat.

Hyperthyroidism

The first sign of a potential hyperthyroid problem may be an enlarged thyroid gland, a condition called goiter. Other symptoms may include unexpected weight loss despite a greater intake of food, increased heart rate and blood pressure, nervousness and trembling, feeling too warm and sweating excessively, more frequent bowel movements, and muscle weakness.

The most common form of hyperthyroidism is Graves' disease, which was brought to national attention when both Barbara and George Bush developed it during his presidency. No one knows for certain what causes Graves' disease, but some experts believe genetic factors affecting the immune system may play a part in its development. What is known is that it is seven times more common in women than in men.

The most noticeable external symptom of Graves' disease may be bulging eyes; internally the body develops antibodies that bind to the cells of the thyroid gland, causing the gland to secrete an excessive amount of thyroid hormones. Graves' disease can be difficult to diagnose, especially in older people, because the symptoms can also be attributed to other conditions such as heart disease and menopause.

There are three treatment options for hyperthyroidism—drinking radioactive iodine to destroy part of the thyroid gland and reduce the production of thyroid hormones; drug therapy with propylthiouracil (PTU) or methimazole to block the production of thyroid hormones; and surgery to remove all or part of the thyroid gland. The choices depend on the severity of the condition and the patient's age and health status.

Hypothyroidism

Underactivity of the thyroid gland, or hypothyroidism, creates a situation that is the opposite of hyperthyroidism. Metabolism is slowed, producing an overall sluggishness. Other symptoms include fatigue, reduced heart rate, intolerance to cold, muscle aches, constipation, dry skin and hair, and lowered libido. Women may have heavy periods and a deepening of the voice. The condition can easily be mistaken for depression and other disorders. Hypothyroidism, however, is easily diagnosed with a blood test.

A daily dose of a synthetic thyroid replacement hormone will usually reverse symptoms within a few months. The treatment is safe and relatively inexpensive but must continue indefinitely.

A person with hypothyroidism needs regular tests to check the level of thyroid hormone in the blood and consultations with the doctor to maintain a proper dosage of the medication.

THE ENDOCRINE SYSTEM

The glands of the endocrine system produce hormones and distribute them on cue from the brain, triggering the chemistry of sexual development, digestion, and responses to physical and mental stress. When any part of the system gets out of balance, illness results.

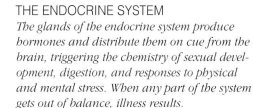

The hypothalamus *controls the secretions of the pituitary gland and regulates body temperature, thirst, hunger, and libido.*

The pituitary gland *regulates the activities of other glands, stimulates bone growth, and determines sexual development.*

The thyroid gland *uses iodine from the blood to create two hormones, which are released at a signal from the pituitary gland.*

The parathyroid glands *sit behind the thyroid and produce the hormone that controls the levels of calcium and phosphorus in the bones.*

The adrenal glands *produce steroid hormones, which regulate sugar, salt, and water in the body, and the hormones adrenaline and noradrenaline, which arouse you to action when threatened.*

The ovaries *produce the female hormones estrogen and progesterone.*

The pancreas *makes enzymes for digestion and the hormones insulin and glucagon, which help cells use glucose.*

The testes *produce the male hormone testosterone.*

DIABETES

When a person has diabetes (medically called diabetes mellitus), the pancreas either fails to produce enough insulin, or the body cannot use the insulin that is produced to metabolize glucose, or blood sugar, the body's major fuel. The excess glucose builds up in the blood and some is excreted by the kidneys. It also triggers excessive thirst and frequent urination, and prompts the body to speed up metabolism of stored fat, a process that further upsets body chemistry.

WARNING SIGNS FOR DIABETES

The American Diabetes Association estimates that 7 million Americans suffer from Type 2 diabetes (pp.282–283) and don't know it. Early diagnosis is important because untreated diabetes can lead to such serious conditions as heart disease, stroke, blindness and other eye problems, nerve damage, kidney failure, and infection. The first column of symptoms below and blurred vision are also signs of Type 1 diabetes.

- Frequent urination
- Increased thirst
- Extreme hunger
- Unexplained weight loss
- Extreme fatigue
- Blurred vision
- Tingling or numb feet
- Frequent vaginal infections in women
- Frequent skin infections

Diabetes in middle age

There are two types of diabetes. Type 1 diabetes, also known as insulin-dependent or juvenile-onset diabetes, usually develops before the age of 30. In Type 1 diabetes, the pancreas produces too little insulin for normal metabolism; treatment involves regular insulin injections to keep the body supplied.

Type 2 diabetes, also called non-insulin-dependent or adult-onset diabetes, is more common than Type 1, affecting more than 13 million Americans. It usually develops after the age of 40 in overweight people with a family history of the disease. In Type 2 diabetes, insulin production may actually increase, but the body can't use it; blood sugar levels rise and diabetic symptoms begin (p.281).

Treatment

Because Type 2 diabetes is related to overweight, modifying the

---

LIVING WITH DIABETES

Although diabetes is a serious disease, millions of people have learned to control it and to lead full, productive lives.

KEEPING TABS ON THE DISEASE

To make sure that their blood sugar remains in the normal range, diabetics can learn to monitor their condition at home with a small portable machine (see photo below).

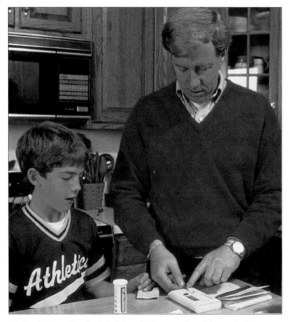

A diabetic checks his blood glucose level by pricking a finger and letting a drop of blood be read by an electronic device that displays the results on a screen.

Maintaining blood sugar levels within a normal range (see facing page) is essential to prevent or minimize complications of diabetes. It's especially important to recognize the signs that your blood sugar has dropped too low, a condition called hypoglycemia that may result from an insulin overdose. Symptoms may include nervousness and shakiness, extreme weakness and fatigue, hunger, confusion, headache, pallor, profuse perspiration, clammy skin, blurred or double vision, and rapid pulse. The immediate remedy is to eat something sweet like candy, honey, a lump of sugar, orange juice, or fruit, followed by some kind of protein, which will help to sustain the release of glucose. Discuss any hypoglycemic episodes with your doctor so that you can analyze what happened and prevent their recurrence.

ESTABLISHING A ROUTINE

It's essential that you understand how your medication, the different foods you eat, and the types of exercise you perform interact and affect your blood sugar patterns.

Start with an established schedule of meals, exercise, and medications. Then learn how to compensate for changes in the routine. Eating too much or too little, skipping your medication, and changing your exercise program can all affect your blood sugar level, as can stress and travel. Nonetheless, you can learn to adjust your diet and activity to stay in balance.

diet and starting a regular exercise program can sometimes restore the body's sensitivity to insulin and correct the problem before it becomes more serious. If diet and exercise alone fail to control blood sugar levels, the doctor may prescribe an oral medication. For some people with Type 2 diabetes, however, oral medications simply don't work and daily insulin injections become necessary.

Any case of diabetes requires careful monitoring of blood sugar levels by the patient and his doctor. Regular consultations with the doctor and a dietitian are also important in controlling the disease.

Because diabetes can lead to many serious complications, it's important that the patient learn to manage the disease skillfully and confidently (see *Living With Diabetes*, below). Regular eye examinations are also a must (see p.289).

BLOOD GLUCOSE HIGHS AND LOWS

The amount of glucose in your blood changes throughout the day. Normal ranges are given below

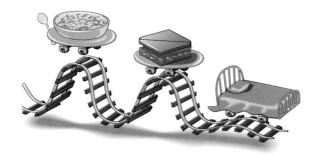

Time of Test	Normal Ranges*
Before breakfast	70-105
Before lunch and dinner	70-130
One hour after eating	Less than 180
Two hours after eating	Less than 150
2 A.M. to 4 A.M.	More than 70

Blood glucose is measured in units called milligrams percent.

THE RIGHT DIET

You should consult with a dietitian and establish a realistic diet that takes into account your likes and dislikes. In general, you will probably follow the same diet recommended by nutritionists for everybody—one low in fat and sugar, high in whole grains, fruits, and vegetables, moderate in protein, and little or no alcohol. In the past, sugar was forbidden; this has been modified to allow small amounts as part of your carbohydrate allowance.

It's important to establish a regular meal pattern that may include snacks or more frequent, smaller meals than usual.

Diabetics should carry extra food to get through a long trip when they may miss meals. They should also check their blood glucose levels frequently en route and take appropriate action. The stress of a trip can upset normal blood sugar patterns, and crossing more than four time zones can throw you seriously off schedule. Discuss how you can compensate with your doctor.

PAMPERING YOUR FEET

Problems with the circulatory and nervous systems can affect a diabetic's feet. You may lose feeling in them and not notice an injury right away.

You should wash your feet daily with mild soap and warm water, dry them carefully, and inspect them for such potential danger signs as redness or other discoloration; cracked, peeling, or dry skin; ingrown, thickened, or discolored toenails; and swelling, tenderness, and warmth, which are indications of infection. Care for simple problems yourself, but take more threatening conditions such as an ingrown toenail or a large uncomfortable callus or corn to your doctor for treatment.

Always wear shoes that fit properly; a diabetic cannot risk crowding his feet and causing blisters or sores. Also, check inside your shoes for nails or pebbles; your feet may not feel such irritants.

IN CASE OF EMERGENCY

Diabetics should wear a medical alert bracelet or tag to inform health care personnel of their condition. In the event of hypoglycemia or an accident, such information will help you get appropriate medical treatment.

PRESERVING YOUR EYESIGHT

Because everyone's eyes change as they get older, it's important to know which changes are a normal part of aging and which problems are warning signs of more serious that can be successfully treated if they are detected at an early stage.

AGE-RELATED CHANGES

Sooner or later, everyone begins to experience some degree of difficulty in seeing close objects clearly. This condition, known as presbyopia, is brought on by the gradual loss of elasticity in the lens of the eye, which causes the process of changing focus to become slower and more difficult. Eyestrain is often a symptom of presbyopia, which is correctable with reading glasses.

Another age-related vision change occurs when the pupils of the eyes no longer can open as wide as they used to, nor adapt to light and dark as readily. The result is that you cannot see objects as clearly as you did before. In addition, you may begin to have trouble distinguishing between different pastel and neutral colors. The solution is simple: plenty of light. A 60-year-old needs seven times as much light as a 20-year-old does to see the same object clearly.

FLOATERS

Tiny dots, wavy lines, cobwebs, or other objects that move across your field of vision are known as floaters. They are microscopic clumps or strands of cellular debris produced by the degeneration of the eye's vitreous humor (a clear gelatinous fluid that occupies the eye's cavity and gives it shape).

Most visible when you are looking at a plain background such as a blank wall or a clear blue sky, floaters appear to be right in front of your eye, but they are actually drifting in the vitreous humor and casting their shadows on the retina, the light-sensing inner back layer of the eye. Although floaters are usually harmless, in some cases they may be a symptom of a torn or detached retina (see p.287).

While there is no medical treatment for floaters, most of them tend to become less noticeable over time. You may be able to temporarily push them out of your line of vision by rolling your eyes, thus stirring up the vitreous humor.

WHEN TO SEE AN EYE DOCTOR RIGHT AWAY

The following symptoms may be indications of serious eye problems; they require immediate attention by your ophthalmologist.

- Blurred, cloudy, dimming, or otherwise distorted vision that persists even when you are wearing your prescription eyeglasses or contact lenses
- A sudden onset of floaters in your field of vision
- Difficulty in focusing your eyes
- Seeing sudden flashes of light
- The sensation of a film or a shadow moving over your eyes
- An abrupt wavy, watery quality to your vision
- Double vision
- A continually narrowing field of vision
- Loss of your central or peripheral vision
- Hypersensitivity to light
- Constantly tired or painful eyes
- Excessive tearing or any other discharge from the eyes
- Unusually red or swollen eyes or eyelids, with no apparent cause
- Persistently dry, itching, or burning eyes

EYE TICS

The involuntary twitching of your eyelids can be annoying, but the condition usually isn't serious. Although the cause of eye tics is unknown, some people have reported that their onset appears to be precipitated by fatigue and stress; others, by the need for a change in their eyeglass prescription. The fluttering, which typically continues for several seconds at a time, can sometimes be relieved by gently massaging the affected eyelid.

DRY EYES

The insufficient production of tears to keep your eyes wet and comfortable and make good vision possible is a relatively benign problem of middle age. So-called dry eyes can cause stinging, scratchiness, burning, and hypersensitivity to smoke, conditions that may make wearing contact lenses difficult or impossible.

Dry eyes can develop in both sexes at any age, but post-menopausal women tend to be the most susceptible. The lack of adequate moisture can be remedied with "artificial tears" (non-prescription eyedrops), which can be used as often as needed.

If you suffer from dry eyes, conserve what natural tears you have by wearing wraparound glasses outdoors and using a humidifier indoors. Because dry eyes may also be a side effect of certain drugs or associated with a form of arthritis, check with your doctor if you experience them.

HOW YOUR EYE LETS YOU SEE

Only about 1 inch in diameter, the eye acts like an incredibly complex three-dimensional movie camera, instantaneously recording every aspect of the world around you.

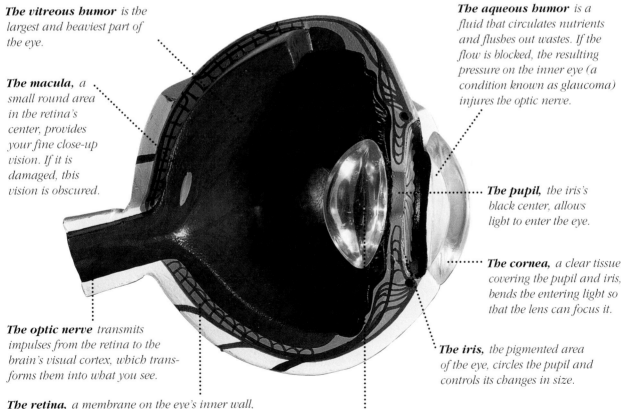

The vitreous humor *is the largest and heaviest part of the eye.*

The macula, *a small round area in the retina's center, provides your fine close-up vision. If it is damaged, this vision is obscured.*

The aqueous humor *is a fluid that circulates nutrients and flushes out wastes. If the flow is blocked, the resulting pressure on the inner eye (a condition known as glaucoma) injures the optic nerve.*

The pupil, *the iris's black center, allows light to enter the eye.*

The cornea, *a clear tissue covering the pupil and iris, bends the entering light so that the lens can focus it.*

The optic nerve *transmits impulses from the retina to the brain's visual cortex, which transforms them into what you see.*

The iris, *the pigmented area of the eye, circles the pupil and controls its changes in size.*

The retina, *a membrane on the eye's inner wall, processes the images entering through the lens and transmits them to the optic nerve. If the retina suffers a tear or a hole, the vitreous humor can flow in behind the retina and detach it from the wall.*

The lens, *a soft tissue behind the pupil, focuses incoming light on the retina. Cataracts result when the tissue solidifies and loses its transparency.*

Profile

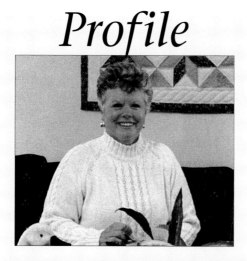

"CATARACT SURGERY WAS A MIRACLE" TO MARIE HERRICK

For years, New Jersey resident Marie Herrick hadn't been able to see very well with her eyeglasses. Although she had her prescription changed several times, her vision only worsened.

Finally Herrick consulted an ophthalmologist, who told her that she had cataracts in both eyes that could easily be removed surgically. But because all surgery carries some risk, he advised her to put it off until her condition began to interfere with her lifestyle. One day Herrick was driving on a highway and couldn't read the overhead signs. "I panicked and got off at the wrong exit. That's when I knew it was time."

In Herrick's initial surgery, the cataract in one eye was removed, and a lens implant was inserted. After the operation, her doctor covered the eye with a protective shield and a bandage. The day the bandage came off, "it was like somebody had taken a glass cleaner to a very dirty windshield," she says. "I couldn't believe the color of the grass!"

A year later Herrick had surgery on her other cataract. "To me, cataract surgery was a miracle," she says. "Before, I couldn't make out my grand-daughters' features. Now I can."

CATARACTS

A clouding and hardening of the once crystal-clear lens of the eye, a cataract is painless and usually develops very gradually, beginning as a small hazy spot in the lens. As the cataract grows, the person's vision slowly dims.

To help forestall the development of cataracts, do not smoke and protect your eyes from the sun's ultraviolet waves by wearing sunglasses (see p.289) and a hat with a brim that shades your eyes.

Surgery is the only effective treatment for cataracts. The most commonly performed operation involves excising the cataract from the thin transparent capsule of the lens and replacing it with an implant. An outpatient procedure, it generally takes less than an hour, is simple and painless, and usually requires only local anesthesia.

Afterward, you may need to wear eyeglasses to fine-tune your vision. A few months (or sometimes even years) after your surgery, a secondary membrane will usually develop behind the implant; your doctor can remove it with a laser.

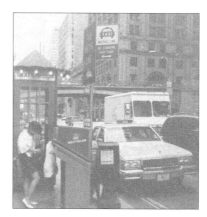

Cataracts. *Incoming light is increasingly blocked, resulting in cloudy, blurred vision.*

GLAUCOMA

A major cause of blindness, glaucoma is a disease in which an increase in pressure within the eye damages the optic nerve. Because the condition produces no symptoms, early diagnosis and treatment are crucial. About 25 percent of all glaucoma victims are not aware that they have the disease until it is too late to save their eyesight.

There are many different types of glaucoma, but all of them can usually be detected during your annual eye examination by an ophthalmologist or optometrist. The damage already caused by glaucoma cannot be reversed, but the earlier it is diagnosed, the easier it is to preserve your vision.

Treatment depends on the type of glaucoma you have. People with the most common type, primary or chronic open-angle glaucoma, generally take a daily drug in eyedrop or pill form that either increases the eyes' fluid drainage or decreases the amount of fluid produced. When medication cannot alleviate the condition, surgery (often using lasers) may help.

MACULAR DEGENERATION

The macula, the central and most sensitive part of your retina, enables you to see details. In macular degeneration, the middle part, but not the outer edges, of the images coming through the lens are blurred or obliterated. Reading or other close work may be possible only with the use of "low vision" aids such as large-print reading material, magnifying eyeglass lenses, telescopes, hand or stand magnifiers, and closed-circuit television reading machines.

There are two kinds of macular degeneration. The less common "dry" type, for which there is no treatment, is caused by an abnormality of pigment cells and results in moderate vision loss. The more serious "wet" type is marked by an abnormal growth of new blood vessels that leak blood and serum into the retina. The result is bulging and distortion that can severely scar or even destroy the macula. Laser surgery to seal off the leaking membranes and destroy the new blood vessels may slow or halt its spread. But even with treatment, poor vision often results.

RETINAL DETACHMENT

A serious but painless medical emergency that requires immediate treatment, retinal detachment occurs most often in nearsighted people or in those who have undergone cataract surgery. The condition is caused by the separation of the retina from the back inside wall of the eye, a process that typically begins after a tear or a hole in the retina allows the vitreous humor to seep under the retina and begin lifting it up.

The symptoms of impending retinal detachment include seeing flashing lights and multiple floaters and experiencing blurred vision. If a partial detachment begins to take place, you may see a shadow moving across the area of your eye where sight is being lost.

Vision can almost always be saved if the tears or holes in the retina are repaired prior to detachment or before any detachment has reached the macula. Laser photocoagulation (p.289) and freezing (cryopexy) are among the treatment options; in advanced cases, more complex surgical procedures may be necessary.

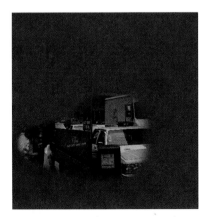

Glaucoma. As the pressure on the optic nerve increases, the brain receives only a partial image.

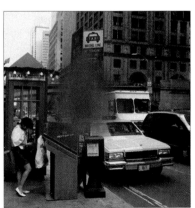

Macular degeneration. Damage to the macula causes a central blind spot to grow.

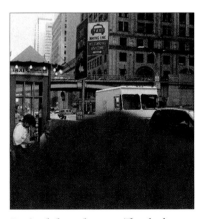

Retinal detachment. The dark patch indicates where the retina has pulled away from the eye wall.

Laser surgery is the most common treatment for diabetic retinopathy. Before beginning the procedure, the surgeon places a special contact lens on the patient's eye, which gives him a magnified stereoscopic view of the area to be treated.

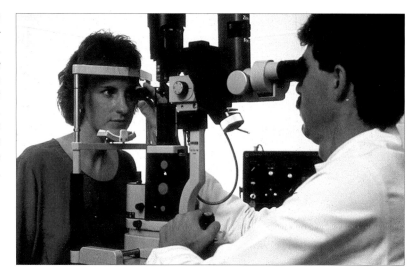

Choosing Eyewear

Eyeglasses

If your only vision problem is presbyopia (p.284), you may be able to use over-the-counter reading glasses, which generally cost about a fifth of the price of prescription lenses. They are usually marked with a number from 1.00 to 4.00, signifying their magnification power.

Nearsighted people who develop presbyopia often use bifocals, which combine lenses for reading at the bottom with those for distance vision at the top, thus eliminating the need to carry two pairs of glasses. "Invisible" bifocals come without the demarcation line between the two types of lenses but are much more expensive.

People who only need reading glasses may prefer half glasses, while those who also need help with middle vision may decide on trifocals.

No matter what kind of reading glasses you buy, however, you still need to have regular eye checkups in order to screen for other, more serious vision problems.

Contact Lenses

Some people alternate between wearing eyeglasses and contact lenses; others wear contact lenses exclusively. Always buy contact lenses from an ophthalmologist or optometrist. The fee should include a complete examination and fitting, instructions for their use and care, and follow-up exams for as long as a year afterward.

Several types of contact lenses are available. Hard lenses correct vision best; they are also the least expensive and easiest to clean. Your eyes will take longer to adjust to them, however—it may be 2 weeks before you can wear them all day long. Gas-permeable lenses are similar to hard lenses but are more comfortable because they have openings that let in oxygen and carbon dioxide, thus allowing the cornea to "breathe."

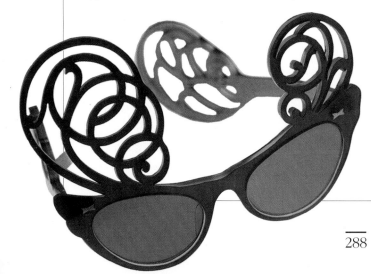

DIABETIC RETINOPATHY

People who have diabetes are at risk of diabetic retinopathy, a type of retinal damage caused by weakening of the blood vessels that nourish the retina. As the vessels deteriorate, they may leak fluid or blood, scarring the retina and blurring vision. These blood vessels are also likely to develop fragile offshoots that eventually break, producing hemorrhages that can leave tiny scars marking areas of lost vision. If the condition worsens into the proliferative phase, the vessel offshoots will grow over the retina and into the vitreous humor, swelling and bleeding and obscuring sight.

The longer you have had diabetes, the higher your risk of getting diabetic retinopathy. Regular eye checkups are important for early detection; treatment begins with control of the diabetes to maintain the correct level of blood sugar. Some people may be helped with photocoagulation, a type of laser surgery that seals the leaking blood vessels, halting the bleeding and producing microscopic scars that bond the retina to the eye's back wall (see photo, facing page). If the vitreous is so full of blood that eyesight is impaired, the surgeon may perform a vitrectomy, a procedure in which the vitreous is removed and replaced with a clear saline solution.

Soft lenses are the most comfortable contact lenses because they are made of a water-absorbent plastic that molds itself to the cornea. They are more fragile, however, and require more upkeep.

Extended-wear contact lenses can be worn around the clock for a week or more at a time. These special soft lenses may be the best choice for those people who cannot manage the daily care of regular lenses because of some physical condition. Disposable extended-wear lenses, which are worn for about a week, and daily-wear disposable lenses, which are worn for up to 2 weeks, may be other options.

SUNGLASSES

Not just a fashion statement, sunglasses help shield your eyes from the sun's ultraviolet (UV) rays, which, over time, can damage the lens, retina, and cornea. Wear sunglasses all year round whenever you go outside during the day.

Your sunglasses should block at least 75 percent of visible light and as much UV radiation as possible. Those labeled as meeting the standards of the American National Standard Institute (ANSI) are best. Have sunglasses made up in your prescription or attach clip-ons to your regular eyeglasses. If you purchase over-the-counter sunglasses, make sure that they don't distort colors, shapes, or lines.

Buy sunglasses large enough to block light from above, below, and the side. Gray or green lenses distort color least, but brown and amber lenses are also acceptable. For driving, gradient lenses, which are darker at the top than at the bottom, make it easier to read the information on the dashboard (see also p.171).

DIFFICULTIES WITH HEARING

A lthough hearing loss is common in older people, it is not inevitable, and the problem varies from person to person. About 15 percent of all Americans over the age of 55 have diminished hearing. By age 75, nearly 40 percent are affected.

TYPES OF HEARING LOSS

There are two general types of hearing loss: conductive, in which sound waves are somehow blocked from reaching the inner ear, and sensorineural, in which sound waves reach the inner ear but are not accurately converted for transmission to the brain.

Conductive hearing loss can be caused by earwax buildup, fluid in the middle ear, an infection such as swimmer's ear, or a spongy bone growth in the middle ear. Drugs or surgery can usually remedy conductive problems.

Sensorineural hearing loss, or presbycusis, is associated with aging, exposure to loud noises, disease, poison, or drugs (too much aspirin, for example). Sensorineural hearing problems are permanent, often progressive, and to date untreatable. A person with this type of hearing loss, however, is most likely to be helped by a hearing aid.

Sensorineural hearing loss affects men more often and more severely than women. The condition, which usually occurs in both ears, is caused by the deterioration of the hairlike nerve cells in the cochlea, a snail-shaped cavity in the inner ear. These nerve cells convert sound vibrations into electrical signals that are sent via the auditory, or otic, nerve to the brain, which interprets the signals as sound.

Damage to the nerve cells usually affects high-frequency sounds first. Having trouble understanding a child's high-pitched voice, for example, is an early sign of sensorineural hearing loss.

Diagnosis

There are some simple ways to check if you have a hearing impairment. Rub several strands of your hair between your fingers and listen for the rustling noise they make. Try to hear a dripping faucet. Hold a manual-wind watch to your ear to catch the sound of ticking or rub leather shoes together and notice the whispering noise.

If your hearing is diminished, see your doctor or an ear specialist (otologist or otolaryngologist) for an evaluation. There are many treatable conditions that may be causing the problem. If your doctor thinks that you can benefit from a hearing aid, he may refer you to an audiologist (facing page). Federal law requires a medical evaluation by a physician before buying a hearing aid, but this may be waived for adults.

COPING WITH HEARING LOSS

Hearing loss may be so gradual that you don't realize right away that you need new listening techniques to understand what people are saying. The following ideas may help.

■ Pick up visual clues and the emotional content of what is being said by watching the speaker's expression.

■ Ask companions to move to a quieter room or to turn down the radio when the background noise distracts you. People will be flattered that you want to hear what they have to say.

■ Ask your family and friends to speak clearly (no mumbling) in a normal tone of voice (no shouting).

■ Explain to your family and colleagues that you must be able to see them if you are to understand them (no shouting from another room or talking with their mouths behind the newspaper). Also remind them to alert you when they want your attention by tapping you on the shoulder or giving you a sign.

■ Use the amplification equipment in movie houses and legitimate theaters; it can be rented for a modest fee.

BUYING AND CARING FOR A HEARING AID

Properly fitted and adjusted, hearing aids can put people with hearing loss back into active conversation with colleagues, family, and friends. Although these devices don't correct hearing as dramatically as eyeglasses do vision, they make the higher range of tones louder and more perceptible.

Hearing aids must be fitted by an audiologist, a specialist with a graduate degree in hearing evaluation and certification from the American Speech-Language-Hearing Association. The audiologist will find the most suitable model for you, teach you how to use it, and make adjustments as necessary. Becoming accustomed to a hearing aid takes time and practice.

A hearing aid, which has a projected 5-year life span, can be expensive. Insist on a 30-day trial period so that you are sure the device is helpful before you buy it.

Keep a hearing aid dry, removing it during exercise that makes you perspire heavily, for example. Protect it from temperature extremes and harsh chemicals (like aftershave lotion). Before going to bed, remove your hearing aid, turn it off, and take out the batteries so that they will last longer. Clean the exterior of your hearing aid with a soft cloth.

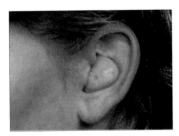

In-the-ear model

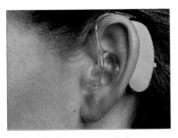

Behind-the-ear model

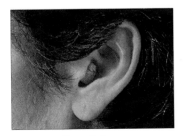

Ear-canal model

Basic hearing aid designs are shown above and at left. Modern hearing aids, some using digital technology, can be programmed to adjust to different sound situations and to amplify high-frequency sounds more than low-frequency ones.

RINGING IN THE EARS

Tinnitus, or ringing in the ears, is another common problem in older people. This constant annoying hum, buzz, or roar in your ears can be brought on by a buildup of earwax, an ear infection, an antibiotic, or the overuse of aspirin, or there may be no apparent cause. It can also be a symptom of a more serious problem such as a tumor, reduced circulation in the neck, or nerve damage.

If surgery or a change of drugs can't remedy the underlying condition that causes tinnitus, allergy medications may help. But often nothing works, and you have to learn to live with the noise. Some long-time sufferers find that they can block out the ringing in their ears by playing the radio softly. Another option is a tinnitus "masker," a device worn like a hearing aid that continually transmits a more pleasant masking sound. Biofeedback and relaxation exercises may also be useful because they can teach you how to relax despite the constant and inescapable ringing.

VERTIGO

Ear disorders can bring on vertigo, or dizziness, because the inner ear plays a crucial role in maintaining your sense of balance. Like tinnitus, vertigo may have no discernible cause, or it may be a symptom of a medically treatable condition such as a drug side effect, a middle ear infection, or a tumor.

If you have recurring attacks of vertigo, you should see a doctor. Antihistamines can sometimes give relief; in more resistant cases, an anti-motion-sickness drug may be more successful.

PROBLEMS THAT CAN AFFECT YOUR LUNGS

As you grow older, your lungs may become stiffer and less efficient at exchanging the carbon dioxide produced by the body for the oxygen that fuels it. This may result in an increased susceptibility to respiratory problems in some people.

ASTHMA

This chronic disease stems from hyperactive airways that over-react to normally harmless substances and circumstances. Normally, the tiny muscles that control the airways constrict in the presence of harmful substances to keep them from entering the lungs. In asthma, however, a tightening of the airways can be triggered by allergens, cold air, exercise, fumes, and even stress, producing such symptoms as coughing, shortness of breath, and wheezing. As the attack progresses, the airways become inflamed and create abnormal amounts of thick, sticky mucus.

If the attack is severe and does not respond quickly to treatment, call a doctor at once or get to a hospital emergency room. Don't panic, however; anxiety can worsen an attack.

Treatments for asthma are designed to prevent attacks as well as to stop them once they have begun. Among the more common medications prescribed are corticosteroids, which help to reduce inflammation, and bronchodilators, which relax the muscles in the airways to keep them open.

Cromolyn, which may make the lungs less sensitive to asthma triggers, helps prevent attacks in some people, but is not helpful during an asthma flare-up.

If you suffer from asthma, you should identify and avoid your particular asthma triggers. Above all, do not smoke and avoid second-hand smoke.

CHRONIC BRONCHITIS

An inflammation of the lining of the bronchial tubes, chronic bronchitis develops when the bronchial walls become progressively thickened, rigid, and constricted. As a result, the bronchi's mucous membranes are permanently inflamed and infected, and the airways fill with a sticky phlegm that induces a chronic cough. The condition is usually brought on by smoking, although some cases evolve from repeated attacks of acute bronchitis.

Bronchodilators, available as pills or aerosol sprays, can relax and open the airways. For severe attacks, antibiotics may also be used. Because you should bring up as much mucus as possible, medicines that suppress coughing are not recommended. Your doctor may suggest that you practice "controlled coughing"

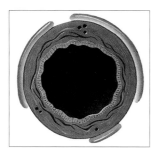
Stage 1. Mild asthma

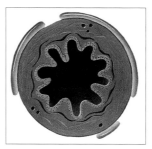
Stage 2. Moderate asthma

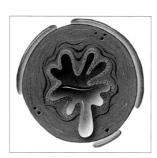
Stage 3. Severe asthma

THE STAGES OF ASTHMA
As the lung's air passages thicken with mucus, less and less air can pass through, breathing becomes increasingly labored, and attacks occur more frequently.

THE RESPIRATORY SYSTEM

Your lungs flank your heart and are attached to it by the pulmonary veins and arteries. Through these connections, the oxygen you breathe in is transferred to the bloodstream and carbon dioxide waste is removed from it.

The trachea, or windpipe, passes the air you inhale into the two main bronchial tubes, one for each lung.

The bronchioles, the smallest bronchial tubes, pass oxygen into the alveoli.

Capillaries receive oxygen from the alveoli.

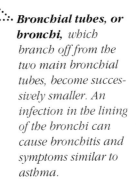

The alveoli, the network of tiny air sacs in the lungs, take in carbon dioxide from a parallel network of capillaries. Emphysema can occur if many alveoli are destroyed or damaged.

Bronchial tubes, or bronchi, which branch off from the two main bronchial tubes, become successively smaller. An infection in the lining of the bronchi can cause bronchitis and symptoms similar to asthma.

TIPS FOR BETTER BREATHING

If you have asthma or emphysema, here are some ways to help you breathe easier.

■ Inhale slowly and deeply into your diaphragm, not the upper chest, and exhale through pursed lips (see p.102).

■ Have your doctor or respiratory therapist show you how to use the postural drainage positions to clear the lungs of excess mucus, as well as how to practice controlled coughing, which helps dislodge and bring up mucus.

■ Don't smoke tobacco; stay away from those who do; and avoid all other types of smoke.

■ Get pneumonia and influenza vaccinations, and call your doctor at the first sign of a cold or other respiratory infection.

■ Take outdoor trips only when air quality is good; stay in an air-conditioned environment when pollution and seasonal allergens are prevalent.

■ Build up your endurance and strength by taking short daily walks.

■ Increase your resistance to infection by eating a balanced diet and getting adequate rest.

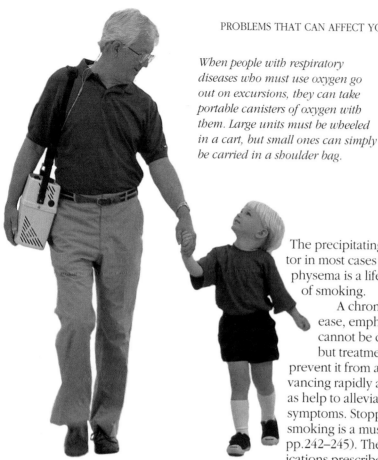

When people with respiratory diseases who must use oxygen go out on excursions, they can take portable canisters of oxygen with them. Large units must be wheeled in a cart, but small ones can simply be carried in a shoulder bag.

in order to make your coughs produce more mucus.

People who have chronic bronchitis should be careful to avoid potential sources of irritation and infection, such as tobacco smoke, air pollution, and dusty working conditions. A doctor may prescribe antibiotics during a cold to prevent a bacterial infection.

EMPHYSEMA

Progressive irreversible damage over the years to the small air sacs in the lungs causes emphysema. The decrease in the amount of healthy tissue makes the lungs increasingly less efficient, and the person begins to suffer from breathlessness. The other symptoms of emphysema are difficulty in exhaling and a deep cough.

The precipitating factor in most cases of emphysema is a lifetime of smoking.

A chronic disease, emphysema cannot be cured, but treatment can prevent it from advancing rapidly as well as help to alleviate the symptoms. Stopping smoking is a must (see pp.242–245). The medications prescribed include most of those used to treat asthma (see p.292). In addition, antibiotics are used to eliminate any lung infection. Doctors may also recommend exercises designed to strengthen the muscles used in breathing.

PNEUMONIA

Not a single disease but a group of diseases, pneumonia is a serious infection or inflammation of the lungs that results in the air sacs becoming filled with pus, thereby reducing the amount of oxygen the body can take in.

Bacterial pneumonias, which include pneumococcal pneumonia and Legionnaires' disease, can come on gradually or suddenly. Among the symptoms are shaking chills, chattering, severe chest pain, a fever as high as 105°F,

coughing that brings up reddish-brown or green phlegm, profuse sweating, and an increase in the person's breathing and pulse rate.

Mycoplasma pneumonia is sometimes referred to as walking pneumonia because it tends to be realatively mild and people often try to maintain their normal routines despite their symptoms. Caused by mycoplasma bacteria, this type of pneumonia is quite contagious, often infecting entire families. Chills and fever are among its early signs; the major symptom is a violent cough that produces a small amount of white sputum.

Viral pneumonias, which most commonly occur in people with heart disease or other types of pulmonary illness, generally have mild initial symptoms that are similar to those of the flu (see pp.248–249). As the pneumonia progresses, however, the body's temperature may shoot up, coughing may worsen, substantially more mucus may be generated, and breathing may become increasingly difficult.

The fourth group of pneumonias has a variety of causes. One pneumonia, brought on by the *Pneumocystis carinii* organism, is almost always associated with the AIDS virus. Several other pneumonias can result from the inhalation of food, liquid, gases, dust, fungi, or other foreign bodies, or from bronchial obstructions such as a tumor.

If you experience any of the symptoms of pneumonia, get medical help as soon as possible. Treatment usually involves antibiotics along with therapy to ease the symptoms—oxygen to facilitate breathing, for example, and medication to relieve chest pain. Recovery can take some time, so be patient and get plenty of rest to avoid relapses.

PLEURISY

An inflammation of the pleura, the two-layered membrane surrounding the lungs and rib cage, pleurisy is often triggered by some other lung inflammation. In its early stages, the surfaces of the membrane rub against each other, causing chest pain that is aggravated by coughing; there may also be pain in the abdomen, neck, and shoulders. As the disease progresses, fluid may seep out between the membranes, producing a condition called pleural effusion. The pain disappears, but breathing becomes more difficult.

Pleurisy usually responds well to treatment aimed at the underlying illness. It is important to cough up any mucus before it can accumulate; clasping a pillow to the chest can help reduce the pain while coughing.

TUBERCULOSIS

A contagious infectious lung disease, pulmonary tuberculosis used to be far more common than it is today. Recently, however, it has re-emerged, largely because of the AIDS epidemic. Tuberculosis may be difficult to diagnose; its symptoms—chronic cough, extreme fatigue and weakness, unexplained weight loss, and lack of appetite—are similar to those of many other conditions. See your doctor if you have any of these symptoms. She can determine whether you have the disease with a skin test and cultures of sputum and other tissues (see pp.228–229).

The treatment of tuberculosis depends on the nature of the case. For some people, no therapy is needed, just close medical

LUNG CANCER

The leading cause of cancer death in the United States, lung cancer produces such warning signs as bloody sputum, a persistent cough, chest pain, and recurring pneumonia or bronchitis.

Cigarette smoking is the major cause of lung cancer. The best way to prevent it is not to smoke. Even if you have been smoking for years, stopping now will reduce your risk (see pp.242–245).

If caught early, lung cancer can be cured with surgery. In most cases, however, the cancer has already spread by the time it is detected. In these situations, radiation therapy and chemotherapy are often needed, in addition to surgery.

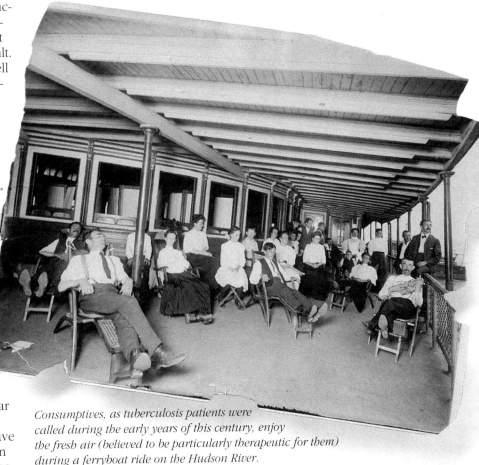

Consumptives, as tuberculosis patients were called during the early years of this century, enjoy the fresh air (believed to be particularly therapeutic for them) during a ferryboat ride on the Hudson River.

supervision. For others, 6 months or more of the drug isoniazid may be prescribed. Those with more advanced infections or drug-resistant TB may require prolonged treatment with a combination of medications.

Most cases of tuberculosis can be treated effectively, generally outside the hospital. Patients are not usually infectious to others once therapy has begun.

CIRCULATORY SYSTEM DISORDERS

*Y*our heart and blood vessels maintain your health by delivering essential nutrients throughout the body and facilitating waste disposal. At the same time, the lymphatic system circulates an infection-fighting fluid to the tissues. Various conditions and diseases may, however, adversely affect both systems' functioning.

HYPERTENSION

Called the silent killer because there are usually no symptoms, hypertension, or persistent abnormally high blood pressure, affects an estimated 50 million Americans. Since even mildly high blood pressure puts individuals at serious risk of heart disease and stroke, it is crucial to detect and treat it as soon as possible.

A simple test that is routinely performed in your doctor's office can reveal hypertension. Two readings are made: the systolic pressure, taken when the heart contracts and blood pressure is higher; and the diastolic pressure, taken in the pause between heartbeats, when the pressure is lower (see chart below).

BLOOD PRESSURE CLASSIFICATIONS
Both blood pressure measurements—the systolic (higher) and the diastolic (lower)—are taken into account when determining whether you have or are at risk of hypertension. A reading between 140/90 and 159/99 is considered to be the first of four progressively worse stages of hypertension.

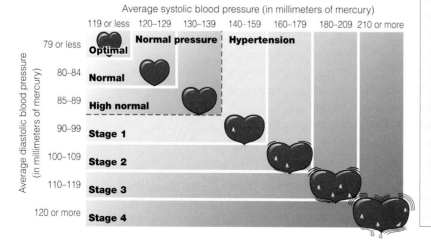

Average systolic blood pressure (in millimeters of mercury)

Average diastolic blood pressure (in millimeters of mercury)		119 or less	120–129	130–139	140–159	160–179	180–209	210 or more
	79 or less	Optimal	Normal pressure		Hypertension			
	80–84	Normal						
	85–89	High normal						
	90–99	Stage 1						
	100–109	Stage 2						
	110–119	Stage 3						
	120 or more	Stage 4						

DRUGS THAT REGULATE BLOOD PRESSURE

■ **Alpha-blocking** drugs block receptors that promote blood vessel constriction and also suppress the effects of norepinephrine, a hormone that increases blood pressure as part of a person's fight-or-flight response.

■ **Angiotensin-converting (ACE) inhibitors** prevent the formation of angiotensin II, which constricts blood vessels and allows the body to retain sodium and excess fluid.

■ **Beta blockers** block the receptors for adrenaline-like chemicals that stimulate the heart and cause the blood vessels to tighten or spasm.

■ **Calcium channel blockers** reduce the amount of calcium in the muscle cells of the blood vessels so that they can't constrict. This allows the vessels to expand, easing flow and reducing blood pressure.

■ **Diuretics** (water pills) increase the kidneys' excretion of sodium and fluid in order to reduce blood volume, thereby lessening the pressure on the blood vessel walls.

■ **Vasodilators** dilate the arteries to promote blood flow and reduce blood pressure.

THE HEART: HOW THE BODY'S GREAT ENGINE SUSTAINS LIFE

Situated in the middle of the chest between the lungs, the heart is a powerful cone-shaped muscle weighing between 7 and 15 ounces. In an average day, this perpetually moving pump will beat more than 100,000 times and circulate more than 2,000 gallons of blood throughout the body.

CROSS SECTION OF THE HEART

The sinus node, *the heart's pacemaker, regulates the heartbeat by transmitting electrical impulses to the heart muscles. A malfunction can cause arrythmias— heartbeats that are too fast, too slow, or irregular.*

The left atrium *moves the newly oxygenated blood into the left ventricle.*

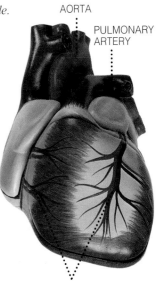

FRONT VIEW OF THE EXTERIOR OF THE HEART

AORTA

PULMONARY ARTERY

The right atrium *receives blood that is returning to the heart, then sends it to the right ventricle.*

The right ventricle *takes in the venous blood from the right atrium and pumps it into the pulmonary artery (see illustration at right). From here, the blood is transferred to the lungs to be oxygenated, after which it flows into the left atrium.*

**The major coronary arteries— ** *the right, the left main, and its branch, the circumflex artery— provide the blood the heart itself needs in order to function. Plaque in the arteries can result in angina pectoris or atherosclerosis. If the blood supply to any of these arteries is obstructed, the person suffers a heart attack.*

The left ventricle *pumps blood into the aorta, the body's largest artery (see illustration at right). From here, the blood is dispatched through all the subsidiary arteries in the body. If one or both ventricles are unable to pump out all the blood they receive, congestive heart failure occurs.*

Hypertension usually has no discernible cause, but factors such as smoking, overweight, alcoholism, physical inactivity, and a family history of hypertension are known to increase its risk. Adopting a healthy lifestyle may help, but treatment with drugs is often necessary.

CORONARY ARTERY DISEASE

Cardiovascular risk factors

Although coronary artery disease remains the nation's number-one killer, a great deal has been learned in recent years about its prevention, which begins with your identifying how much you are in danger. Risk factors are divided into two groups: those that can't be changed and those that can. The first group includes being male, being over 55 years old, and having a family history of heart attacks.

THE ROLE OF CHOLESTEROL IN HEART DISEASE

Despite what you have heard, cholesterol isn't all bad; in fact, it is essential for cell formation, hormone production, and other vital processes. But too much cholesterol in the blood can harden arteries and increase the risk of heart attack and strokes. Most cholesterol is synthesized in the liver; your diet partially determines how much is made.

To reduce your risk of heart disease, physicians usually recommend keeping your total cholesterol level, or count, below 200. People whose count is between 200 and 239 are considered to have a slightly increased risk; those with a count of 240 or more, a higher risk. A low-fat, high-fiber diet may lower cholesterol levels. If that is not enough, drugs can help.

To travel through the blood, cholesterol is attached to a lipoprotein. Some physicians believe the ratio of your total cholesterol to your HDL (high-density lipoprotein) cholesterol, the "good" cholesterol, is a more accurate measure of risk than your total cholesterol count. To get this figure, divide your total count by your HDL count. For example, if your total count is 210 and your HDL is 76, you have a ratio of almost 2.8. A ratio below 2.8 is considered to be low risk; a ratio between 2.8 and 5 is neutral; and a ratio above 5 signals high risk. But keep in mind that while your total cholesterol count and your HDL ratio are significant barometers, other factors like smoking may compound your risk.

As **VLDL (very-low-density lipoprotein)** *enters a capillary, it releases triglyceride, a fat, to cells on the vessel walls; then it deflates and separates into LDL and HDL particles.*

LDL (low-density lipoprotein) *carries cholesterol to cells farther along in the bloodstream. If the cells are already sated, the cholesterol will float free and may collect on the artery walls as plaque.*

HDL (high-density lipoprotein) *may come to the rescue by "vacuuming up" this surplus cholesterol and taking it to the liver where it is either reprocessed or converted into bile acids and eliminated.*

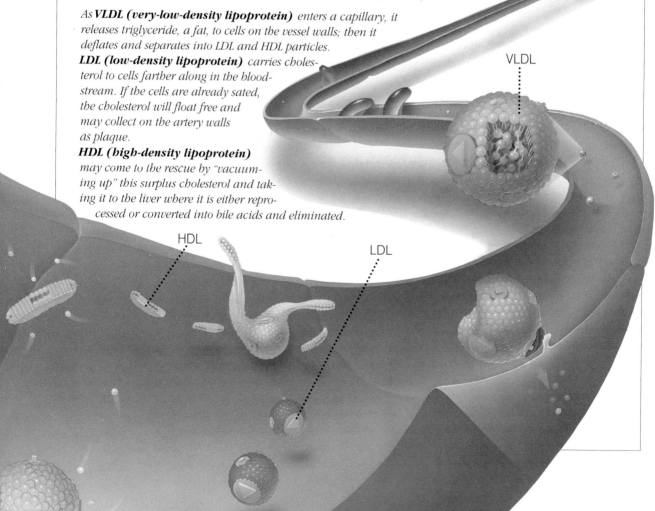

VLDL

HDL

LDL

The second group of risk factors—those that can be changed—includes hypertension, high cholesterol and triglyceride levels, diabetes, excess weight, alcoholism, and smoking. You can reduce or eliminate these risk factors by adopting a diet low in fat and salt, losing weight, exercising regularly, stopping or limiting alcohol intake, and quitting smoking.

Angina pectoris

When narrowed coronary arteries cannot supply enough oxygen to the heart muscle, angina pectoris results. Variously described as pain, heaviness, or tightness in the chest, neck, or arm areas, the feeling usually occurs when the heart needs increased amounts of blood—during or after physical activity or emotional stress, after a meal, or in cold weather.

Medications to help angina either reduce the heart's need for oxygen or increase the blood supply to the heart muscle. Your doctor may prescribe them singly or in combination. Nitrates, available as nitroglycerin tablets or in skin patch form, are the drugs most frequently used. They dilate the blood vessels, reducing blood flow back to the heart and lowering blood pressure.

People with angina may need to change their lifestyles. Check with your doctor about adopting a low-fat diet and starting an aerobic exercise program. You should also stop smoking, avoid emotional upset as much as possible, and reduce stress (see pp.180–181).

If the artery causing the angina becomes so obstructed that you are in danger of a heart attack, your doctor may suggest cardiac catheterization. In this procedure, a thin tube is threaded through

the artery and a dye visible to X-rays is injected to locate the exact site where the narrowing has occurred. A decision can then be made, usually in consultation with other medical experts, as to whether surgery, angioplasty (see pp.300–301), or drug treatment is best for you.

Atherosclerosis

A major cause of coronary artery disease, atherosclerosis is a buildup of cholesterol and other fatty deposits, fibrous tissue, and calcium (which are collectively referred to as plaque) on the inside of the artery walls. As a consequence, the artery is narrowed, normal blood flow is inhibited, and the danger of a complete obstruction, usually by a blood clot, is increased. If the blood flow in a coronary artery becomes totally blocked, the result may be a heart attack.

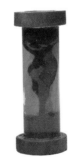

This many-times-larger-than-life model of an artery shows how plaque can constrict—and ultimately block—the body's blood flow.

HEART ATTACKS

When a blood clot or, less commonly, a spasm completely closes off a coronary artery already narrowed by atherosclerosis, a heart attack occurs. Without prompt treatment, the portion of heart muscle nourished by the artery dies from lack of oxygen.

If a clot is the cause of the blocked artery, clot-dissolving

(continued on page 302)

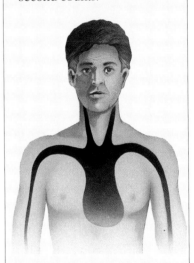

THE WARNING SIGNS OF A HEART ATTACK

If you or someone you know experiences any of the symptoms that are listed below, get medical assistance immediately. Every second counts.

■ Uncomfortable pressure, fullness, squeezing, or pain experienced in the center of the chest and lasting for 2 or more minutes. The sensation may occur for no apparent reason or may be brought on by exertion or stress.

■ Searing pain in the chest that radiates to the shoulders, neck, or arms.

■ Severe chest pain that is accompanied by light-headedness, fainting, sweating, nausea, or shortness of breath.

■ Pain in the lower jaw that is not dental pain, together with shortness of breath.

■ Pain in the neck, in the left arm, or the right arm.

■ Severe indigestion or stomach pain.

SURGICAL TECHNIQUES THAT HELP AND HEAL THE HEART

Made possible by the development of the heart-lung machine, which came into widespread use in the mid-1970's, coronary artery bypass surgery (see box, facing page, above) is one of the most commonly performed heart operations. But the surgery is not for everyone. Balloon angioplasty (see box, facing page, below) may be a better option for many individuals. Less invasive than surgery and usually performed under a local anesthetic, the procedure is primarily used on people with one or two narrowed or clogged coronary arteries, and sometimes in case of a heart attack (see p.302).

THE HEART-LUNG MACHINE

One of the lifesaving marvels of modern medicine, the cardiopulmonary (or "heart-lung") bypass machine takes over the functions of a patient's heart and lungs whenever surgery that requires the heart to be stopped temporarily is performed. The machine pumps an average of 6 liters of blood per minute through the patient's blood vessels.

The photograph below shows the machine in use during an operation. The schematic diagram at right depicts how the bypass machine works.

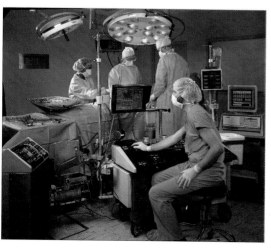

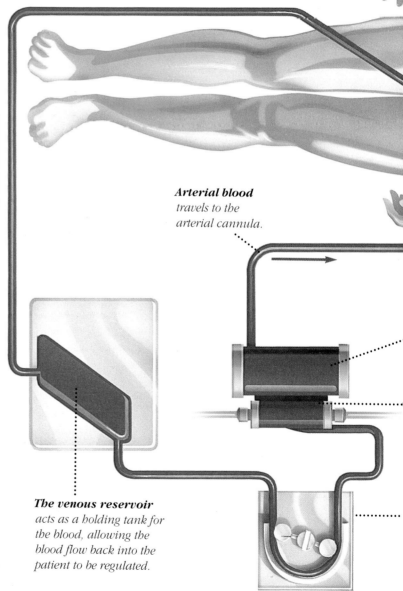

Arterial blood *travels to the arterial cannula.*

The venous reservoir *acts as a holding tank for the blood, allowing the blood flow back into the patient to be regulated.*

CORONARY ARTERY BYPASS SURGERY

Using sections of the patient's leg vein or chest artery, one to five or more bypasses can be constructed to restore or facilitate blood flow in the heart. In the triple bypass, right, a surgical team has created three alternate routes around the blocked or narrowed parts of the coronary arteries to enable the blood to pass freely from the aorta into the heart muscle.

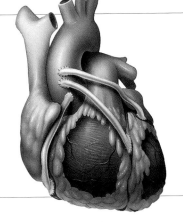

The venous return catheter *collects the patient's blood and drains it into the venous reservoir.*

The arterial cannula *returns the oxygenated blood to the patient.*

The oxygenator *mimics the function of the lungs by adding oxygen to the blood and removing carbon dioxide.*

The heat exchanger *cools the blood to keep the patient's body temperature lowered. When the operation is completed, the exchanger warms the blood to normal body temperature before the patient's heart is restarted.*

The arterial pump *mimics the function of the heart by propelling the blood through the oxygenator and back into the patient.*

BALLOON ANGIOPLASTY

A guide wire with a catheter attached to it is inserted into an artery. To keep the wire on course, its progress through the artery is continuously monitored by X-rays or ultrasound. Once the wire reaches the blockage or constriction, it is eased into the area and then the catheter is pulled over it. Air or liquid is pumped into the catheter, inflating the balloon and compressing and breaking up the plaque. The inflating procedure is repeated until the artery has been sufficiently widened; then the catheter and the wire are withdrawn.

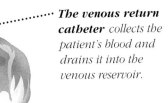

LIVING WITH A HEART CONDITION

Most heart attack patients are encouraged to begin rehabilitation within a day or two, building up from doing simple exercises while sitting on the edge of the bed to taking short walks around the hospital floor.

Once at home, the patient should begin a cardiovascular-conditioning program designed by his physician to improve his endurance and strength, foster weight control, and enhance his self-confidence and sense of well-being. It's important not to overdo, however. If you experience pain or feel light-headed, nauseated, or unwell, rest for a few minutes; if the symptoms persist, call your doctor.

The rehabilitation process also involves adjusting to the psychological impact of the attack as well as to any necessary lifestyle changes. Don't hesitate to discuss any aspect of your life with your doctor, including sex. It's normal to feel some anxiety and fear, but the likelihood that sexual intercourse will cause another attack is extremely slight. In fact, research shows that sexually active heart attack patients enjoy a reduced risk of future heart attacks.

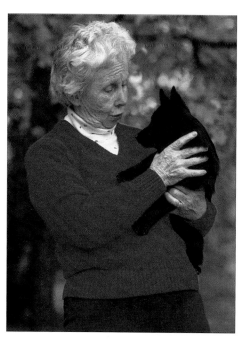

Many physicians recommend pets for their heart patients. Taking care of a pet has been shown to help reduce blood pressure, heart rate, and stress levels. According to one study, heart patients who owned pets had a higher survival rate 1 year after their hospitalization than those who didn't.

drugs will be used. These drugs are most effective when they are administered in the first few hours of an attack. In some cases, doctors will use balloon angioplasty (see p.301) to renew the blood flow in the artery.

Patients may also be given aspirin and heparin, which prevent a clot from growing larger or from re-forming after being dissolved. Morphine may be administered to relieve pain, and oxygen may be given to increase the blood's oxygen content.

The medical team will also be on the alert for cardiac arrhythmia, an irregular heartbeat, which can be fatal (see p.304). Doctors can usually restore the heart's regular beat with medication, but in more severe situations a defibrillator, a machine that delivers an electric shock, must be used.

CONGESTIVE HEART FAILURE

When the heart is not able to pump enough blood to meet the body's needs, congestive heart failure may develop. Symptoms can vary from hardly noticeable to disabling.

The heart's reduced pumping ability produces a buildup of pressure in the veins, forcing fluid into the surrounding tissues. When the failure occurs in the left side of the heart, the lungs become congested, causing breathlessness. When it happens in the heart's right side, there is swelling (edema) in the legs, ankles, and other parts of the body. Often, however, both sides of the heart are affected.

These and other symptoms of congestive heart failure, such as constant fatigue, dizziness, and wheezing, usually can be controlled with medication. Digitalis

THE WONDERS OF ASPIRIN

Although aspirin has long been America's most widely used drug, people usually don't think of it as being "serious" medicine. Even scientists have only recently begun to understand the remarkable potential of this venerable household staple.

Benefits

■ Aspirin helps prevent blood from clotting by interfering with blood platelet functioning. As a result, it can reduce the number of deaths that occur once a heart attack has taken place as well as lower the risk of second attacks. Aspirin may also lessen the possibility of occlusive strokes, those produced by a clot in an artery that supplies blood to the brain. Recent studies show that healthy adults may benefit from aspirin too: individuals who took an aspirin every other day substantially reduced their risk of a heart attack or a stroke.
■ Aspirin use may help decrease the risk of colon cancer by significant amounts; it may also have a similar benefit on other digestive tract cancers such as those of the esophagus, stomach, and rectum. This effect may stem from aspirin's ability to inhibit the production of prostaglandins, hormone-like chemicals that may be implicated in tumor formation.
■ Aspirin may help forestall the development of cataracts, gum disease, miscarriages, migraines, peripheral vascular disease, and hypertension in pregnant women. There is evidence that it may be useful in treating viral diseases as well.

Drawbacks

Along with aspirin's benefits can come serious side effects, including ulcers and stomach bleeding. Asthma sufferers may find that aspirin makes their condition worse. People with kidney problems may also be adversely affected and should consult their doctors to see if they can take aspirin safely.

High doses of aspirin may increase the likelihood of a hemorrhagic stroke, which is caused by a ruptured blood vessel bleeding into the brain. High doses also inhibit the body's own mechanism for preventing blood from clotting after an injury.

Dosage

According to recent research, very small amounts of aspirin—30 mg, a little less than half a baby aspirin (81 mg) every day—work just as well as larger doses in reducing the risk of heart attack or stroke, but with minimal side effects. Aspirin, however, can't take the place of a healthy lifestyle—regular exercise, eating a low-fat, high-fiber diet, and quitting smoking—in reducing heart disease risk. And because of aspirin's potential for serious side effects as well as for adverse interactions with other medications, no one should consider taking aspirin regularly without consulting a physician.

can strengthen the contraction of the heart muscle and slow any acceleration of the heart rate. Diuretics can reduce the heart's workload by helping the body get rid of excess water and salt. Vasodilators can make blood flow more easily by widening the blood vessels.

To help ease the strain on their hearts, people with congestive heart failure should avoid salt (which helps the body retain fluids) and caffeine (which can adversely affect the heart's rhythm), lose any excess weight, get adequate rest, and eat smaller but more frequent meals.

In certain cases, congestive heart failure can be corrected with surgery or medication.

RHYTHM DISTURBANCES

Disturbances in the heart's rhythm, known as arrhythmias, are caused by a malfunction in the heart's electrical impulse system. There are three main types of arrhythmias: tachycardias, in which the heart speeds up to more than 100 beats a minute; bradycardias, in which it slows to less than 60 beats a minute; and various types of irregular heartbeats. Everyone's heart occasionally goes faster, slower, or skips a beat. If, however, the abnormal rate is produced by an arrhythmia, you may experience breathlessness, dizziness, fainting spells, or a fluttery feeling in the chest. Severe arrhythmias can be life threatening.

Arrhythmias are treated with drugs, including digitalis, beta blockers, and calcium channel blockers, or with a surgical implant. A pacemaker sends timed electrical impulses to the heart in order to stimulate a normal rhythm. A defibrillator implant (see photo above) can be placed in people whose arrhythmias put them at risk of cardiac arrest.

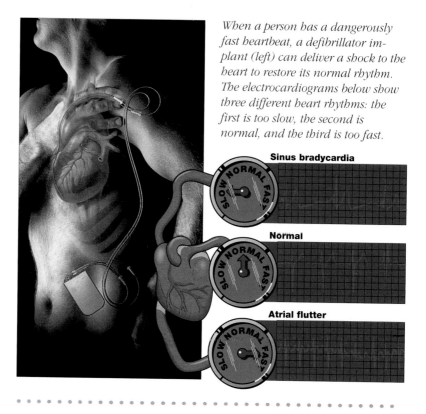

When a person has a dangerously fast heartbeat, a defibrillator implant (left) can deliver a shock to the heart to restore its normal rhythm. The electrocardiograms below show three different heart rhythms: the first is too slow, the second is normal, and the third is too fast.

Sinus bradycardia

Normal

Atrial flutter

CIRCULATION PROBLEMS

Varicose veins

A common vascular problem, varicose veins are swollen, twisted veins occurring mainly in the legs. Most of them are unattractive but medically harmless. The symptoms of varicose veins include aching legs, itching, swelling, bleeding, and open sores (usually near the ankles).

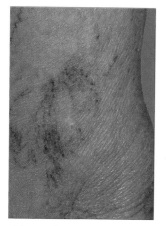

A leg with varicose veins before undergoing the sclerotherapy procedure.

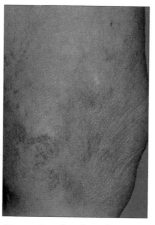

Six weeks after the sclerotherapy, most of the varicose veins have disappeared.

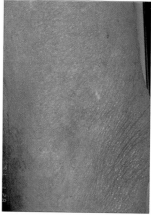

Fourteen weeks after the sclerotherapy, there is no sign of the varicose veins.

SCLEROTHERAPY
A cosmetic treatment for superficial varicose veins, sclerotherapy involves injecting a chemical solution into the veins that makes them shrink. The benefit is usually temporary, and side effects can include skin discoloration and sores.

To alleviate some of the discomfort, try wearing support hose, taking regular walks, elevating your legs whenever you sit or lie down, avoiding sitting or standing for long periods, and controlling your weight. Sometimes doctors use sclerotherapy (see facing page, below) to treat the condition; in severe cases, the veins are removed surgically.

Phlebitis

A painful inflammation of the veins (usually in the legs) caused by infection or injury, phlebitis is associated with blood clots. See your doctor at once if you think you have it. Moist heat and non-steroidal anti-inflammatory drugs (NSAID's) can relieve the pain. If the deeper veins are involved and blood clots are present, immediate treatment with a blood thinner is necessary to prevent the clots from traveling to the lungs.

Aneurysm

A grossly distended section of an artery, an aneurysm is produced when there is a weakness in the artery wall. High blood pressure can cause it or make it worse. If an aneurysm is not surgically corrected, the artery can rupture, resulting in rapid hemorrhaging and possibly death.

Aneurysms generally occur in the abdominal aorta, the blood vessel that delivers blood to the lower body. Often there are no symptoms, but a large aneurysm may produce pain in the stomach and lower back. Diagnosis is confirmed by an X-ray, ultrasound, or a CT scan.

The symptoms of a brain aneurysm may include headaches, a drooping eyelid, a dilated pupil, or double vision. In the majority of cases, however, there are no symptoms. The aneurysm can be

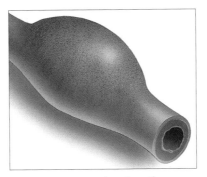

An aneurysm results when the blood flow presses against a weak or damaged area in the arterial wall and makes it balloon out.

located with an angiogram, a procedure in which a dye is injected into the bloodstream to make vessels in the brain visible on X-rays. If such an aneurysm bursts, a person suffers a cerebral hemorrhage, a type of stroke (see pp.272–275).

Raynaud's phenomenon and disease

Characterized by coldness, blueness, numbness, tingling, and pain in the fingers and toes, Raynaud's phenomenon is caused by spasms of the small arteries in those extremities in response to cold, emotional distress, or nicotine. The blood supply is reduced, turning the skin white and the blood remaining in the area blue because of lack of oxygen.

Slowly warming the hands and feet usually relieves the condition. Calcium channel blockers may be effective too, but self-help measures may be better: avoid the cold, wear thermal socks and gloves, and don't smoke.

Raynaud's phenomenon is usually associated with connective tissue diseases such as lupus or scleroderma. When there is no discernible primary cause, it is known as Raynaud's disease.

FAST FACTS

■ Moderate drinkers (one drink a day for women, two for men) have 20 to 40 percent less heart disease than nondrinkers, according to a number of studies.

■ Adults with fevers below 102°F may be better off without medication, according to some researchers, because a fever helps the immune system fight disease.

■ It's true. People with arthritis often are able to predict a storm; their condition somehow makes them more sensitive to the low atmospheric pressure and high humidity that precede it.

■ People with high blood pressure—or any heart ailment—should avoid hot tubs, saunas, and steam rooms; the intense heat can cause dizziness, fainting, and even a heart attack.

■ Men on a healthy diet that included nuts, particularly walnuts, experienced more of a reduction in their risk of heart disease than did men on the same diet but without nuts.

■ Contrary to popular myth, cracking your knuckles in childhood (or even in adulthood) does not result in arthritis.

BLOOD DISORDERS

Anemia

A condition that develops when the blood has too few or abnormal red cells, anemia produces such symptoms as pale skin, fatigue, and weakness. Anemia also exacerbates the effects of other illnesses, including coronary artery disease.

The most common type, iron-deficiency anemia, is caused by a decrease in iron, a key element of red blood cells. Other anemias include pernicious anemia, the result of insufficient vitamin B12; two inherited anemias—sickle cell, which afflicts mostly black people, and thalassemia, affecting persons of Mediterranean descent; and aplastic anemia, a bone marrow malfunction.

Treatment depends on the anemia's underlying cause. Individuals with vitamin deficiency anemias, for example, can usually be helped by increasing their intake of the vitamin. Sometimes blood transfusions may be given.

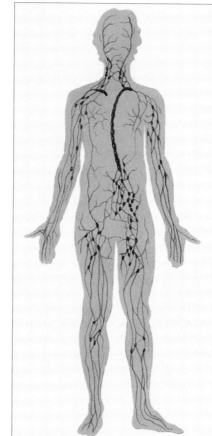

THE LYMPHATIC SYSTEM

The main part of the lymphatic system consists of a circulatory network that delivers lymph, a colorless fluid filled with infection-fighting lymphocytes, to all the body tissues. Lymph nodes, bean-shaped organs in the network, filter the fluid as it passes through them. The neck, underarms, groin, and abdomen contain clusters of these nodes, which are also called lymph glands. Swollen lymph glands often indicate the presence of infection or disease.

The lymph nodes, as well as other elements of the lymphatic system—the tonsils, thymus gland, spleen, and bone marrow—also play an important role in the immune system network (see facing page).

Leukemias

The cancers of the blood, bone marrow, and lymph system known as leukemias create large numbers of abnormal white blood cells that crowd out healthy cells, reduce the body's ability to fight off infection, and interfere with organ function.

The symptoms of leukemia may include unexplained weight loss, fatigue, fever, swollen lymph nodes, infections, bleeding, bone pain, night sweats, and pressure under the left ribs due to an enlarged spleen. Occasionally there are no symptoms. A blood test provides the only sure diagnosis.

Anticancer drugs that kill the invading cells are the usual treatment; in some cases, bone marrow transplants are also used.

THE LYMPHOMAS

Hodgkin's disease

One of the more controllable cancers, Hodgkin's disease attacks the lymphatic system, causing such symptoms as painless swelling of the lymph nodes (most noticeable in the nodes of the neck, underarm, or groin), fatigue, fever and chills, night sweats, appetite and weight loss, and severe itching. If the disease is detected early, radiation therapy is the main treatment, either alone or with chemotherapy. In more advanced cases, the patient is prescribed combinations of chemotherapy drugs. Some drugs may be given orally; others, injected. Bone marrow transplants may also be used.

Non-Hodgkin's lymphomas

Because they are similar to Hodgkin's disease, cancers designated as non-Hodgkin's lymphomas produce many of the same symptoms; in addition, the person may experience edema, abdominal swelling or pain, nausea, and vomiting.

Non-Hodgkin's lymphomas are much more common than Hodgkin's disease. They affect mostly older people and persons whose immune systems have been suppressed by disease or organ transplants. Treatment includes combinations of chemotherapy drugs, radiation therapy, surgery, and sometimes a bone marrow transplant.

THE IMMUNE SYSTEM: THE BODY'S SHIELD AGAINST DISEASE

Composed of a network of organs and blood cells, the immune system preserves health and promotes healing by defending the body against bacteria, viruses, fungi, and cancerous cells. Its organs include the lymph nodes, thymus gland, spleen, and bone marrow. Among the major blood cell defenders of the immune system are the T-cells, which are subdivided into helpers, killers, and suppressors. Helper T-cells act as facilitators by coordinating all of the immune system's interlocking elements.

In the battle between your immune system and disease, your system wins most of the time. When it doesn't, your doctor can prescribe medication both to ease your symptoms and to help the immune system defeat the illness.

AIDS AND THE IMMUNE SYSTEM

Unfortunately, neither the immune system nor modern medicine has as yet an effective weapon for overcoming acquired immune-deficiency syndrome (AIDS). It is caused by the human immunodeficiency virus (HIV), which is found in blood, semen, and other body fluids and can be transferred from one person to another during sexual intercourse, blood transfusions, sharing of intravenous needles, or from an infected mother to an unborn child. Taking up residence in the T-cells, the virus multiplies, killing the helper T-cells and gradually overwhelming the entire immune system. The breakdown in immunity goes through several stages until it produces full-blown AIDS.

AIDS produces various symptoms that result from the destruction of the immune system rather than a single disease. Patients typically incur so-called opportunistic infections that the body normally is able to fight off.

AIDS PREVENTION AND TREATMENT

AIDS is not just a young person's disease. Ten percent of the AIDS patients in this country are over the age of 50, and that number is growing. Because the condition is often misdiagnosed in older people, treatment may be delayed.

The only sure way to protect yourself from sexual transmission of HIV is to abstain from sex or to maintain a monogamous relationship with someone who is not infected. You can also practice "safer" sex by using a condom. If you are not sure that you or your partner is free of the virus, you should both take blood tests that are used to detect HIV antibodies.

The search for an AIDS cure continues. In the meantime, antiviral drugs such as zidovudine (AZT) and other medications are used to treat or delay symptoms.

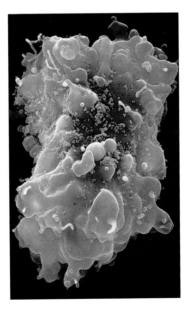

Once HIV infiltrates a white blood cell, it takes over the cell's reproductive apparatus and turns out a seemingly endless supply of viruses. In this magnified picture, the blue specks are new HIV particles emerging from the membrane of a helper T-cell.

DYSFUNCTION IN THE DIGESTIVE SYSTEM

Advances in technology, such as endoscopy, three-dimensional imaging, and less invasive surgical techniques, have in the last 20 years made the diagnosis and treatment of digestive problems more exact, more comfortable, and far less risky than they ever were before.

HERNIAS

Not necessarily painful or dangerous, a hernia is a protrusion of an organ or tissue through an abnormal opening. Although hernias can emerge in various locations, many occur in the abdominal wall when a portion of small intestine pushes through the muscle covering the abdominal cavity. Men are especially vulnerable to hernias in the groin, or the inguinal canal, sometimes causing the scrotum to swell. Other symptoms of an inguinal hernia include a tender lump in the groin area and pain when bending over or lifting something heavy.

Femoral hernias are more common in women. They develop where the upper part of the thigh meets the abdomen, along the narrow canal that carries the main blood vessel, the femoral artery, into the thigh. The symptoms of a femoral hernia are similar to those of an inguinal hernia—discomfort while bending over or lifting—but the tender lump is somewhat lower.

Most hernias can be treated successfully with surgery. The procedure involves pushing the protruding intestine back into the abdomen and repairing the weakened or torn muscle to prevent the same thing from happening again. Full recovery from the operation takes about a month.

If a hernia suddenly becomes very sore or the area over the hernia becomes swollen and feels hot, go to a hospital emergency room immediately. Occasionally a hernia twists and cuts off the blood supply to the intestine, a condition called strangulation that requires emergency surgery to prevent damage to the intestines.

Hiatal hernias

A weakness in the muscle of the diaphragm can cause another type of hernia, a hiatal hernia, in which a part of the stomach pushes through the opening where the esophagus passes through the diaphragm.

Approximately half of all people over the age of 50 will develop a hiatal hernia. Because they seldom produce symptoms, most remain undetected or are found only by accident. Sometimes a hiatal hernia causes heartburn, or uncomfortable acid reflux into the esophagus, and subsequent inflammation. In such cases, the sufferer can prevent recurrences by avoiding overeating, never lying down right after a meal, sleeping with the head of the bed elevated, abstaining from smoking and alcohol, using antacids to reduce stomach acidity, and (if appropriate) losing weight.

GASTRITIS

An inflammation of the stomach lining, gastritis can be caused by smoking, alcohol abuse, overuse of certain medications—anti-inflammatory painkillers such as aspirin, ibuprofen, and corticosteroids, for example—or an infection by the *Helicobacter pylorum* bacterium. Symptoms may include pain in the upper abdomen, nausea, and vomiting.

Most cases of gastritis are mild and pose no danger. Even so, the condition can be uncomfortable. If an attack is related to smoking or drinking, it's important to stop these activities before they cause further irritation. If medications are at fault, ask your doctor for less irritating alternatives. In the

THE GASTROINTESTINAL SYSTEM

In order to function properly, the human body needs a regular supply of nutrients. The gastrointestinal, or digestive, system processes the food you eat and the liquids you drink with a variety of enzymes and digestive juices and makes their nutrients available to your body. Any breakdown in this process can seriously affect your health.

The esophagus, *a muscular tube that moves food from your mouth to your stomach, can become blocked or inflamed.*

The stomach *begins processing the food you eat and stores it for gradual release into the small intestine. It can be the site of inflammation and ulcers.*

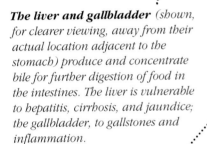

The liver and gallbladder *(shown, for clearer viewing, away from their actual location adjacent to the stomach) produce and concentrate bile for further digestion of food in the intestines. The liver is vulnerable to hepatitis, cirrhosis, and jaundice; the gallbladder, to gallstones and inflammation.*

The pancreas *produces digestive enzymes as well as insulin. When it fails to produce adequate insulin, diabetes results.*

The colon, rectum, and anal canal, *which dispose of the digestive system's waste products, are subject to polyps, inflammation, diverticular disease, and cancer.*

The small intestine, *where food from the stomach is broken down further and nutrients are passed into the bloodstream, is subject to hernias and ulcers.*

meantime, antacids may provide some relief. If more help is needed, your doctor may prescribe medications like cimetidine, ranitidine, and famotidine, which decrease the amount of acid produced by the stomach, or sucralfate and misoprostil, which help strengthen the lining of the stomach while protecting it from digestive acids. If your doctor finds that you have a bacterial infection, he will prescribe some form of antibiotic.

PEPTIC ULCERS

Sores in the lining of the stomach or duodenum, the part of the small intestine that connects to the stomach, are called peptic ulcers. Their most common symptom is a burning, aching, or gnawing sensation somewhat like hunger pangs in the middle of the upper abdomen.

What precipitates these ulcers is unclear, but it is the effect of acid on the cells of the upper in-

testinal tract that creates the sores. Contrary to popular thinking, stress does not appear to cause ulcers, although it can make clearing up an existing one harder. Cigarette smoking does increase the risk of ulcers and can make healing one more difficult.

Surgical treatment for ulcers used to be quite common. The development of new drugs over the last 15 years, however, has led to a dramatic decrease in the need for surgery. With early detection and proper medication, most ulcers can be cured within 6 weeks; longer-term treatment may be prescribed to reduce the risk of a recurrence. It is a myth that milk is particularly helpful for people with ulcers.

Medications for dealing with ulcers are similar to those for gastritis (p.309). Most doctors now believe that *Helicobacter pylori* bacteria are a major factor in cases of recurring ulcers and prescribe antibiotics to control them.

· · · · · · · · · · · · · · · · · · · ·

DIVERTICULAR DISEASE

Diverticula are small sacs of tissue that protrude outward through the muscular wall of the intestine; they are most common in the colon and may be exacerbated by constipation. The term diverticulosis refers to the presence of the diverticula.

There are two main symptoms related to diverticular disease: intestinal bleeding and diverticulitis. Diverticula usually bleed painlessly and intermittently. When you see blood in a stool, this may be the reason; check with your doctor to make sure the cause is not more serious.

Diverticulitis develops when one or more of the diverticular pouches become infected and inflamed. The inflammation can cause painful swelling and muscle spasm, as well as fever. An attack of diverticulitis is usually successfully treated with antibiotics and a restricted diet. In se-

vere cases, surgery may be needed to deal with complications.

To prevent diverticulitis, eat a high-fiber diet, drink plenty of nonalcoholic, noncaffeinated liquids, and exercise regularly. Such a regimen, which is designed to make the stool soft, bulky, and easy to pass, can also reverse diverticular problems that have already developed.

People who know they have diverticula should avoid foods with small seeds or hard particles—tomatoes, strawberries, raisins, and cracked wheat bread, for example—as well as foods that produce intestinal gas, such as beans, cabbage, and onions. Try not to strain when moving your bowels; if you are troubled by constipation, ask your doctor about stool softeners.

TESTS FOR GASTROINTESTINAL PROBLEMS

Thanks to modern technology, doctors today can use sophisticated tests to diagnose digestive problems. The most common diagnostic tools are discussed below and at right.

Abdominal ultrasound scanning. As a handheld ultrasound instrument is moved across the patient's abdomen, reflected sound waves are displayed in a two-dimensional image on a screen. The scan detects cysts, tumors, gallstones, and thickening of the bowel wall.

Barium enema. A barium solution, which acts as a contrast agent, is introduced into the colon to allow X-ray examination of the interior for inflammation, ulcers, polyps, and tumors.

Barium swallow, or upper GI series with small-bowel follow-through. After fasting overnight, the

patient drinks barium (a chalky substance often flavored with chocolate or strawberry) suspended in water and then lies on an X-ray table, which will be tilted at different angles during the procedure. A radiologist follows the barium through the patient's digestive system on an X-ray monitor to detect inflammation, ulcers, tumors, esophageal reflux, and other abnormalities. Individual X-rays of significant findings are made during the process, which can take from half an hour to 6 hours, depending on how much of the gastrointestinal tract is to be studied.

Colonoscopy. Inserting a flexible tube containing light-carrying fiber-optic bundles (an endoscope) through the anus of a partially sedated patient, a doctor can view the entire length of the colon, take tissue for biopsy, and remove polyps. The patient may be asked to eat no solid food for

INFLAMMATORY BOWEL DISEASE

The term inflammatory bowel disease refers to two recurring gastrointestinal disorders: Crohn's disease and ulcerative colitis. Crohn's disease, also called ileitis or regional enteritis, can cause inflammation anywhere along the intestinal tract, especially the lower part of the small intestine and upper colon. Sometimes people with Crohn's disease also develop intestinal fistulas (abnormal channels). Ulcerative colitis is a chronic condition characterized by tiny ulcers and abscesses in the lining of the colon and rectum.

Both types of inflammatory bowel disease produce similar symptoms, including diarrhea, fever, and abdominal pain. The causes of these diseases are not clear, but infections, genes, and emotional stress have all been suggested as possible culprits.

The course of both diseases varies greatly. Some people have no symptoms for long periods of time, while others have recurrent flare-ups of painful, sometimes bloody, diarrhea and fever.

Therapy is designed to control inflammation, restore nutrients lost during severe diarrhea, and prevent complications. Medications prescribed for inflammatory bowel disease include corticosteroids and anti-inflammatories as well as agents such as azathioprine to suppress the body's immune system. In severe attacks, hospitalization—and sometimes surgery—may be required.

Patients with inflammatory bowel disease, especially those with ulcerative colitis, are at a higher risk of developing cancer of the colon than other people. This danger increases as the duration and severity of the inflammatory bowel disease increases. Special efforts should be made to detect these cancers early and treat them promptly.

IRRITABLE BOWEL SYNDROME

Also known as spastic colon, irritable bowel syndrome is a common gastrointestinal disorder. The condition is characterized by abdominal distress that comes

---

2 days and have an enema before the test. The patient lies on his side throughout the procedure, which is uncomfortable but not painful. The test takes from 30 minutes to 2 hours to complete.

Upper GI endoscopy. Using an endoscope, the doctor can view the upper part of the digestive tract, take tissue for biopsy, and even stop bleeding from an ulcer or a dilated vein. The endoscope is inserted through the mouth and threaded into the esophagus, stomach, and duodenum. Performed after overnight fasting and under some sedation, the procedure can usually be done on an outpatient basis.

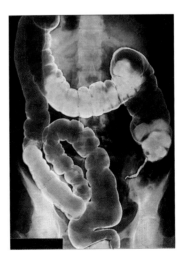

Two high-tech images (far left) show a tumor at the junction of the esophagus and stomach. The large picture is an ultrasound image, and the inset is an endoscopic view. A barium-enema X-ray (left) allows a clear view of a patient's colon.

and goes, alternating bouts of constipation and diarrhea, and indigestion that occurs in the absence of any known disease. Other symptoms include bloating, excess gas, a feeling of incomplete bowel evacuation, and occasional mucus in the feces.

Although the cause of irritable bowel syndrome is unknown, it appears to result from abnormal muscle contractions within the abdominal wall. There is also evidence of a link to emotional stress. People with the condition can help themselves by practicing biofeedback and other relaxation techniques and by eating a high-fiber diet when constipation is the problem and a low-fiber diet when diarrhea is the problem. Antispasmodic drugs or antacids may offer some relief.

COLON POLYPS

Growths that project from the lining of the intestine into the digestive tract, colon polyps usually produce no symptoms (except perhaps bleeding) and are relatively harmless. One type, the adenomatous polyp, however, can develop into cancer and should be taken out early. Polyps can be removed by electrocauterization during a colonoscopy. Where there are many adenomatous polyps, that section of the colon may have to be cut out.

COLON CANCER

One of the most common forms of cancer, colon cancer is often relatively far advanced before any recognizable symptoms—rectal bleeding, blood in the stool, and a change in bowel habits, for example—are experienced.

For that reason, it's vital to be on the lookout for the warning signs of colon cancer. The American Cancer Society recommends that everyone over the age of 40 have an annual rectal examination. People over 50 should also have an occult blood test every year and a sigmoidoscopy (pp.228–229) every 3 to 5 years. Any problems should be followed up with more extensive examinations, such as a colonoscopy and a barium enema X-ray (p.310).

People with a personal or family history of cancer or polyps are at increased risk for colon cancer. Since most cases develop from adenomatous polyps, it's important that these growths be detected early and removed promptly before they become malignant. People with inflammatory bowel disease are also at risk for colon cancer. In addition, there is some evidence that a high-fat and/or low-fiber diet may increase colon cancer risk, while a diet high in fruits, vegetables, and grains may lower risk.

Depending on the stage at which it is detected, colon cancer is treated with various combinations of surgery, radiation therapy, and chemotherapy.

HEPATITIS

There are several types of liver inflammation that are called hepatitis. The most common kinds are caused by viruses. Acute hepatitis A, for example, is caused by the hepatitis A virus. Highly infectious (it used to be called infectious hepatitis), it is transmitted mainly by contaminated food or water. Symptoms include yellowing of the skin and eyes (jaundice), lack of appetite, nausea and vomiting, alterations of taste and smell, and low-grade fever. Almost everyone with hepatitis A recovers completely with rest, a healthful diet, and abstinence from alcohol.

Acute hepatitis B, caused by the hepatitis B virus, has similar symptoms. Hepatitis B used to be called serum hepatitis because it was frequently transmitted by contaminated blood. Blood screening, however, has dramatically decreased the chances of getting hepatitis B through a blood transfusion, and a vaccine can protect vulnerable people like hospital workers. Hepatitis B is now mainly a sexually transmitted disease that, like hepatitis A, clears up in most people with rest, a healthful diet, and abstinence from alcohol. Up to 10 percent of hepatitis B cases develop into chronic hepatitis.

Hepatitis C, formerly called non-A, non-B hepatitis, is another blood-borne strain of the disease. A new test is now available to blood banks for screening donated blood for both hepatitis B and C viruses. Hepatitis C can also develop into chronic hepatitis.

People with chronic hepatitis may have few if any symptoms (chronic persistent hepatitis), or they may experience fatigue, lack of appetite, nausea and vomiting, low-grade fever, and jaundice (chronic active hepatitis). People with chronic persistent hepatitis may not need treatment, but they should be careful not to spread the disease. Chronic active hepatitis is a serious progressive disease that can lead to liver failure, cirrhosis, and death. Some cases of chronic active hepatitis respond well to alpha interferon, a genetically engineered protein that fights viral infections. In severe cases, however, a liver transplant may be the only option.

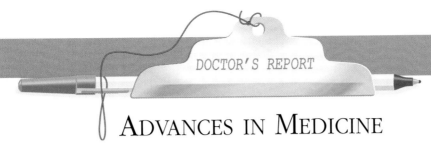

ADVANCES IN MEDICINE

Medical tools today allow doctors to directly view the interior of a patient's body from almost any perspective. A diagnosis can be made with remarkable accuracy, and in some cases, the screening device can guide doctors in correcting the problem. For a patient, these new procedures are far less invasive and debilitating than the exploratory surgery that used to be necessary.

COMPUTERIZED AXIAL TOMOGRAPHY (CT OR CAT SCAN)

A scanner sends low-dose X-rays through the body at different angles while a computer translates them into cross-sectional images, which are projected onto a television screen. A CT scan can pick up aneurysms, bleeding, and other abnormalities in the brain; tumors, internal abscesses, and other abdominal disorders; injuries of the kidney, liver, and spleen; and a variety of other problems. The patient lies on a movable table that slides into the scanner's round opening. The scan may last 30 minutes or more.

MAGNETIC RESONANCE IMAGING

A painless procedure, magnetic resonance imaging, or MRI, produces more detailed images of the soft tissues of the body than any X-ray. The patient, wearing ear plugs to block out a knocking noise, lies on a table inside a large cylinder, which is actually a giant magnet. (Some patients may experience claustrophobia.) Using a magnetic field and radio waves, an MRI reads the internal structure of the body and converts it into an image. Doctors can view a detailed cross-section of the spinal cord, the brain, blood vessels, and other structures to detect abnormalities.

ENDOSCOPIC SURGERY

Using fiber-optic tubing that allows direct viewing of the inside of the body, surgeons are able to perform a number of procedures without making a major incision or incapacitating the patient for more than a few days. Endoscopic surgery, or endoscopy, has many purposes—taking tissue for biopsy, removing polyps in the colon, repairing torn cartilage in joints, or taking out the gallbladder (see photo, p.315). Special endoscopes are used to gain access to different parts of the body—a bronchoscope is put through the mouth to view the bronchial tubes; a laparoscope goes through an incision in the navel to view the abdomen; an arthroscope, also inserted through an incision, views joints.

LASER SURGERY

First used as a surgical tool by ophthalmologists in the 1960's, the concentrated light of a laser beam can cut and seal tissue as well as a scalpel, and sometimes with more precision. Still key in the treatment of such eye problems as retinal damage, glaucoma, and macular degeneration, lasers are being used more and more in other procedures such as removing skin growths and abnormal cervical tissue, stopping gastrointestinal bleeding, and unclogging blocked arteries in the legs. There is a potential danger in laser surgery, however, of injuring normal tissue.

CIRRHOSIS

By doing severe injury to the organ's cells, cirrhosis gradually destroys the liver and eventually causes death. Scar tissue builds up around the damaged cells and prevents the liver from performing its normal functions of aiding digestion, monitoring blood sugar levels, storing nutrients, and filtering wastes from the blood. Alcohol abuse is the most frequent cause, but cirrhosis can also develop as a complication of hepatitis or other diseases or from exposure to toxic chemicals.

A person whose cirrhosis results from alcohol abuse can slow the progress of the disease by giving up alcohol. Although liver damage cannot be completely reversed, abstinence from alcohol can prevent further deterioration of the organ. There is no established therapy for cirrhosis; treatment is designed to alleviate the symptoms as they occur. Often the only chance for a patient's survival is a liver transplant.

JAUNDICE

The yellowish tinge of jaundice develops in the skin when blood levels of bilirubin—a substance produced when the body breaks down hemoglobin—are too high. The yellow pigment travels throughout the body, causing the discoloration.

Jaundice has many causes: cirrhosis, hepatitis and other liver disorders, obstructed bile flow due to gallstones, cancer, anemia, pancreatitis, and certain drugs. Treatment depends on the cause.

GALLSTONES

As the name implies, gallstones are solid deposits that collect in the gallbladder. They can vary in size—from microscopic to several inches in diameter (see photo below)—and in shape and number. Some gallstones produce no symptoms. Others may obstruct the bile duct or the cystic duct that leads from the gallbladder to the bile duct, causing painful spasms and inflammation.

Gallstones that produce no symptoms need no treatment. There are several options for dealing with troublesome ones. For many patients, traditional removal of the gallbladder is the best procedure, although it involves major surgery and requires 5 to 10 days in the hospital and a lengthy recuperation. In a new type of surgery called laparoscopy (see photo on facing page),

the gallbladder can be removed without making a large abdominal incision and an eventual scar. The cut is often made near the navel, where it is hardly noticeable. The patient spends one night in the hospital and is back on her feet within a few days.

Gallstones can be crushed with external shock waves (a procedure called lithotripsy), so that the residue is expelled naturally. Another alternative is to dissolve the gallstones with drugs. On rare occasions, gallstones are removed from the bile duct by an endoscope threaded through the mouth, esophagus, stomach, and duodenum into the bile duct. Each method has advantages and disadvantages, which you should discuss with your doctor.

Cholecystitis

Often a complication of gallstones, cholecystitis is an inflammation of the gallbladder. Acute cholecystitis, or sudden inflammation, develops when a gallstone gets stuck in the cystic duct. Its symptoms include a sharp, severe pain over the gallbladder in the upper right of the abdomen that can spread into the back or shoulder. The pain subsides with treatment or when the stone passes into the duodenum or is

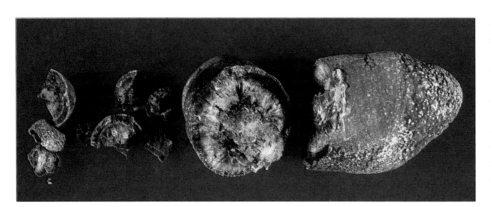

Gallstones are solid lumps that develop in the gallbladder when there is an imbalance in the chemistry of the bile; they often consist mainly of cholesterol. They are shown life-size at left.

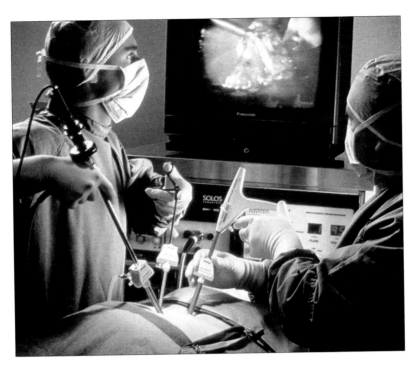

dislodged and falls back into the gallbladder. A patient with acute cholecystitis should get in touch with his doctor immediately; treatment usually involves removing the gallstone by crushing it with shock waves or employing endoscopic surgery.

Chronic cholecystitis can develop from repeated attacks of the acute condition. It is usually treated by removing the gallbladder itself.

In the laparoscopic removal of a gallbladder shown at left, doctors perform endoscopic surgery by manipulating their tools through small incisions and watching their progress via a fiber-optic tube on a television screen.

SAFE JOURNEYS WITH CHRONIC AILMENTS

You needn't give up travel just because you have a chronic disease. With careful planning, you can manage a trip with a minimum of fuss and still be prepared for an emergency.

■ Whatever your chronic condition, first discuss your travel plans and the health factors you need to consider with your doctor. You may also get useful information from a travel medicine clinic associated with your local medical center.

■ Buy some kind of medical identification to carry or wear, such as a Medic Alert tag, which tells your condition and gives a toll-free phone number to call for your medical history. Medical identification bracelets and tags are available from the Medic Alert Foundation, P.O. Box 1009, Turlock, CA 95381, 800-344-3226.

■ If you will be traveling outside the United States, make sure your medical insurance covers foreign medical expenses. If necessary, you can buy supplemental insurance for the trip.

■ Carry a letter from your doctor on letterhead stationery describing your condition, with specific details about your medications and their dosages. This gives background to a new doctor and explains to customs officials why you have extra syringes, batteries, or drugs.

■ If you have a pacemaker, do not go through an airport metal detector, which may reprogram the pacemaker. Carry all pertinent information about your pacemaker with you, including the manufacturer, model number, and the name and telephone number of the doctor who monitors it.

■ People who depend on supplemental oxygen should make arrangements with the airline well in advance for in-flight oxygen as well as supply sources in the airport during any stopovers. (To eliminate this problem, try to get a nonstop flight to your destination.) You will need a letter from your doctor authorizing your request. Passengers cannot use their own oxygen tanks on board a plane, and each airline has its own policy about checking through an empty tank.

■ To minimize stress and maximize your health for a trip, spend several weeks ahead of time getting as fit as you can by eating wisely, exercising consistently, and getting enough sleep.

MALFUNCTIONS IN THE
URINARY SYSTEM

Collecting and disposing of the body's liquid wastes, the urinary system also helps to regulate salts and other substances in the blood. As you grow older, your problems with this efficient and finely tuned system may increase.

URINARY TRACT INFECTIONS

More common in women, urinary tract infections cause a frequent urge to urinate that results in burning, painful urination. Antibiotics will usually clear up the symptoms in a day or two, but they may need to be taken for several weeks to ensure a cure.

To prevent urinary tract infections, drink at least six to eight glasses of liquid daily, empty your bladder often, wipe yourself from front to back, and urinate after intercourse to rinse away any bacteria in the urethra.

INCONTINENCE

Although people who experience urinary incontinence are often embarrassed to talk about it, the problem is not shameful, nor is it inevitable. Recent research shows that 65 percent of those affected can be cured or greatly helped.

Urge incontinence, in which you have almost no time between the urge and the need, is the most prevalent type of incontinence. Drugs can relieve it; so can self-help methods (see box, right).

Stress incontinence, the involuntary loss of urine when you exercise, cough, laugh, or pick up something heavy, has several effective treatments. One, for women whose incontinence is caused by a dropped bladder, is to reposition the bladder with a pessary, a mechanical lift inserted into the vagina. Other cases can be alleviated with medication or, if the problem is structural, with surgery. Certain techniques can help too (see box, below).

Overflow incontinence, when the bladder remains full because of a blockage or weak bladder muscles, results in small amounts of urine being leaked frequently. Causes may include certain drugs, an enlarged prostate, or other illnesses. Treatment involves correcting the underlying problem.

BLADDER CANCER

The most obvious symptom of bladder cancer is blood in the urine, often accompanied by an increased need to urinate. Diagnosis is confirmed with a biopsy of the bladder tissue. Bladder cancer is highly curable if it is detected early. Surgery is the usual treatment, alone or with chemotherapy or radiation.

SELF-HELP FOR INCONTINENCE

■ Practical measures that help with urge incontinence include not drinking water or other liquids before you leave the house or go to sleep, placing a chamber pot or other receptacle near the bed, and wearing easily removable clothes.

■ Weight loss and exercise can improve continence by relieving pressure on the bladder and firming up muscles.

■ Kegel exercises can cure stress incontinence that is caused by weak pelvic muscles. Ask your doctor about them. Basically, they involve contracting the muscles that halt urine flow 10 to 20 times every 3 or 4 hours.

■ Behavior modification techniques that teach scheduled urination (done under medical supervision) can greatly alleviate both urge and stress incontinence.

KIDNEY STONES

Crystallized salts and minerals that clump together in the urinary tract or the kidney develop into kidney stones. If one of them blocks the flow of urine, excruciating pain in the lower back, stomach, and groin results.

Treatment depends on the stone's size and location. A small one near the bottom of the ureter will usually exit on its own. In other cases, lithotripsy, a nonsurgical procedure (see photo, right), can be used. Some stones can be removed through a catheter equipped with a snare-like device. If all else fails, surgical removal may be necessary.

The best way to avoid the formation of kidney stones is to

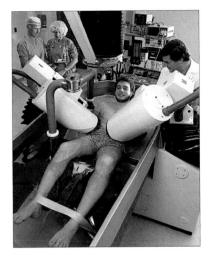

After the patient is given a local anesthetic and is immersed in water up to his shoulders, the lithotripter pulverizes his kidney stone by bombarding it with hundreds of shock waves.

drink about eight glasses of water a day. Your doctor may also recommend changes in your diet or preventive medication.

KIDNEY FAILURE

When the kidneys are unable to filter waste from the blood, kidney failure results. The condition may be acute, occurring suddenly and needing immediate care, or chronic, a steadily increasing interference with kidney function.

The symptoms of kidney failure include fluid retention, decreased urination, gastrointestinal bleeding, seizures, and coma. Treatment involves medication, restriction of fluid intake, and dialysis, a procedure in which a machine temporarily takes over the removal of waste products.

Patients with chronic kidney failure may develop hypertension; experience weight loss, vomiting, fatigue, decreased urination, and itching; and acquire a yellow-brown tinge to their skin. Chronic kidney insufficiency is not usually curable, but medication can slow its advance. If it progresses to complete kidney failure, permanent regular dialysis or a kidney transplant will be necessary to prevent death.

KIDNEY CANCER

In the initial stages, kidney cancer has vague symptoms; there may be blood in the urine and pain in the flank region. If detected early, the disease's cure rate is generally high. Surgical removal of the tumor or the entire kidney is the usual treatment.

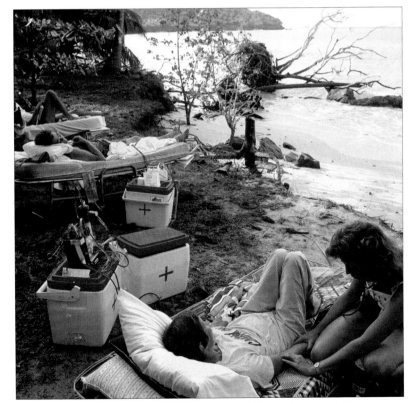

Today many dialysis patients can lead normal lives. Above, portable dialyzers provide needed treatments at an outing on a secluded beach.

Possible Problems for Mature Men

A small gland called the prostate is the most vulnerable organ of the male reproductive system. Enlarging naturally with age, it is often the cause of discomfort and sometimes the source of a silent cancer. Although it is rare after age 35, testicular cancer still can strike men of any age.

PROSTATITIS

An inflammation of the prostate gland, prostatitis is typically caused by bacteria from the urethra. Its symptoms include painful and increased urination, sometimes accompanied by fever, chills, discharge from the penis, and pain in the lower abdomen, back, and rectum. Antibiotic drugs will usually clear up the infection, although men who once suffer prostatitis are often subject to recurring attacks.

ENLARGED PROSTATE

Aging in men is normally accompanied by a gradual increase in the size of the prostate, a condition called benign prostatic hypertrophy (BPH). An enlarged prostate may cause no symptoms until around the age of 60, when up to one-half of all men experience some problems. The most common are a delay in the start of urination (you may have to stand for a while before the urinary stream starts) and a stream that may be very slow or dribbling. More frequent urination, particularly at night, is another sign of an enlarged prostate.

Until recently, the standard treatment for men with severe symptoms was surgery to remove the excess tissue pressing against the urethra. In the most common procedure, the surgeon passes an instrument into the bladder through the urethra and penis that carves away the prostate from within, leaving a hollow shell that gradually shrinks back to form a passageway for urine flow. During the convalescent period, patients must drink plenty of water to flush out the bladder and speed healing, avoid straining when using the toilet, and stay away from all heavy lifting. Full recovery from such surgery may take months, but sexual functioning is usually not impaired.

Doctors now have other treatment choices for an enlarged prostate. In some cases, medications can shrink the gland enough to relieve pressure on the urethra. New, faster-healing surgical procedures have also been developed. You should discuss the pros and cons of each therapy option with your doctor.

PROSTATE CANCER

With 200,000 new cases a year, prostate cancer is the most prevalent male malignancy and exceeded only by lung cancer as a cause of cancer mortality in men. The cause is unknown, but advancing age and a family history of prostate cancer increase your risk.

Early detection of prostate cancer is difficult because you are likely to feel no symptoms until the cancer is far advanced and has spread to other parts of the body. The American Cancer Society recommends that men over 40 have a digital rectal exam every year; this test, while certainly useful, often identifies benign growths but misses cancerous ones. A blood test to measure levels of prostate-specific antigen (PSA), a protein produced by the prostate that may become elevated when cancer is present, offers another possible indication of cancer. Ultrasound screening is a third test that is used to detect possible cancer. None of these tests are foolproof; only a biopsy can give a diagnose.

Most prostate cancer grows very slowly; the average age of men at the time of diagnosis is 73.

THE MALE REPRODUCTIVE SYSTEM

Men have no climacteric like a woman's menopause; the decrease in production of the male hormone testosterone and the enlargement of the prostate gland happen gradually and without notice until something goes wrong—usually with the prostate gland and, rarely, with the testicles.

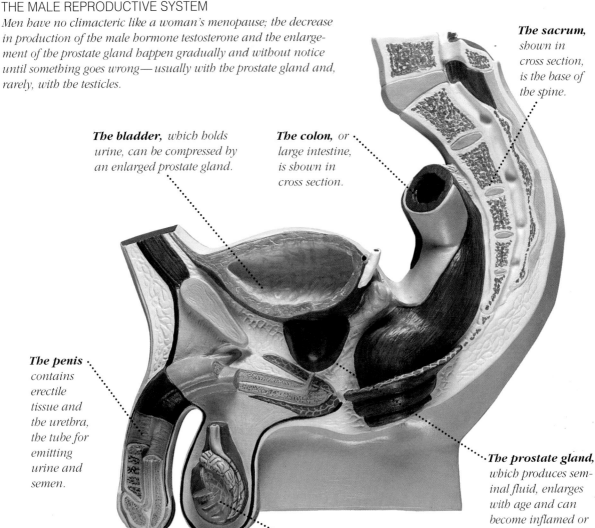

The sacrum, *shown in cross section, is the base of the spine.*

The bladder, *which holds urine, can be compressed by an enlarged prostate gland.*

The colon, *or large intestine, is shown in cross section.*

The penis *contains erectile tissue and the urethra, the tube for emitting urine and semen.*

The prostate gland, *which produces seminal fluid, enlarges with age and can become inflamed or harbor malignant tumors.*

The testicles *produce sperm and the hormone testosterone.*

When prostate tumors occur in younger men, however, they often grow aggressively and require prompt medical attention.

The symptoms of advanced prostate cancer are similar to those of prostatitis or an enlarged prostate: weak or interrupted urine flow, difficulty urinating, and increased frequency of the need to urinate, especially at night. Other signs include bloody urine, painful or burning urination, and pain in the lower back, pelvis, or thighs.

Treatments include surgery, alone or with radiation or chemotherapy. Patients may also be given hormones to shrink the tumor, which relieves pain and may keep the cancer from enlarging.

TESTICULAR CANCER

Testicular cancers are most common in young men, but some types also occur in older men.

There are usually no symptoms in its early stages. The first sign may be a bump on the testicle's surface, which you should discover in your monthly self-examination.

Testicular cancer is treated by surgical removal of the affected testicle. The removed testicle can be replaced with a lifelike prosthesis, and most men continue to enjoy normal sexual function. In severe cases, surgery is followed by radiation therapy, chemotherapy, or a combination of both.

POSSIBLE PROBLEMS
FOR MATURE WOMEN

. . . .

*M*enopause does not signal the termination of a woman's relationship with her gynecologist. She still needs regular screening tests for breast cancer and cervical cancer. Also, other problems, which are uncomfortable or interfere with her sexual life, can develop in her reproductive system.

ATROPHIC VAGINITIS

An inflammation of the vagina caused by drying of the tissue, atrophic vaginitis is a painful condition experienced by some post-menopausal women. Reduced supplies of the hormone estrogen after menopause can leave the walls of the vagina drier, thinner, less elastic, and more prone to irritation. The symptoms of atrophic vaginitis may include vaginal soreness, burning, or itching, painful intercourse, and slight bleeding after intercourse.

Estrogen replacement therapy (p.239) can help relieve all the symptoms. Regular sexual activity will keep the vaginal tissues supple, but intercourse may continue to be painful because of irritated tissue. In that case, a water-soluble lubricant may be beneficial.

UTERINE PROLAPSE

Sometimes the ligaments that hold the uterus weaken with age, allowing it to prolapse, or slip out of place. You may feel a bulge in the walls of the vagina, experience heaviness and discomfort when bearing down, and have stress incontinence (loss of control of the bladder when you cough or laugh too hard), as well as other difficulties in urination and defecation.

Treatment, including Kegel exercises to strengthen the pelvic muscles, is similar to that for stress incontinence (p.316). For a woman who is not sexually active, a vaginal pessary, a rubber ring that is inserted into the vagina to support the uterus, may correct the problem. Surgical repair is another option.

CERVICAL CANCER

Thanks to the widespread use of the Pap test, cervical cancer is usually found in an early, curable stage. Although the disease is associated with young women, older women should continue to have regular Pap tests since there is a long delay between the onset of precancerous changes in the cervix and the actual develop-ment of the disease. Later symptoms of this cancer include bleeding or unusual vaginal discharge.

Treatment for cervical cancer usually involves surgery or radiation therapy, either alone or in combination. In its earliest stages, cervical cancer may be treated on an outpatient basis with cryotherapy (freezing), electrocoagulation (intense heat), or laser surgery. More advanced cervical cancer requires a hysterectomy.

. . . .

OVARIAN CANCER

Called a "silent" killer because it often has no symptoms until its later stages, ovarian cancer requires ongoing vigilance. It is most common in women in their fifties and sixties. One clue to the disease may be an enlarged abdomen caused by an accumulation of fluid. Other vague symptoms, particularly in older women, may include abdominal pain, gas, and bloating.

There has been significant progress in successfully treating ovarian cancer—even advanced cases—in recent years. Depending on the stage of the disease, a combination of surgery (to remove the diseased ovaries, uterus, and/or fallopian tubes), radiation, and chemotherapy is recommended. Taxol, a substance originally derived from the bark of a yew tree, and bone marrow transplants may help in advanced cases.

THE FEMALE REPRODUCTIVE SYSTEM

With the childbearing years behind her, a postmenopausal woman may still face problems with her reproductive system. Ranging from dry tissue in the walls of the vagina, which may require no more than the right lubricant, to difficult-to-diagnose cancers, these health hazards require regular checkups.

The fallopian tubes *are where eggs are fertilized. The egg then travels through the tube to the uterus, where pregnancy is established.*

The ovaries *produce estrogen and other female hormones and release eggs every month during the reproductive years.*

The uterus, *or womb, is where a fetus grows during pregnancy.*

A prolapsed uterus *(shown below) can slip far into the vagina. In this position, it crowds other organs and puts uncomfortable pressure on the bladder.*

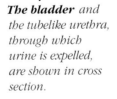

The cervix *is the neck of the uterus.*

The rectum and anus *are shown in cross section.*

The bladder *and the tubelike urethra, through which urine is expelled, are shown in cross section.*

The vagina *is the channel through which a man's sperm travels to fertilize the woman's egg and through which a baby is delivered.*

ENDOMETRIAL CANCER

One of the dangers of estrogen replacement therapy is the possibility of developing endometrial cancer, or cancer of the lining of the uterus. For that reason, many doctors prescribe progesterone as well as estrogen so that women continue to have monthly menstrual periods during which endometrial tissue can be expelled.

Endometrial cancer, which usually occurs only in postmenopausal women, is one of the most curable cancers, especially if detected early. Its symptoms include a bloody or other unusual vaginal discharge. Doctors use hormone therapy to treat precancerous changes of the endometrium; endometrial cancer calls for surgery and radiation treatments.

BENIGN LUMPS IN THE BREAST

During her monthly breast self-examination (p.227), a woman may feel lumps from time to time. Nearly 90 percent of them are no cause for concern. Most are small fluid-filled sacs, or cysts, which form in response to hormonal changes just before menstruation each month and disappear right after. These cysts, referred to as benign fibrocystic condition, occur in half of all women and become more noticeable near menopause.

A less common but equally benign breast growth is a fibroadenoma, a firmer and larger lump that must be biopsied to be identified. A fibroadenoma can safely be left alone. If it causes discomfort or is large enough to distort the shape of the breast, however, it can be removed surgically, often as an outpatient procedure.

A mammogram can help determine whether a lump is benign, as can aspirating fluid from the lump with a needle. Frequently, however, a biopsy is necessary to confirm or rule out cancer.

BREAST CANCER

One out of every nine women will get breast cancer during her lifetime. Most at risk are women over the age of 50; those whose mothers, grandmothers, or sisters have had the disease; those who have never had children; and those who first became pregnant after the age of 30.

The signs of breast cancer are changes in the breast that persist, including a lump, thickening, swelling, dimpling or irritation of the skin, or distortion, retraction, scaliness, pain, or tenderness of the nipple. Many breast cancers are first detected during breast self-examination (p.227). Others are found during a doctor's examination or on a mammogram (pp.228–229). A biopsy can confirm if a lump is malignant. Most biopsies are now performed on an outpatient basis, which allows the patient and her doctor time to discuss the results and the available options before taking action.

The surgical options for a woman with breast cancer have changed dramatically in recent decades (see below). Radical mastectomy—taking the whole breast, the pectoral muscles, and the lymph nodes—is no longer considered necessary. Surgery, however limited or extensive, may be followed by chemotherapy as well as radiation treatments to make sure that any residual cancer cells are destroyed. More advanced cancers, which may require more extensive surgery, are usually followed by radiation, chemotherapy, hormone therapy, or a combination of therapies. These therapies also may be used in advanced inoperable breast cancer.

TYPES OF
BREAST
CANCER
SURGERY
*Mastectomy,
surgical removal
of all or part of
the breast, is the
primary treat-
ment for breast
cancer. The type
of procedure
used depends
on the size and
location of the
tumor and the
extent of the
cancer.*

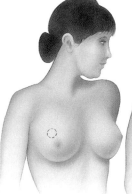

A lumpectomy,
*the least invasive,
removes only the
tumor and some
surrounding tissue.*

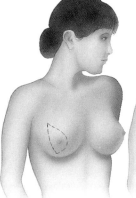

A partial mastectomy
*removes the tumor, more
of the surrounding
tissue, and the skin that
covers the tumor.*

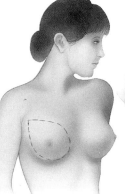

A simple mastectomy
*removes the breast but
leaves the lymph nodes
and the supporting
pectoral muscles.*

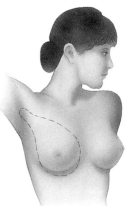

**A modified radical
mastectomy** *removes
the breast and lymph
nodes but leaves the
pectoral muscles.*

LIVING WITH CANCER

Many more people are cured of cancer today than ever before. Fifty percent of Americans with cancer are alive 5 years after their original diagnosis, and a growing number are still living 10 years and more beyond their diagnosis date.

BETTER TREATMENT CHOICES

For many people who do battle with the disease, conditions have greatly improved. A number of cancers that are found early can be treated conservatively to preserve function in the affected organ. Many patients with cancer of the larynx, for example, retain their voice boxes and the ability to speak. Very few patients with colorectal cancer have to cope with permanent colostomies anymore. When bone cancer is found early enough, doctors can often treat it by removing and replacing a section of bone rather than by amputating a limb. New types of surgery for prostate cancer can often preserve a man's potency.

Doctors have also found better ways to pinpoint radiation treatment to more specific areas of the body, sparing healthy organs from unnecessary damage. The new drug combinations used in chemotherapy reduce some of the unpleasant side effects, such as nausea, vomiting, fatigue, and hair loss.

PATIENT INVOLVEMENT

No longer kept in the dark about their disease, patients are urged to participate in decisions about their treatment after they have heard all the pros and cons of the choices. Patients are also encouraged to take steps to make the therapies less traumatic. Learning relaxation techniques, for example, will ease many of the anxieties of being ill. Eating small amounts of food more frequently will keep you nourished and may prevent nausea. Taking afternoon naps may allow you to work full-time without becoming overtired.

Cancer pain can also be better controlled by having patients self-administer analgesics or, in the hospital, having staff give pain medication when it's requested rather than according to a set schedule. Severe pain can be controlled with intravenous pain medications delivered on a continuous basis.

FACING A HOSTILE WORLD

Despite the improvements in treatment, cancer survivors must still cope with a societal stigma about cancer. Being fearful of contagion (totally unfounded because cancer is not an infectious disease) and not knowing what to say to someone who has just fought off a deadly disease may make some friends and colleagues avoid a person who has had cancer.

Federal law now protects a cancer survivor's job, but it can't help with getting promotions or landing a new job when employers won't believe that you are well enough to do the work or worry that you will become ill again. Qualifying for health insurance after you have undergone cancer treatment may also be difficult. Although it may be expensive, you should be able to find coverage through an insurance broker familiar with this problem.

For survivors and for their families and close friends, support groups can supply helpful information as well as comfort from people who understand the experiences you have been through and the problems you are facing. To find a suitable support group, ask your doctor for recommendations or contact the local office of the American Cancer Society, which also offers several rehabilitation and family education programs of its own.

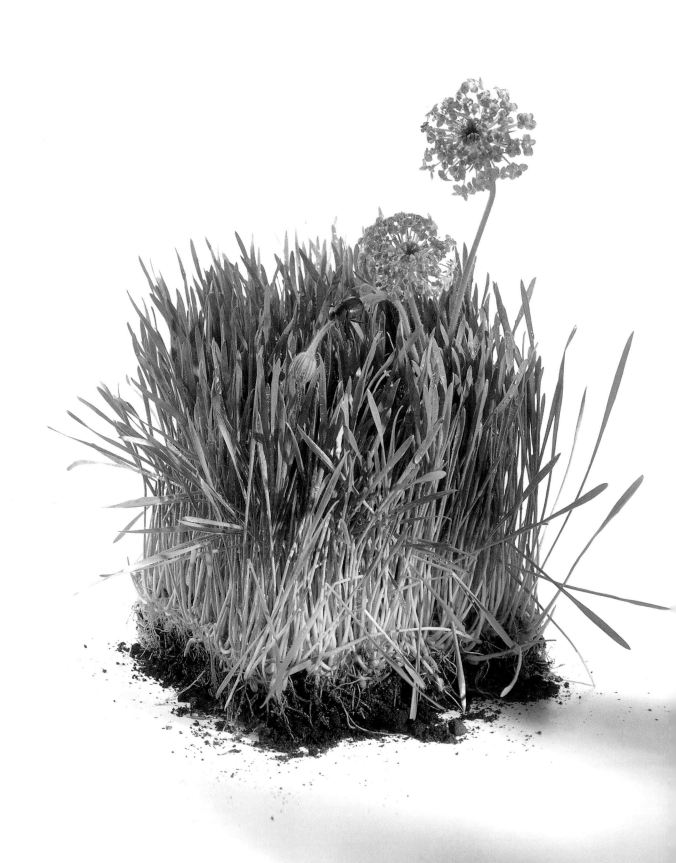

Chapter 8

DEALING WITH YOUR ENVIRONMENT

▦ KEEPING YOUR HOME SAFE AND SECURE *326*

▦ MAKING SURE YOUR WATER IS GOOD FOR YOU *330*

▦ CHECKING INDOOR AIR POLLUTION *332*

▦ RADIATION IN YOUR HOME *336*

▦ AVOIDING TOXIC HOUSEHOLD PRODUCTS *338*

▦ THE DANGERS IN YOUR OWN BACKYARD *342*

▦ BLOCKING OUT NOISE *344*

▦ THE PROBLEM OF OUTDOOR AIR POLLUTION *346*

▦ HOW WEATHER AFFECTS YOU *348*

▦ DRIVING SAFELY THROUGH THE YEARS *350*

Keeping Your Home Safe and Secure

. . . .

Even healthy people become more accident prone as time goes on—you need more light to see clearly, your bones are more fragile, and your reactions are slower. You can prevent some mishaps, however, by rethinking home safety precautions.

SURVEY YOUR LIVING QUARTERS

Some parts of a house present more hazards than others. Stairs, for example, are the site of many serious accidents every year. Bathrooms and kitchens also offer many potential dangers (see *A Home Safety Checklist,* facing page). Fewer mishaps occur in the living room, den, or bedrooms, but you still might trip over exposed electrical wires or slip on polished floors.

Outdoors be sure that your entryways are well lighted and that you have sturdy railings by any steps. If the outside lights are on timers, they can help you see your way when you return home late. Mark or decorate glass doors at eye level so that you or your guests won't walk into them.

. . . .

RULES FOR HANDY PEOPLE

People who do their own home maintenance and repairs should keep safety in mind when they use tools or work in out-of-the-way parts of the house. Each year thousands of people fall off lad-

ders or stools and require emergency care. Always use a ladder tall enough and strong enough for the job. Never stand on the top three rungs of a ladder or the top two steps of a stepladder. Put a ladder's feet on firm and level ground at least a quarter of the ladder's height from the wall. Keep household traffic away and lock any doors under the ladder. Have a helper hold the bottom of the ladder while you climb up. Don't use aluminum ladders near electrical wires in wet conditions—they conduct electricity, and you could get a lethal shock.

Check the lawn for rocks and other objects that could fly up at you while running the power mower. Wear ear protectors when you use loud equipment like leaf blowers, mowers, or saws.

Be sure your workshop has adequate ventilation before using solvents, paints, and stains. Store flammable products in metal containers away from heat sources. Label poisonous products. Wear goggles for any work in which dangerous liquids or sharp pieces might hit your eyes. Wear filter masks when sanding, painting, or working with irritating chemicals.

FIRE PREVENTION

The primary cause of household fires is faulty or misused home heating equipment. Clean and check the heating system annually. Don't use an unvented kerosene or gas heater (they are illegal in many communities). If you use portable heaters, set them well clear of furniture and drapes. Buy only heaters that shut off automatically when tipped over. Be sure your fireplace or wood stove conforms to local fire laws (ask for an inspection). Store trash and other combustible materials at least 3 feet away from your furnace and water heater. Have your chimney and heating system flue inspected and cleaned at least once a year.

Home electrical systems can also cause fires. A blown fuse or tripped circuit breaker is the first sign of overloaded circuitry. Before replacing a fuse (always with a fuse of the same amperage) or resetting the circuit, make sure you know what caused the failure—too many appliances on a single circuit or a faulty appliance, for example—so that you can remedy the dangerous situation. If you feel a hot spot in the wall, assume that your circuitry is overloaded and unplug your appliances. Call the fire department to be sure a fire isn't already smoldering, then have an electrician identify and remedy the problem. Extension cords are potential hazards; use as few as pos-

A HOME SAFETY CHECKLIST

Stairs	• Provide lighting at the bottom and top of stairs; put switches on both levels. • Keep the stairways inside and outside the house in good repair, with firm handrails and no wobbly steps. • Mark the edges of basement and attic stairs (especially the first and last steps) with contrasting strips of tape or rubber so that you won't miss a step. Post signs on doors opening onto stairs. • Clear staircases of clutter that you or someone else may trip over. • Carpet frequently used stairs to cushion falls, making sure that the installation is secure.
Bathroom	• Make sure that bathroom electrical outlets are ground fault interrupters (GFI's), which protect you from shock when you are wet (they are now required in many building codes). • Keep electrical appliances away from the sink, tub, and shower. • Use only nonslip bath mats and rugs on the floor. • Install nonskid strips on the bottom of the tub and/or shower. • Install handrails near the toilet and the tub. • To prevent scalding, set the water heater temperature no higher than 120°F. • Label all medicine bottles clearly and flush their contents down the toilet when a prescription expires.
Kitchen	• Be sure a gas stove is properly vented to the outside. • Store flammable items away from burners. • To avoid burns while cooking, turn pot handles in on the stove and always use pot holders. • Never wear garments with long, loose sleeves while cooking. • Maintain a sharp edge on knives (dull knives cause accidents). • Keep cabinet doors closed to avoid bumping your head or hitting your shin. • Wash but don't wax the floor (waxed floors are slippery). • Buy a sturdy step stool to stand on when reaching high cupboards (chairs tip) or invest in a long-handled clamp for taking items off high shelves.
Living Room	• Be sure bulb wattage matches lamp capacity (don't put a 100-watt bulb in a socket designed for a 60-watt bulb). If you need more light for reading or close work, buy lamps designed for more powerful bulbs. • Keep the fireplace screen or glass doors closed whenever there is a fire. Keep flammable materials at least 3 feet from the fireplace. • Tape down area rugs or stabilize them with nonskid padding. • Tack electrical cords to baseboards along the floor and to the woodwork around doors to keep them out of the way. Don't run cords under rugs; if they fray and become an electrical hazard, you won't notice.
Bedroom	• Make sure that the switch on your bedside lamp is easy to reach from bed and that the night table is large enough to hold your glasses, a telephone, and other necessities comfortably. • Keep emergency numbers by your telephone (or program them into a telephone that stores numbers). • Clear the path from your bed to the door of obstacles and clutter.
Hallway	• Check that all carpeting is smooth and tacked down securely. • Make sure the light switch is convenient to reach (a switch with a light in it is also a help). • Keep the path from bedrooms to bathroom free of obstacles and clutter. A low-wattage hall light will make middle-of-the-night trips to the bathroom safer. • Install a smoke detector near the bedrooms.

sible and make sure each is the correct gauge for the appliance. Check all your lamps and electrical appliances periodically and replace frayed cords or damaged plugs as needed.

Smokers can start fires if they are careless about extinguishing their cigarettes, cigars, and pipes. Provide a smoker with a deep fireproof ashtray that is broad and sturdy enough not to tip over. Insist that no one in the household—family member or guest—ever smoke in bed.

Smoke detectors are your best insurance against being surprised by fire, particularly at night. Units with ionization sensors may start bleating every time you use the oven, but the newer photosensitive detectors aren't fooled by normal kitchen vapors. Install a smoke detector on each level of the house, high on a wall or on the ceiling, away from windows, doors, and vents. Test the units regularly and replace the batteries twice a year (do it when you turn your clocks back in the fall and forward in the spring).

You should also keep multipurpose fire extinguishers on each level of the house and make sure you know how to use them (see p.328).

DEALING WITH A FIRE

Be prepared to fight different types of fires with the appropriate extinguising material. Don't throw water on a grease fire, for example; smother it with salt, baking soda, or a Class B fire extinguisher instead.

Fires spread quickly and allow little time for escape. You and your family should agree upon a fire alarm signal to use. You should have two exit routes for each room in the house, and the family should practice using them in regular fire drills. During a fire, if one door is hot, take the alternate route. Upstairs bedrooms may need folding escape ladders for climbing out a window as a second exit. Keep your escape windows in working order and your hallways free of clutter for an easier exit.

INSTALLING A FIRE EXTINGUISHER

The most likely places for a home fire—kitchen, fireplace, and garage—should be equipped with suitable fire extinguishers. Class A extinguishers put out paper, wood, cloth, or trash fires; Class B, fires from oil or flammable liquids; Class C, electrical fires. An extinguisher rated BC is a good choice for the kitchen, garage, and workshop, where grease and electrical fires are likely. Other parts of the house may best be served by an ABC "all-purpose" extinguisher. Buy a model that is light enough to lift and use easily and that has a UL (Underwriters Laboratory) or FM (Factory Mutual) seal.

Install fire extinguishers near room exits to give yourself a way out if you can't quench a fire.

HOME SECURITY

Some people don't feel safe in their homes without an electronic alarm system. The best ones, for which you pay an installation charge and a monthly fee, automatically call a security agency to alert the police when any of the sensors are tripped. Since there are many alarm systems on the market, ask your local police for recommendations. Completely burglar-proofing your home—even with an alarm system—may be impossible, but a few simple security measures can go a long way toward discouraging intruders and preventing the loss of things you love.

Locking up

Secure *all* the entrances to your home. Many burglars walk right in the front door because the lock

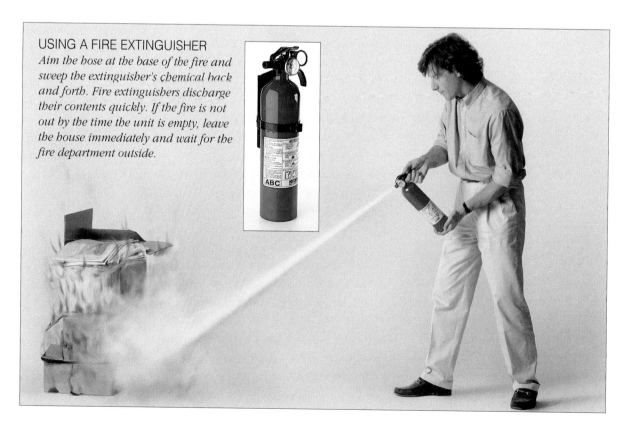

USING A FIRE EXTINGUISHER
Aim the hose at the base of the fire and sweep the extinguisher's chemical back and forth. Fire extinguishers discharge their contents quickly. If the fire is not out by the time the unit is empty, leave the house immediately and wait for the fire department outside.

is easy to pick or remove or the door itself is flimsy. Solid doors equipped with dead-bolt locks and wide-angle peepholes instead of glass panels offer the surest protection. Sliding glass doors should be equipped with locking metal rods in the sliding channel. Be sure all your accessible windows have locks, and if you live in a high-crime neighborhood, consider putting grates or steel shutters on all the basement and first-floor windows. Get in the habit of always locking up.

Smart moves

Make it hard for a burglar to figure out whether or not you're at home. Use timed floodlights or porch lights to light up your property. Keep trees and shrubs trimmed so that prowlers have no place to hide as they try to get into the house. Choose see-through fences for the same reason.

Don't tempt burglars by putting expensive items on display near a window. Mark your valuables so that they can be identified if they are stolen. Many police departments lend out engraving tools and give you a window sticker that tells thieves that your possessions are registered.

Keep an inventory of your valuables. If you are burglarized, you will have an easier time establishing a claim with your insurance company if you can show receipts, model numbers, and snapshots of the missing items.

Friendly allies

Neighbors are good protection against burglars. People who are familiar with your regular routine will notice something unusual and let you know. An effective way to discourage break-ins is to form a block watch group. Burglars don't want to be noticed.

They will usually avoid neighborhoods where they see a lot of traffic between houses.

Dealing with a burglary

When you discover a theft, don't touch anything. Call the police. If you hear an intruder, leave the house quietly if you can and call the police from a neighbor's house. If you can't leave, hide or pretend to be asleep.

. . . .

HOW TO HAVE A WORRY-FREE VACATION

If you carefully secure your home and valuables before you leave and take measures to make the house appear lived in, you can relax and enjoy your holiday.

■ Put cash, jewelry, and other valuables in a safe-deposit box.
■ Lock all windows, doors, and other possible points of entry.
■ Set timers to turn lights on and off in an irregular sequence. Also use timers to turn on a television or a radio to increase the illusion that someone is home.
■ Ask a trusted neighbor to pick up your mail and newspapers and to reset the blinds and curtains.
■ Don't announce that you're away on your telephone answering machine. Set the machine to pick up on the second ring and simply ask callers to leave a name, number, and message. Otherwise, lower the phone bell so that it can't be heard outside.
■ Arrange for someone to keep the lawn mowed.
■ Lock up ladders and tools a burglar could use to break into your house.
■ Keep empty garbage and trash cans out of sight.
■ Leave a locked car in the driveway or ask a neighbor to park there while you're away.

FAST FACTS

■ Protect yourself from lightning. If you are caught in the open outdoors during a thunderstorm, kneel on the ground away from trees, metal fences, and water. Stay in a closed car, but get out of an open vehicle such as a tractor or golf cart. Indoors, stay off the telephone and unplug electrical appliances.

■ Lead crystal decanters are no place to store brandy or wine; lead can leach from the glass into the liquid. The longer alcoholic beverages remain in crystal containers, the higher the lead content. Port wine stored in a lead crystal decanter for 4 months can reach a level of 3,500 micrograms of lead per liter—233 times the Environmental Protection Agency guidelines for drinking water.

■ Residential smoke detectors, first widely used in the 1980's, contributed to a 20 percent drop in home fire deaths during that decade, according to the United States Consumer Product Safety Commission.

■ A manual lawn mower is healthier for you than a power mower: it is quiet, causes no pollution, and using it burns between 420 and 480 calories an hour.

Making Sure
Your Water Is Good for You

. . . .

American drinking water is among the best and safest in the world, thanks to drinking water quality standards established by the federal government. But no system is perfect, and adherence to guidelines varies.

WATER SOURCES AND WATER QUALITY

The quality of your drinking water depends in part on where you live—in the city, in the country, near an industrial plant or a landfill—and whether you get your water from a well, spring, lake, pond, or reservoir.

Contrary to popular belief, city water is usually purer than small town water or water from a private system. Small towns often can't afford the sophisticated water treatment plants that cities can. And in rural areas, private water systems don't always conform to local health codes.

Water from lakes, rivers, ponds, and reservoirs may be polluted with chemicals such as oil, gasoline, nitrates, and pesticides, as well as with microorganisms that can cause a wide range of illnesses.

Water from underground sources can also be polluted. A spring or shallow well can be full of algae, decaying plant matter, insects, and animal waste products. Deep-drilled (artesian) wells can be contaminated not only by microorganisms but also by nitrates, pesticides, radionuclides, oil, and industrial products and wastes. Because of these possibilities, it's a good idea to monitor any activity in your area that could affect your water source.

. . . .

CONTAMINANTS FROM PLUMBING

If your plumbing or the pipes that connect you to the local water delivery system are old, you may have problems with lead, asbestos, and other harmful substances leaching into your drinking water through the pipes. It's always wise, even if you have new plumbing, to let your cold water tap run for a few minutes the first time you use it in the morning or after any period of disuse. That way, residues that have accumulated can be flushed out. Never cook with or drink water from the hot water tap— hot water dissolves lead more rapidly than cold water and can, as a result, contain much higher levels of lead.

CHECKING THE SAFETY OF YOUR WATER SUPPLY

According to the experts, your safest source of drinking water is still the kitchen tap—provided that your supplier meets all the requirements of the Safe Drinking Water Act and you have not received notices of any violation.

If you're concerned about your water supply, here's how you can determine whether it meets Environmental Protection Agency (EPA) standards:

■ Request the latest water quality report from your water supplier. For help in interpreting the numbers, call the EPA's Safe Drinking Water Hotline at 1-800-426-4791.

■ Look through local newspapers for articles on water pollution, new construction, and land planning decisions that may affect your water supply.

■ If you suspect a problem with your drinking water, notify officials at your local health department. If they don't provide water testing, ask them to help you select which tests to have done and to recommend a state-certified laboratory in your area to do them (or check the Yellow Pages). Or find out if the public health or ecology departments of any local universities offer testing. Tests should cost between $15 (for lead) and $1500 (for dioxin). Be wary of firms that offer "free" tests. These are usually the introduction to a sales pitch for expensive water-purifying equipment.

A CONSUMER'S GUIDE TO BOTTLED WATER

	Source	Advantages	Disadvantages
Club soda	Tap water.	Most pollutants are filtered from the water, and minerals are added for flavor.	Most club soda is high in sodium—30 to 65 milligrams per 8 ounces.
Distilled (or purified) water	Tap water.	All minerals (including sodium) are filtered out.	Beneficial minerals are also removed. Purified water stored in plastic bottles may absorb chemicals leached from the plastic.
Mineral water	Usually spring water.	Most pollutants are filtered from the water, and beneficial minerals are often added.	Mineral water may not be any better for you than filtered tap water, but it is definitely more expensive.
Seltzer	Tap water.	Most pollutants are filtered from the water.	Manufacturers sometimes add sweeteners such as sucrose or corn syrup.
Spring water	Natural spring or underground reservoir.	The water contains a generally high level of beneficial minerals.	The water is only as pure as its source. Some springs contain toxic organic chemicals and heavy metals. Even premium brands have been found to contain pollutants.

HOME WATER FILTERS

Although the EPA contends that in most instances home water filters are unnecessary, many people use them. The major types of filters are described below. No single device can eliminate every contaminant, however, and all filters need regular upkeep to prevent bacterial contamination.

■ *Carbon filters* (see photo, top right). Relatively inexpensive, carbon filters remove organic chemicals, odors, and bad tastes, but not usually lead. Make sure you choose the type of carbon filter that fits your particular needs.

■ *Distillers.* This type of filter boils water until it turns into steam, then allows it to recondense. The process gets rid of lead, other heavy metals, and microorganisms—but not organic chemicals. Distillers are generally expensive and require the most maintenance and energy use.

■ *Lead filter cartridges.* Your best choice if lead is your only problem, these filters are relatively inexpensive and very effective if changed frequently.

■ *Reverse osmosis filters* (see photo, bottom right). These units use a porous membrane and a carbon filter to screen out most contaminants. The process wastes a great deal of water, and some units store purified water in holding tanks, where it can stagnate.

■ *Water softeners.* Used with hard water, softeners filter out calcium, iron, and magnesium, minerals that limit sudsing and leave stains or deposits. Because softeners make your water more corrosive, they can increase any leaching of lead from plumbing.

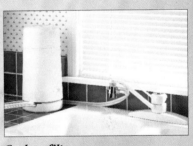
Carbon filter

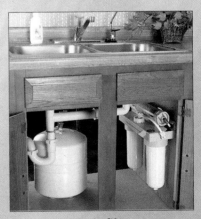
Reverse osmosis filter

CHECKING INDOOR AIR POLLUTION

The Environmental Protection Agency lists indoor air quality among the leading environmental health threats in the United States—ahead of such serious issues as hazardous waste dumps, toxic pesticides, impure drinking water, and unsafe sewage. Aware of the problem or not, people spend an average of 90 percent of their lives indoors.

DEFINING THE PROBLEM

Doctors recognize that indoor air pollutants can damage the lungs and cause allergic and other reactions, but identifying the specific substance causing sickness in a particular patient is often difficult. Pollution-related illnesses can mimic the symptoms of the flu, allergies, and other diseases. And some people are more vulnerable to indoor air pollutants than others. Exposure to carbon monoxide, for example, may give one person a headache but cause another to have a heart attack.

Whether or not you are particularly susceptible to these pollutants, you should be aware of the potential health consequences for some people.

THE CAUSES OF INDOOR AIR POLLUTION

Energy-conscious homeowners who have made their houses airtight with caulking and weatherstripping have also, inadvertently, exacerbated whatever indoor pollution their homes may be subject to. Before homes were so carefully weatherproofed, natural ventilation through cracks, loose window and door frames, and other openings completely changed the air in a house every hour. In today's well-sealed buildings with both heating and cooling systems, the air may not totally change for 4 to 25 hours.

The major sources of bad indoor air are often by-products of modern technology. The most serious pollutants that you are likely to face at home are discussed in-

---

SICK BUILDING SYNDROME

If allergic symptoms—migraine headaches, sinus pain, sneezing, coughing, and fatigue—flare up when you are at work and subside when you leave, you may be suffering from sick building syndrome.

When homes and office buildings were made airtight in the 1970's to cut down on energy bills, they also locked in stale, unhealthy air. Climate-controlled office buildings with windows that can't be opened often have ventilation systems that are inadequate to the challenges of modern office technology. Electrical equipment such as photocopiers and laser printers can give off ozone. Glue, rubber cement, inks, typewriter ribbon, and correction fluid release toxic vapors. Carpeting and uphol-

stered furniture contain volatile organic chemicals such as formaldehyde. Maintenance workers often use strong cleaning chemicals. All these fumes can spread throughout a building via the ventilation system.

The antidote to sick buildings is fresh air. If a building has air that negatively affects a number of the people who work in it, the management should be petitioned to check the ventilation system. Often a malfunctioning system can be repaired and adjusted to circulate more fresh air through the building and solve the problem. When occupants of the building suffer severe reactions, however, the management may have to consider replacing the building materials and furnishings that are causing the illness.

dividually on pages 334–335. Radon, a radioactive gas that occurs naturally in soil, water, and natural gas in some parts of the country and can seep into houses, is discussed on pages 336–337.

CLEARING THE AIR

Controlling the sources of pollution is the first step to fresh indoor air. Keep your heating and cooling systems and their flues well maintained and clean. Reduce the number of toxic chemicals employed in your home and be sure you use and store them properly. Confine smokers to the porch or a single room.

Ventilation can be an effective antidote to indoor pollution. Open windows strategically at opposite ends of the house to create crosscurrents that will draw fresh air into the whole building. An exhaust fan in the kitchen and another in the bathroom will remove humidity as well as pollutants, discouraging mold and fungi. An attic exhaust fan, used in summer for cooling, will also draw fresh air through the house.

People with allergies, asthma, heart disease, or any condition made worse by air pollution may benefit from using an electronic air cleaner. A unit that serves the whole house can be installed in the return-air duct of a warm-air heating system or a central air-conditioning system. A less expensive alternative is a room-size unit that can be plugged into an electical outlet. Air cleaners can filter out such airborne pollutants as pollen, dust, bacteria, viruses, mold spores, mite pellets, and animal dander, but they can't remove dangerous gases. They must be cleaned regularly in order to stay effective.

Another option is a central vacuum cleaner system, which has a vent to the outside for dust and locates the dirt canister safely out of the way in the basement; it can cut down on interior dust, pollen, animal dander, and mite pellets.

If you have room air conditioners, keep the filters clean (some can be washed; others need replacing) to discourage the growth of molds. You should clean humidifiers regularly (daily for some) to prevent the dispersal of mold spores and mineral dust.

CALLING IN A PROFESSIONAL

Some forms of indoor pollution are difficult to handle safely by yourself. If you have gas heat or gas appliances, call your local utility company when you suspect a leak. Open a window for ventilation, then leave the house without delay; leaking gas is volatile and easily ignited.

If there are smells in the house that you can't identify, or if people in the house are suffering illnesses that may be pollution related, you may want to hire a testing service to evaluate your indoor air.

Also, before you start a remodeling project in an older house, you should have an expert look at the materials that you will be tearing out to see if asbestos is involved. If asbestos must be disturbed, you should hire a professional to do the job.

To find reliable experts and services in your area, consult your state or local health department or the Environmental Protection Agency (EPA). The EPA publishes a state-by-state directory of people who are trained and experienced in diagnosing and handling indoor pollutants.

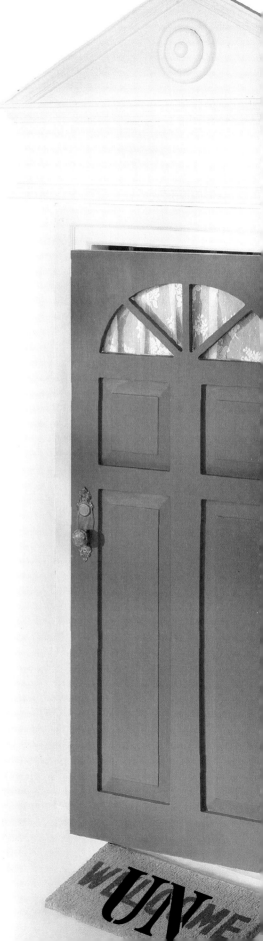

THE SOURCES OF INDOOR AIR POLLUTION

The major pollutants that you are likely to encounter in your home are discussed individually below. The letter keys in the illustration indicate where each may be found in a typical house. Living in an apartment doesn't exempt you from these poisons; they may be present in any kind of home.

Ⓐ Asbestos

Prolonged exposure to asbestos fibers can cause lung cancer, other lung diseases, and respiratory problems. Banned from most new products, asbestos is a threat only when its fibers become airborne and are inhaled. Houses that were built more than 20 years ago may have asbestos-containing materials in floors, ceiling tiles, exterior siding and roof shingles, and the insulation around heating pipes and electrical wires. Until they begin to deteriorate with age or are disturbed during remodeling or cleaning, these materials usually present no danger. If you must remove asbestos materials, hire a professional to do the job (p.333).

Ⓑ Carbon monoxide

A colorless, odorless, and tasteless gas, carbon monoxide (CO) accounts for half the fatal poisonings in the United States each year. The gas can be detected with sensors similar to smoke alarms. Undetected, it causes symptoms ranging from headaches and irritability to nausea and vomiting. Prolonged exposure in confined areas causes coma and death. To keep it out of your house, have your heating and hot-water systems and their flues inspected and cleaned annually. Vent all your gas appliances to the outside. Never burn chemically treated wood or charcoal in the fireplace. Never idle the motor of your car in the garage.

Ⓒ Formaldehyde

A common source of indoor air pollution is formaldehyde, a strong-smelling gas used in the building-material adhesives that bond the particle board and plywood often found in paneling, floors, kitchen counters, and kitchen cabinets. Formaldehyde is also used in no-iron fabric finishes, upholstery, and carpeting and was formerly used in home insulation. Exposure to its fumes causes headaches, eye irritation, asthma and other breathing problems, and possibly cancer.

The best defense against formaldehyde in your home is to improve ventilation. You can also

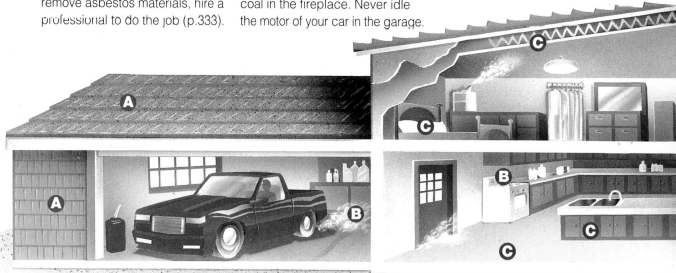

In addition to the pollutants keyed in above, you should be aware of other threats to indoor air quality. Humidifiers should be scrubbed (see p.333). Newly dry-cleaned clothes should be aired by an open window to dissipate the chemicals. Cleaning supplies should be used only in ventilated areas.

seal reeking particle board and plywood with polyurethane varnish, vinyl wallpaper, or vinyl floor coverings. Sometimes, however, subflooring or walls contain such high levels of formaldehyde that you may finally have to replace them to eliminate the fumes.

Formaldehyde emissions from building materials usually decrease with time. It takes about 8 years, however, for the fumes to dissipate from pressed-wood products. To check the level of formaldehyde in your home, buy a dosimeter from an industrial health and safety supply company and measure the fumes yourself or consult with the EPA or your local health department.

D Pesticides

Americans use some 350 million pounds of pesticides inside their homes and on their lawns and gardens every year. Many contain extremely toxic and long-lived chemicals. Until 1987, for example, chlordane, which persists in soil for decades and has been connected to cancer, chronic liver disease, and other health problems, was commonly used to kill termites in the ground around homes. Chlordane and other toxic chemicals in the soil can seep through cracks in the basement walls or flooring. If you smell a chemical odor that you don't recognize in the basement, you may want to have your basement air tested (p.333).

E Tobacco smoke

Not only does smoking cigarettes, cigars, or pipes cause emphysema, bronchitis, lung cancer, and other diseases, but it also fills the room with carbon monoxide emissions, benzene, ammonia, nicotine, and carcinogenic tars. Well-documented evidence now shows that people who smoke put others besides themselves at risk. Nonsmokers, particularly young children, in the same room with smokers also suffer ill effects from breathing these chemicals. If you smoke, the only way to reduce the health threat to yourself—and to the people you live, socialize, and work with—is to give up the habit (see pp.242–245).

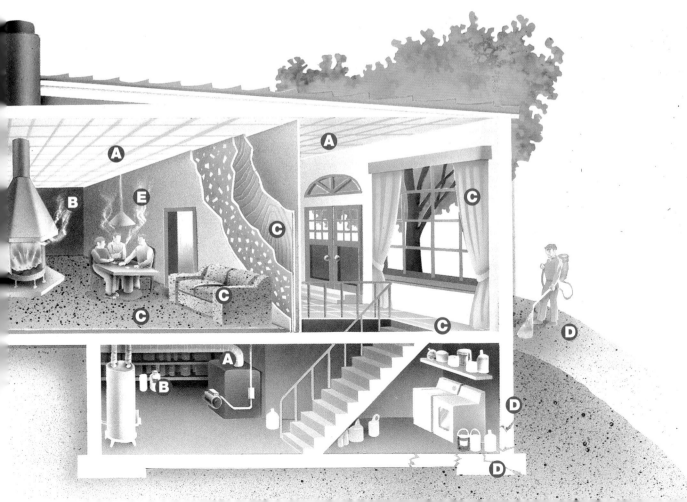

RADIATION IN YOUR HOME

*R*adiation—electromagnetic energy—is everywhere. It reaches you from the sun, from the
earth as a by-product of certain elements, and
from man-made objects and systems. While some of
your exposure to radiation is beneficial, certain kinds
can be harmful to your health.

MAGNETIC FIELD EMISSIONS FROM HOUSEHOLD APPLIANCES

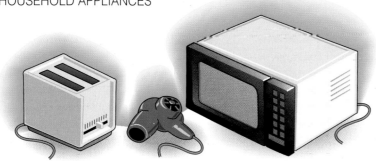

The magnetic fields of household appliances vary considerably, depending on
product design and manufacturer. If the appliance has different speeds, magnetic
fields may be higher when the appliance is operated on a high setting. Some
experts claim there may be health risks at 3-milligauss levels, but studies are
inconclusive.

Appliance	Magnetic Field (in milligauss)		
	At 6 inches[†]	At 1 foot	At 2 feet
Coffeemakers	4–10	*–1	Insignificant
Color TV's	Not available	*–20	*–8
Electric blankets (at 2 inches[†])	0.09–2.7	NA	NA
Electric conventional ovens	4–20	1–5	*–1
Electric ranges	20–200	*–30	*–9
Electric shavers	4–600	NA	NA
Fluorescent lights	20–100	*–30	*–8
Hair dryers	1–700	*–70	*–10
Microwave ovens	100–300	*–100	2–30
Portable heaters	5–150	1–40	*–8
Toasters	5–20	*–7	Insignificant
Vacuum cleaners	100–700	20–200	4–50
Video display terminals (color monitors)	7–20	2–6	1–3

*The magnetic field was so small that it could not be distinguished from background mea-
surements taken before the appliance had been turned on.
Source: Environmental Protection Agency, 1992.

MAN-MADE RADIATION

The dangers of very-high-fre-
quency radiation—the kind produced by nuclear energy and
other radioactive sources—are
well known. High-frequency (or
ionizing) radiation can damage
and even kill body cells. What's
less clear is how people are affected by very-low-frequency (or
non-ionizing) radiation, which
occurs in the form of electric and
magnetic fields (or EMF's) that
surround power lines and electrical appliances (see chart, left). Al
though some studies suggest a
link between exposure to low-
frequency radiation and leukemia
and other forms of cancer, there is
still no conclusive scientific evidence. Until more is known, reasonable caution is probably the
best approach.

■ Replace electric blankets made
before 1990 with newer ones
whose electric magnetic field
emissions have been reduced by
85 percent. Or use quilts, com-
forters, and ordinary blankets instead. If you have a waterbed, run
the heater during the day and
turn it off when you get into bed.

■ Keep your microwave oven in
good repair. Check the gasket on
the door periodically to make
sure that it closes properly.

■ When using a video display terminal (VDT), sit at least 28 inches
away from the screen (an average
arm's length).

One source of man-made radiation that should be of less concern is medical X-rays. While it
makes sense to minimize your exposure, the diagnostic benefits of
X-rays usually outweigh the risks.

HOW RADON ENTERS YOUR HOME

The gas seeps into your house through small cracks and openings in your foundation and walls and around pipe fittings, as well as from building materials and exposed soil. Any radon in your water supply is released into your household's atmosphere whenever you turn on faucets or showers.

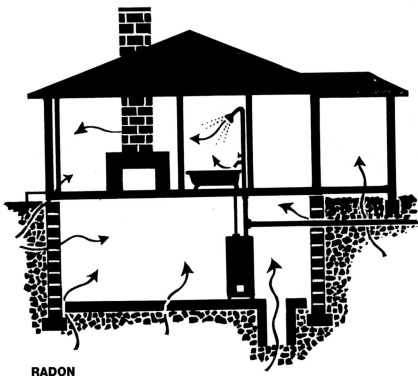

RADON

About two-thirds of the radiation you're exposed to comes from natural sources—the bulk of it from radon, a radioactive gas produced from uranium in the soil, from water that runs through uranium-bearing rock, or from materials made from such soil or rock. Outdoors, radon dissipates in the atmosphere; indoors, where it can accumulate, it becomes a health hazard. This odorless, invisible gas is second only to smoking as a cause of lung cancer. Exposure to both tobacco smoke and radon greatly increases your risk of lung cancer.

Because radon levels depend on a home's specific structure and location, every home should be tested. You can buy an Environ-mental Protection Agency (EPA) –approved or state-certified kit at a hardware store. A test lasting 90 days to 1 year is the most accurate because radon levels fluctuate. If you need results quickly, two successive tests, each lasting from 2 to 7 days, can be done.

To reduce elevated radon levels, patch any cracks in the house or its foundation, cover or vent sumps or other exposed basement areas, and install a system of ventilation fans to move the gas out of the house. To find an EPA-rated contractor, consult your state radon office. For more information, write to the Environmental Protection Agency, Public Information Center, 401 M St. S.W., Washington, DC 20460.

VDT-RELATED INJURIES

While the radiation risks from working at video display terminals (VDT's) have not been determined, other health problems are very evident. Eyestrain, neck and back pain, and repetitive-motion injuries of the hands, such as carpal tunnel syndrome, are all common. There are measures you can take, however, to ease or prevent such problems.

■ Make sure that there is no glare on the monitor screen and that the top of the screen is at eye level, so that you look at the center with a slightly downward gaze. Adjust the screen for brightness, contrast, and focus. You should not have to lean forward to see properly. If you continue to have trouble, ask your ophthalmologist to prescribe special eyeglasses for use with the monitor.

■ Place the keyboard so that you can reach it with your elbows bent at a 90-degree angle. You should not have to bend your wrists to type.

■ Sit up straight, with your back angled backward a few degrees, arms relaxed, feet flat on the floor, in a chair whose height and backrest are adjustable.

■ Limber up your hands regularly: massage one hand with the other and clench and release your fist.

■ Take a break at least every 2 hours. Get up and walk around or do some simple exercises.

AVOIDING TOXIC HOUSEHOLD PRODUCTS

*N*o one knows what consequences the long-term use of toxic household chemicals may have on your general health. If you are especially sensitive, you may develop problems after just one exposure. Other people may not exhibit any reactions. Regardless of their effect on you, however, it makes sense to limit your contact with these products as much as possible.

USING TOXIC PRODUCTS SAFELY

Drain and oven cleaners, furniture and floor polishes, laundry detergents, pesticides, spot removers, and window cleaners all contain dangerous chemicals. To keep your home—and your family—healthy, consider replacing such materials whenever possible with low-tech alternatives (see chart, facing page, and *Getting Rid of Pests*, pp.339–340).

For those tasks that require using heavy-duty commercial household products, follow these safety guidelines:

■ Always read the entire label of a product to ensure that you will use it correctly and take whatever safety precautions may be necessary.
■ Store all materials in their original labeled containers with their lids firmly sealed so that volatile fumes can't escape; keep them in a place out of the reach of children and pets.

■ Buy only as much of a product as you need. Read the directions carefully and don't use more of it than is stipulated. Finish it promptly and clean up thoroughly. If you're not sure how to dispose of any leftover materials and cleaning rags or sponges, call your local waste disposal facility or poison control center.
■ Never combine two or more substances unless the instructions specifically say you should do so. Mixtures—ammonia and chlorine bleach, for example—can be lethal.
■ Use all chemicals in a well-ventilated area so that you won't breathe in their fumes.
■ Check with your local waste disposal department to find out if it schedules special household hazardous waste days, when items such as paints, solvents, motor oil, antifreeze, pesticides, and batteries can be dropped off at a collection point.

HOBBY MATERIALS

Art and craft supplies—acrylics, oil-based paints, paint solvents, shellacs, inks, pastels, photographic chemicals, clay ceramic powders, wood stains, airplane glue, rubber cement, and epoxy and instant-bonding glues—all contain toxic chemicals.

If you are a hobbyist, ask your suppliers for the least toxic materials. Always be sure to work in a well-ventilated area that has been specifically designated for your activity. Wear rubber or plastic gloves, goggles, and masks when

TOOLS FOR NONTOXIC HOUSEHOLD CLEANING

Old-fashioned household products often work just as well as—and sometimes even better than—commercial ones that contain such hazardous chemicals as corrosives, respiratory irritants and toxins, known and suspected carcinogens, and even environmental hazards such as petrochemicals. The following are some safe and inexpensive alternatives.

	Commercial Products	*Alternatives*
All-purpose cleaners	Usually contain ammonia.	Combine 1 teaspoon of liquid soap, borax, or trisodium phospate (TSP, available in hardware stores) with 1 quart of warm water. Add a few drops of lemon juice or vinegar to cut grease. Or use a soap-based commercial cleaning product.
Drain cleaners	Contain lye. May contain hydrochloric acid and sodium hypochloride. Liquid drain cleaners release strong vapors.	Try using a plunger first. Also practice preventive plumbing—use drain strainers to trap food and hair and never put grease down the drain. Once a week, pour 1/4 cup of baking soda and 1/2 cup of white vinegar down the drain. Keep the drain covered tightly for 1 minute, then run hot water for 1–2 minutes.
Furniture and floor polishes	Contain nitrobenzene and phenol. May contain diethylene glycol.	Use any vegetable oil or plain mineral oil, the active ingredient in most commercial polishes. If you prefer a fresh scent, add 1 teaspoon of lemon oil to 2 cups of oil.
Laundry detergents	Contain bleaches and petrochemicals.	Clean natural fibers with soap flakes. To remove perspiration and other odors, add 1 cup of baking soda, white vinegar, or borax, or 1 tablespoon of trisodium phosphate, to each load of wash. Check your supermarket or health food store for nontoxic detergents with natural ingredients.
Oven cleaners	Contain ammonia and lye. May contain potassium hydroxide.	Sprinkle water on the area, then cover with a dusting of baking soda. Scrub with a fine steel wool pad. Wipe off with paper towels. Rinse well and wipe dry.
Silver polishes	Contain ammonia and petroleum distillates.	For silverware: Place a sheet of aluminum foil in a saucepan, cover with 2 or 3 inches of water, add 1 teaspoon each of salt and baking soda, and bring to a boil. Put in the silver for 2 or 3 minutes, then rinse and wipe dry. For jewelry: Fill a glass jar halfway full with thin aluminum foil strips. Then add 1 tablespoon of salt and enough cold water to fill the jar. Drop your jewelry into the jar and cover; remove the jewelry after a few minutes, rinse, and dry. You can also polish silver with a mixture of toothpaste and warm water, applying it with an old soft-bristled toothbrush.
Spot removers	Contain perchloroethylene and toluene.	For chocolate and red wine stains, pour on club soda— liberally and immediately. To remove blood, chocolate, coffee, mildew, mud, and urine stains, soak the garment in a mixture of 1/4 cup borax and 2 cups of cold water. For grease stains, a damp cloth dipped in borax—or a paste of cornstarch and water—is often effective.
Window cleaners	Contain ammonia and blue dye.	Use a mixture of 1/2 water and 1/2 vinegar in a spray bottle.

necessary. Don't eat or drink while you're working—you could inadvertently poison yourself. And, of course, resist the temptation to let the kitchen double as an art studio.

GETTING RID OF PESTS

Fly and roach sprays, flea bombs, and roach and rat poisons don't just kill pests. They expose people and their pets to toxic chemicals such as deet (diethyl toluamide), contained in insect repellents, and dichlorvos, used in commercial fly strips, flea collars,

POISONING EMERGENCIES

Unfortunately, the antidotes listed on household product labels are sometimes inadequate or erroneous. Rather than relying on such information, you're much better off calling your local poison control center in the event of an emergency.

When a poison is swallowed, first aid varies. Describe the substance swallowed and the age and physical condition of the victim. You may be told to induce vomiting by giving the victim syrup of ipecac. For those poisons that will cause more harm if they are brought up, you may be instructed to give the person milk or water to dilute the poison and slow its absorption, or activated charcoal to prevent its absorption. Never attempt to induce vomiting in or give liquids to someone who is unconscious or having seizures; instead, you should get medical help at once.

If a toxic substance has been splashed in the person's eyes, keep flooding the eyes with lukewarm or cold water for at least 15 minutes. For toxic spills on skin, carefully remove the person's contaminated clothing and flood the affected area with water, then cleanse thoroughly with a mild soap and rinse again with water. If the poison has been inhaled, move the victim to fresh air immediately or open all the doors and windows.

In severe cases of poisoning, in which the person is not breathing, knowing how to perform artificial respiration and cardiopulmonary resuscitation (CPR) may prevent a tragedy from occurring.

---

flea bombs, and roach sprays. Pesticides are hazardous during their application; professionally applied ones can linger for days or weeks afterward.

Fortunately, there are effective, less toxic alternatives to chemical pesticides. Begin by making your home inhospitable to pests: Clean thoroughly and store and dispose of food properly. Fill all cracks, holes, and other pest entryways in your house; repair leaky faucets, pipes, and drains to dry up pests' water supply; and eliminate clutter to leave them without places to hide. If they have already invaded your home, here's how you can usher them out.

Ants
To deter ants, wipe them up with a soapy sponge; then spray their entry points with a synthetic pyrethroid liquid or a dust containing boric acid or silica aerogel.

Fleas
To combat fleas, start with a heavy-duty vacuuming, then continue to clean frequently. Be sure to dispose of the vacuum bags promptly; otherwise the fleas will crawl back out. To get rid of fleas in the larval stage, spray your carpets with an insect growth regulator, which will prevent the larvae from developing into adults.

Use a flea comb on your pet, dunking the comb in soapy water to drown the fleas. When you bathe your pet, sponge on an insecticide such as pyrethrum. Wash your pet's bedding frequently and dry it on high heat to kill any flea pupae.

Roaches
To deal with a minor roach problem, use commercial roach traps. For major infestations, sprinkle technical (not medicinal) boric acid in out-of-the-way corners where roaches congregate. The powder clings to the insect and is ingested when the roach grooms itself. A few days later, the roach dies. Because boric acid is also toxic to humans and animals, never use it near food or in places where children or pets might come across it.

A relatively new product, hydramethylnon, is also effective against roaches; it is available in traps that are child and pet proof.

Termites
To dispose of termites, begin by making sure your house's foundation is dry.

Use a desiccating dust containing silica aerogel or a synthetic pyrethroid to kill dry-wood termites. To combat subterranean termites, destroy their earthen tubes, then use either a biological control such as termite-eating ants or apply a borate spray to wood surfaces. In severe cases, wood in contact with the soil may have to be replaced with chemically treated wood or concrete.

Rats and mice
To get rid of rats and mice, bait several mousetraps with peanut butter powdered with corn or oat meal. Place the traps at the animals' suspected points of entry.

REDUCING YOUR EXPOSURE TO LEAD

The terrible effects of lead poisoning on children—culminating in neurological damage, intellectual impairment, and sometimes death—are well known. But adults can be poisoned too. Symptoms may include fatigue, irritability, difficulty concentrating, tremors, headaches, abdominal pain, vomiting, weight loss, constipation, and in severe cases, convulsions, paralysis, and coma. Often, however, there are no symptoms. People with high blood pressure are at particular risk; even slightly elevated blood levels of lead can raise pressure more. A person with extremely high levels of lead may suffer damage in all the body systems.

Because the body can't break down or eliminate lead, most of it is stored in skeletal minerals. Blood levels usually indicate only recent exposure. Past exposures can be detected in pregnant and postmenopausal women, however, when their bodies need to draw on minerals in the skeleton. As they do so, there is a rapid rise in blood lead levels.

Lead poisoning is treated with "chelating agents," drugs that bind with the lead and are excreted in the urine.

GETTING RID OF LEAD INDOORS

Most houses built before 1970 contain lead paint. When it cracks, peels, or flakes, lead dust gets into the air. Don't try to remove the paint yourself; have the job done professionally and stay away until the work is completed.

In homes with plumbing systems that contain lead pipes or lead solder, lead may be leaching into the drinking water (see p.330).

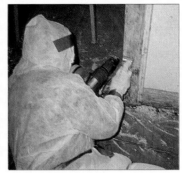

To remove lead paint safely, this worker must wear a protective suit with a respirator filter and hand and foot coverings.

Lead may also contaminate many household items, such as ceramic dishes and cookware. If their lead glaze was not fired at a high enough temperature, lead may leach out into food. Older ceramics and imports pose the greatest risk. And because all lead crystal leaches out lead into whatever it holds, use it for special occasions only, never for storage.

GETTING RID OF LEAD OUTDOORS

Lead is a natural ingredient in soil, but extra lead can accumulate in your backyard in the form of dust from industrial pollution or flaking paint. To avoid carrying this lead indoors on the soles of your shoes, plant ground cover to act as a barrier, and wipe your feet on a doormat before going inside. If a test of your topsoil shows very high levels of lead, have it replaced with clean soil.

TESTING FOR LEAD

Although you can buy inexpensive kits at your local hardware store to test for lead in wall paint, water, soil, and dishes, their accuracy has not yet been proven. Professional testing, especially for lead paint, is recommended.

The Dangers in Your Own Backyard

*W*hether you actively garden or simply commune with nature, you should take a few precautions—among them, protecting yourself from poisonous plants and avoiding bites and stings—whenever you spend time in your backyard.

POISONOUS PLANTS

Merely touching poison ivy, poison oak, or poison sumac can cause a rash, itching, blisters, and a fever. When you develop a rash, rinse the area with water, then apply calamine lotion to relieve the itching. For severe reactions, seek medical treatment.

To rid your yard of these plants, apply an herbicide —making sure to dress properly for the task: wear long sleeves and pants, thick gloves, and heavy shoes. Bury the plants or put them in the trash in sealed plastic bags. Never burn them; the plants' poison will become airborne and can damage your lungs. Afterwards, bathe, wash your clothes, and sponge your shoes.

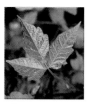
POISON IVY

POISON OAK

POISON SUMAC

Often you don't realize you've touched one of these plants until a rash appears on your skin.

ANIMAL BITES

If an animal bites you, rinse the affected area with water, wash it with soap, apply an antiseptic, and call your doctor; bites can transmit infection and disease. Rabies has become more prevalent in recent years, especially among raccoons and squirrels. Stay away from any animals, wild or domestic, that act strangely.

The treatment for a suspected rabies bite is a series of injections. If you are bitten by a dog, you may be able to forgo the shots if its rabies inoculation is up-to-date. Because an animal bite can also cause tetanus, get a tetanus shot if you haven't had a booster within the last 10 years.

INSECT STINGS AND BITES

Bee, wasp, and hornet stings
To avoid attracting bees, wasps, or hornets, don't wear perfume, aftershave lotion, hair spray, or scented suntan lotion. Dress in white or light, neutral colors. Walk away from buzzing insects or slowly and carefully brush them off—don't swat at them. If you stay calm, they will generally fly away on their own accord.

If you are stung, gently scrape out the stinger—never remove it with tweezers; you may squeeze more poison into the skin. Wash the area with soap and water, then apply an ice pack and a poultice of baking soda or meat tenderizer. If you get multiple stings, see a doctor.

Some people are highly allergic to stings; they should always carry a syringe with a dose of epinephrine (adrenaline) on outdoor excursions so they can inject themselves if they are stung.

Mosquito bites
To forestall the discomfort and itching that result from mosquito bites, make yourself as unappealing to mosquitoes as possible: bathe often and apply repellent to your clothes (not to your skin) in the early morning and evening when mosquitoes feed. Repellents containing deet work well, but people with chronic illnesses and children should use ones with permethrin instead.

If you are bitten by a mosquito, bathe the area with soap and water or apply an antiseptic.

Tick bites
Deer ticks carrying Lyme disease may be the biggest problem in your yard from May through August, especially if you live in the Northeast, Midwest, or California.

The best defense against being

bitten by a tick is to dress properly: wear a hat, a long-sleeved shirt, and long pants tucked into your socks. Spray your clothing with a repellent containing permethrin. When you go back indoors, check your body and scalp for ticks. Remove any tick with tweezers, wash the affected area with soap and water, and apply an antiseptic. Take the tick to your doctor to have it identified.

The symptoms of Lyme disease—headache, fever, and a spreading "bull's-eye" rash—may appear within 1 or 2 weeks, but not everyone develops these early symptoms. Blood tests also may fail to diagnose Lyme disease. Because Lyme disease can cause chronic or recurring arthritis and other problems, some doctors may give a bitten patient antibiotics—the effective treatment—without waiting for symptoms to appear.

Different ticks carry different diseases. If you suffer rashes and fever soon after being bitten, call your doctor. You may be infected with another tick-borne disease.

To prevent tick bites, make your yard uninviting to ticks: cut down brushy areas, remove leaf litter, and keep the lawn mowed.

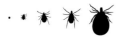

Most incidences of Lyme disease are caused by deer tick nymphs that have been infected in their larval stage; until they become engorged, they are difficult to see. Above, actual sizes of a tick larva, nymph, adult male and female, and an engorged tick.

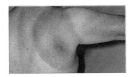

Left, a typical Lyme disease rash.

Profile

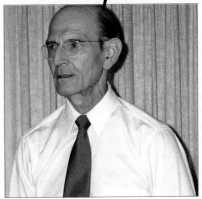

HANS RENNHARD HASN'T LET LYME DISEASE KEEP HIM INDOORS

One day in June 1993, Hans Rennhard, a retired research chemist living in Lyme, Connecticut, removed a black spot from his back. "It was a deer tick, and it was larger than usual because it was engorged with my blood."

Although he'd found deer ticks (the carriers of Lyme disease) on his body before, Rennhard had never developed any symptoms. This time a rash the size of half his hand appeared after 9 days, on a Saturday, when no doctor was available. On Sunday, he became nauseated and had a fever of 102 °F. "By Monday, the rash was the size of my whole hand."

Rennhard's doctor prescribed doxycycline, which is the antibiotic of choice in the treatment of Lyme disease and which, coincidentally, Rennhard had co-invented some years earlier. Rennhard's temperature returned to normal almost immediately, and the rash disappeared completely within a few days.

Having had Lyme disease hasn't stopped Rennhard, an avid gardener, from spending time outdoors, although he takes more precautions than he did before. "I wear white clothes now, so that it's easier to see the black ticks," he says.

BLOCKING OUT NOISE

The contemporary environment is barraged with unwelcome noises. Whether you live near a busy highway or your neighbor has a loud stereo, quiet is becoming a luxury. Noise can directly damage your hearing; the stress it creates can undermine your general health.

ASSESSING THE DAMAGE

More than a third of Americans who suffer serious hearing loss owe the condition to years of exposure to loud noises, often in the workplace, without wearing proper protective gear.

Unless you live very close to an airport or work with a jackhammer or a rock band, however, noise is more likely to cause symptoms of stress than hearing loss. Studies show that stress-related illnesses, such as ulcers, high blood pressure, and cardiovascular disease, can develop from living with too much noise.

Obnoxious noises, loud or soft, can trigger the release of adrenaline, calling into play the body's fight-or-flight response to stress (p.174). Any sound that interferes with

The noise of a jackhammer from 3 feet away registers 120 decibels, very near the threshold of pain.

conversation, hampers your concentration, or disturbs your sleep can set your nerves on edge. What annoys people most is noise they have no control over—a loud radio in the apartment next door, a barking dog, a car's burglar alarm.

Noise can affect the way you relate to the people around you. In one study, a man who dropped the books he was carrying on the sidewalk got much more help from strangers when a neighborhood was quiet than when a lawn mower was operating nearby. Quiet neighborhoods are generally friendlier than noisy ones. People who live on a cul-de-sac, for example, report knowing more of their immediate neighbors than people who live on a highly trafficked thoroughfare.

HOW TO PROTECT YOURSELF

The best protection against noisy situations—using a power saw or a leaf blower, for example—is to wear the protective earmuffs designed for target shooters or factory workers, sold in sporting goods stores. Although acrylic or foam earplugs don't work as well as these professional earmuffs, they are inexpensive and safer than stuffing cotton in your ears, which can cause infections.

To cope with a constant annoying noise, consider buying a small appliance that creates a pleasant sound like ocean waves or rainfall. White-noise machines, often used by therapists to ensure that doctor-patient conversations can't be heard in the waiting

TAKING THE MEASURE OF EVERYDAY NOISE

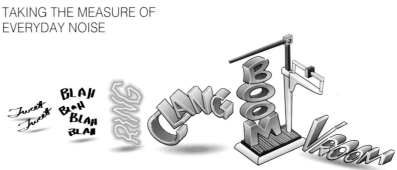

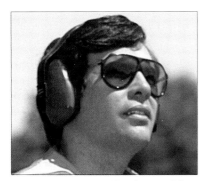

Protective earmuffs, designed for the shooting range, can also blot out the noise of home power equipment.

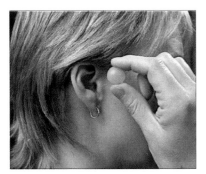

Inexpensive earplugs, available from a drugstore, should be placed at the opening of your ear, not in it.

The relative loudness of sounds is measured in decibels. Persistent 8-hour-a-day exposure to sound levels above 85 decibels is hazardous to your hearing. Because decibels are calculated on a logarithmic basis, an increase of 10 decibels is no small matter: it represents a 10-fold increase in acoustic energy. A 20-decibel increase in noise, for example, corresponds to a 100-fold rise in acoustic energy. Listed below are the average decibel levels for many common sources of noise.

Noise Source	Decibel Level
Shooting range	140–170
Jet engine at close range	140
Threshold of pain	**140**
Customized car stereo with multiple speakers	130
Rock band at close range	125
Thunderclap (nearby)	120
Personal stereo on busy street	115
Chain saw	110
Snowmobile	105
Jet flyover (1,000 feet)	103
Car horn	100
Subway train	100
Garbage disposer	95
Food processor	90
Washing machine	78
Vacuum cleaner	70
Telephone bell	65
Conversation	60
Annoyance threshold	**55**
Refrigerator hum	40
Whisper	30
Rustling of leaves	15

room, produce a sound like radio static. You may find that playing relaxing music is more soothing to you. All of these techniques, however, simply mask offensive noises with more acceptable ones. None reduce sound levels.

NOISE-PROOFING YOUR HOME

Most of the techniques you use to keep cold air out of your home in the winter and hot air out in summer—caulking, weatherstripping, insulating exterior walls, and installing storm windows and storm doors—will also hold outside noise at bay. In addition, solid flat doors keep out more noise than hollow or paneled ones.

To muffle sounds generated inside your home, there are many things you can do. Relocate television sets and stereo speakers so that they are not in direct contact with walls or floors. Choose sound-absorbing furnishings such as thick curtains, dense carpeting, and upholstered furniture. Consider using suspended ceilings and cork or burlap wall panels to mute sound. In the kitchen, keep appliances in good repair and place them on rubber or cork vibration pads so that they'll run more quietly. Keep up the maintenance on your heating, cooling, and plumbing systems and discuss any noise problems with a repair person.

THE PROBLEM OF OUTDOOR AIR POLLUTION

Not long ago, a vigorous walk in the fresh air was considered good health insurance. On a similar walk today, your eyes may water, and you may cough, sneeze, and get a headache. The cause of this discomfort: smoke, smog, harmful gases, and microscopic particles.

CAUSES OF AIR POLLUTION

An increasing problem in larger cities since the 1950's, air pollution, spread far and wide by air currents, also has become prevalent in many suburban and rural areas. Motor vehicles are the primary cause, producing two-thirds of the carbon monoxide in the air, plus over half of the nitrogen oxide and one-third of the hydro-carbon emissions.

Other major contributors to air pollution include fuels that are used to heat homes, office buildings, and factories; emissions from power plants and factories; and agricultural pesticides and herbicides. Some of these pollutants are invisible; others create a haze that lingers in the air over a community. When solid waste such as leaves and trash is burned, pollution is discharged into the air in the form of a highly visible black smoke.

Although most pollution problems are man-made, some result from natural phenomena. Forest fires cause carbon monoxide, carbon dioxide, and hydrocarbons to escape into the air. Volcanic eruptions throw tons of sulfur dioxide into the atmosphere. More common natural events are thermal inversions, which allow pollutants to accumulate in specific areas, sometimes to dangerous levels. Inversions occur when a layer of cool air near the ground is trapped by a layer of warm air that moves in over it. Pollutants begin to build up because the layer of warm air prevents them from rising and dispersing as they normally would. A thermal inversion continues until it is broken up by rain or wind.

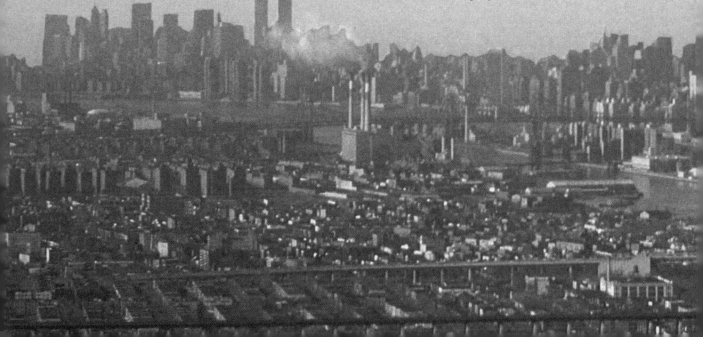

THE EFFECT OF AIR POLLUTION ON YOUR HEALTH

The adverse effects of air pollution are undeniable, especially for people with chronic health problems. Epidemiologists are now making connections not only between air pollution and such respiratory diseases as asthma, bronchitis, and emphysema, but also between air pollution and heart disease, cancer, and immune system malfunctions.

Microscopic particles of soot, thrown into the air by industrial plant emissions and diesel vehicle exhausts, may cause more deaths, according to recent studies, than any other kind of air pollution—mainly among people with respiratory problems. Microscopic particles of nitrogen dioxide and sulfur dioxide, released into the air by the burning of coal or fuel oil, can damage the lungs and respiratory tract.

Ground-level ozone, the major ingredient of smog, is created when nitrogen oxides (from cars and industrial plants) and hydrocarbons (from sources such as refineries and backyard barbecues) combine in the presence of sunlight. Ozone inflames lung tissue, reduces lung capacity, and triggers asthma attacks. (Air pollution also causes the decrease in stratospheric ozone, which shields you from ultraviolet radiation.)

Carbon monoxide, a colorless, odorless gas emitted by motor vehicle exhausts and industrial combustion processes, is particularly toxic to people with heart disease because it impairs the blood's ability to carry oxygen.

. . . .

PROTECTING YOURSELF

Improving the quality of the air is a long-term national environmental problem. Besides joining a local advocacy group to aid in this effort, there are other steps you can take to protect yourself and your immediate environment:

■ On days when weather forecasters report pollution alerts, avoid any strenuous outdoor activity. If you have circulatory or respiratory problems, stay inside, preferably in an air-conditioned room, until the air improves.

■ Reduce or eliminate your use of pesticide sprays on your lawn and garden. Their toxins can pollute the air you breathe. Stay indoors when your neighbors spray; the fumes will migrate to your yard. Try to persuade your neighbors to adopt alternative methods of pest control.

■ Limit your use of gas-powered lawn mowers, which emit smog-causing hydrocarbons.

■ Make sure your car is equipped with up-to-date pollution-control devices and is well maintained. Drive less, join a carpool for commutes, and walk or bicycle more.

> **"And noxious airs begin to crawl along ...into this atmosphere of ours...."**
>
> —*Lucretius, Roman poet (96?-55 B.C.)*

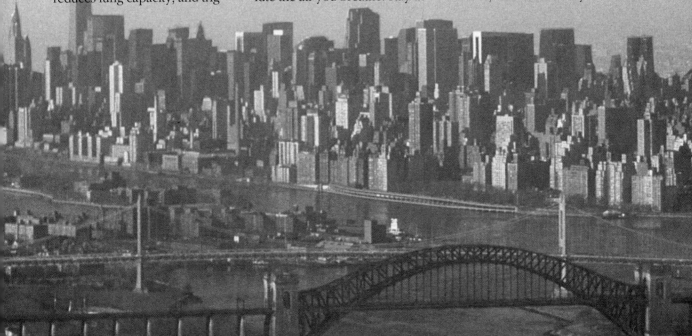

HOW WEATHER AFFECTS YOU

*W*hether you are aware of it or not, you respond to the change of seasons—and even the flow of day into night—in profound physical ways that can influence your energy level, your moods, and your health.

COLD WEATHER

Extreme cold is no easier for an older person to handle than sultry heat. Aging makes people more vulnerable to hypothermia, a serious loss of body heat that can result from continued exposure to temperatures as mild as 60°F (see also p.113).

When you feel cold, take steps to make yourself warmer right away. Indoors and out, dress warmly and stay dry. If you can help it, don't go outdoors on frigid days. When you do, always wear a hat, since you can lose as much as 20 percent of your body heat through your head. Keep the thermostat in your home set at a minimum of 65°F during the day and a minimum of 60°F at night. Ask your doctor about the cold and the drugs you are taking. Some make you less conscious of how cold you are.

HOT WEATHER

As you grow older, your body becomes more sensitive to extremes of temperature. In very hot weather, for example, because your body composition contains less water than when you were younger, you can't cool off as well by sweating.

To avoid problems with heat, relax your pace when the temperature soars. Stay inside during the heat of the day (10 A.M. to 2 P.M.) and use air conditioners or fans. Wear loose, lightweight clothes made of fabrics that breathe. Eat sparingly and drink plenty of liquids (see also p.112).

NATURAL RHYTHMS AND YOUR BIOLOGICAL CLOCK

Circadian, or daily, rhythms affect all living things; human beings are no exception. For the last two decades, scientists have been tracking human circadian rhythms. Their research has helped swing-shift workers to adjust to odd hours (facing page) and doctors to find more beneficial times for some medical treatments. Some examples of your circadian highs and lows are listed below.

■ Body temperature, which normally fluctuates about 2°F during the course of a day, reaches a high in the late afternoon and falls to its low between 4 A.M. and 6 A.M.

■ Your tolerance for pain is highest from 8 A.M. to 10 A.M.

■ Your manual dexterity and eye-hand coordination are at their best between 3 P.M. and 6 P.M.

■ Your blood clots more readily in the morning because blood platelets are stickiest then.

■ Immune cells that fight viruses and cancer are at their peak in the morning.

CIRCADIAN RHYTHMS

Sunlight has a major influence on human behavior because it triggers circadian rhythms (*circadian* means "about a day" in Latin). Most people are naturally inclined to spend days awake and nights sleeping because a group of neurons in the brain, stimulated by the sun, program their bodies to be alert in the morning and sleepy at night.

Circadian rhythms explain why people who work swing shifts, alternating day and night hours on the job, feel tired and have trouble sleeping. Your biological clock can be reset by manipulating light and darkness. Working in brightly lit rooms, for example, helps people who work nights sleep better during the day. Spending daylight time outdoors can help travelers overcome jet lag (p.259).

. . . .

SAD

Seasonal affective disorder (SAD) may affect as many as 10 percent of the people who live in the more northern latitudes. In a human version of hibernation, SAD sufferers slow down with winter's arrival, become depressed, crave carbohydrates, and don't want to get out of bed until spring brings ample daylight back.

In recent years, doctors have tested the connection between these mood swings, seasonal changes, and biological clocks. Experiments show that many SAD sufferers are helped by artificial lights (see *Profile* at right). For people with marginal cases of SAD (essentially just the winter doldrums), taking brisk walks outdoors in morning light may prove surprisingly therapeutic.

Profile

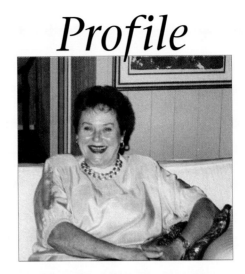

CHARLOTTE CRIDLAND
BEATS A SEASONAL DISORDER

Reading the morning newspaper in front of a box of lights has become a winter routine for speech pathologist Charlotte Cridland. This hour-long ritual was prescribed by doctors at the Oregon Health Science University in Portland, Oregon, where she lives. Cridland suffers from seasonal affective disorder (SAD), a depression brought on by the decrease in sunlight during fall and winter.

Before the light treatments, Cridland rarely went out on winter evenings. She would come home after work, "sleep hard for an hour or two, have dinner (eating everything in sight, especially sweets), and then go to bed." Every winter she gained 10 to 12 pounds, which she worked off in summer.

Neither counseling nor medication helped. Then she volunteered for the university's SAD study and started on light therapy. Cridland says, "I'm eating normally year round, and I enjoy nighttime fun again." She is as surprised as anyone at the simple solution to her problem.

Driving Safely Through the Years

Normal physiological changes and increasing health problems can affect the way you drive as you grow older, so adjust your driving to accommodate them. Also important, at any age, are safe driving practices and security precautions.

VISION PROBLEMS

People often need reading glasses as they get older. By their sixties and seventies, many people also begin to have trouble reading road signs. Visual impairments such as cataracts and glaucoma (see pp.286-287) can compound older drivers' problems. It's important to have your eyes checked regularly; many vision changes come on gradually, without your being aware of them.

While no one's night vision is as good as their day vision, over time, night vision deteriorates. The eyes' ability to accommodate changes in the available light slows down as well. Roads where brightly lit patches alternate with dark ones are especially challenging for older people.

If you must drive at night, give your eyes at least 5 minutes to adjust. Drive more slowly than you would during the day, maintain a greater distance between yourself and the next car, and keep your headlights and windshield clean.

Bad weather and low light present other problems. Whenever you must drive in rain, snow, or fog—or at daybreak or dusk—slow down, increase the space between you and other cars, and turn on your low-beam headlights (you won't see better, but other drivers will see you better). In extreme weather, use your emergency flashers for more visibility or pull off the road and wait for conditions to improve.

SAFE DRIVING

If illness or injury has kept you off the road for a while, or if you are feeling uneasy behind the wheel, check with your doctor to see if there is any medical reason why you should not drive.

Once you get a clean bill of health, consider taking one of the safe-driving courses geared toward older people offered by the American Automobile Association, the National Safety Council, and the American Association of Retired Persons. In at least 33 states and in Washington D.C., you'll be rewarded with insurance premium reductions.

THE SAFEST CAR FOR YOU

■ Choose a light-colored car; it is more visible to other drivers than a dark one. A medium to large car is preferable to a small one because it is more comfortable and easier to get in and out of.

■ For maximum protection, get a car with air bags as well as seat belts.

■ Make sure the car also has a defrosting system for the rear window so that you can avoid getting out to scrape it in icy weather.

■ To see well in all kinds of weather, choose clear, not tinted, windshields.

■ Install a wide rearview mirror that automatically adjusts to the presence of headlights, as well as left and right side mirrors.

How do you know when it's time for you—or someone you love—to move into the passenger's seat? If you have been involved in a number of fender benders or near crashes, if your reflexes have slowed, if you are not as alert to pedestrians or approaching cars as you once were, if you get nervous behind the wheel or become exhausted after a short drive—you may want to consider giving up your license.

SAFETY AND SECURITY PRECAUTIONS

Safe driving practices

■ Don't start the car until you put on your seat belt. The bottom strap goes across your pelvis, never your stomach; the shoulder strap comes down your upper chest, never beneath your arm or across your neck.

■ Be sure you can see the road clearly. If necessary, sit on a cushion.

■ Help your concentration by limiting distractions. Don't eat or smoke at the wheel. Don't drive when you're upset.

■ Allow extra time for a trip so that you won't feel pressured.

■ If another driver is swerving across the road or tailgating you, pull over to let him pass.

■ Stay with the traffic flow—driving either too fast or too slow can cause an accident.

■ Never drink and drive.

Protective measures on the road

■ Keep your doors locked and your windows rolled up far enough so that no one can reach inside your car at stop signs or red lights.

■ Keep your purse, wallet, and other valuables out of sight.

■ Avoid shortcuts through unsafe areas.

■ On a regular route, pick out safe havens such as gas stations, convenience stores, and police and fire stations. If you encounter any trouble— someone following you, for example—drive to one of these spots at once, flashing your lights and blowing your horn to attract attention.

■ Carjackers sometimes bump a car from behind so that the driver will stop and get out. If you suspect this, remain in your car, motion to the other driver to follow you, and drive to the nearest police station or fire station.

■ If your car breaks down and you are not near a telephone, stay in the locked car and wait for help. If someone stops, remain in the car and ask him to get help.

■ Never pick up a hitchhiker.

Avoiding trouble when you park

■ Leave your car in a well-lit and well-traveled area. Lock your doors and roll up the windows, no matter how briefly you intend to be gone.

■ Put packages, radios, and tape decks out of sight, and take your car title, registration, and driver's license with you.

■ If you park in a lot or a garage, give the attendant only the ignition key.

PHYSICAL CHANGES AND HEALTH PROBLEMS

Reflexes get slower over the years. To compensate, widen the space between you and the next car, try not to drive at rush hour, and have someone act as a navigator on an unfamiliar route.

Chronic ailments such as arthritis can limit mobility behind the wheel. To make car handling easier, invest in power steering and brakes and a motorized front seat, and adjust your seat and mirrors to reduce neck movements. Doing exercises to limber up before you drive may help too.

If you take prescription drugs, ask your doctor about side effects that may affect your driving.

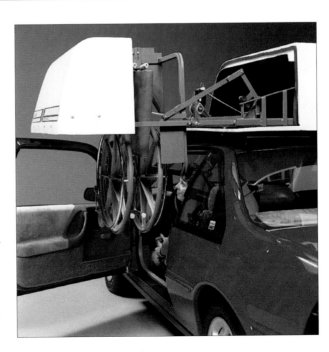

Instead of stowing their wheelchairs inside the car, disabled drivers or passengers can transport them in this cartop-mounted carrier.

CREDITS AND ACKNOWLEDGMENTS

Photographs

Cover: *bottom* David Madison; *remainder* David Arky. **3** *bottom* David Madison; *remainder* David Arky. **7** Colin Cooke. **8** Colin Cooke. **10** *bottom left* J. Howard/FPG International; *bottom right* Boltin Picture Library. **11** *top* Dan Bosler/Tony Stone Worldwide; *middle* Brown Brothers; *bottom* Metropolitan Museum of Art. **13** Lawrence Ivy. **14** Steve Miedorf/The Image Bank. **15** Jerry Valente. **17** Courtesy of the National Institute on Aging, Gerontology Research Center. **19** *left* Jean Pierre Fizet/Sygma; *right* Courtesy of Kelmscott Gallery, Chicago. **20** *left* Courtesy of The Kobal Collection; *right* Michael O'Neill, Inc. **21** Gjon Mili/Life Magazine © Time Warner. **22** *bottom left* Dan McCoy/Rainbow; *inset* Will & Deni McIntyre/Photo Researchers. **24** David Scharf. **25** Courtesy of Helen Boley. **26** Kevin Horan. **27** Co Rentmeester/The Image Bank. **29** Guinness Publishing. **30** Ethan Hoffman/Picture Project, Inc. **31** Alan Reininger/Contact Press Images. **32** Sidney A. Tabak. **34** Colin Cooke. **38–39** Colin Cooke. **40** Ron Chapple/FPG International. **42–43** Colin Cooke. **44** Colin Cooke. **45** Colin Cooke. **46** Colin Cooke. **47** Colin Cooke. **48** By permission of *Ebony* magazine, © 1992 Johnson Publishing Company. **50** Courtesy of Dr. Robert C. Northcutt. **52** © Lisa Masson 1992. **56** Colin Cooke. **57** Colin Cooke. **58** Scott Dorrance. **59** Scott Dorrance. **60–61** Colin Cooke. **65** Colin Cooke. **66** Colin Cooke. **68** Colin Cooke. **70** Colin Cooke. **74** Roy Morsch/The Stock Market. **77** Alan Levenson/*Time* magazine. **78–79** Colin Cooke. **81** Colin Cooke. **83** Colin Cooke. **85** Colin Cooke. **87** Colin Cooke. **88–89** Colin Cooke. **90** Colin Cooke. **92** David Brownell. **93** David Madison. **94–95** Focus on Sports Inc. **98–99** Jan Cobb. **100** Jan Cobb. **101** Blair Seitz/Photo Researchers, Inc. **103** Jan Cobb. **104–105** Jan Cobb. **108** Marc Rosenthal. **112–113** Jan Cobb. **115** Jan Cobb. **116–117** Jan Cobb. **118** Jan Cobb. **121** *left* Diane Johnson; *right* David Stoecklein/Stock Solution. **122** Courtesy of Jo Reynolds. **123** *top* Frank Siteman; *bottom* Enrico Ferorelli. **127** Mark Stephenson/West Light. **128–129** Jan Cobb. **131** Courtesy of Clyde J. Villemez. **132** *left* Tunturi, Inc., by permission; *right* Quinton Instrument Co. **133** *both* Quinton Instrument Co. **134** Bruce Curtis. **135** *top* Bruce Curtis; *bottom* Janeart Ltd./The Image Bank. **137** *top right* Helen Harris Associates/U.S. National Senior Sports Orgnization; *bottom* John Dowling/U.S. National Senior Sports Organization. **138** Colin Cooke. **140** *left* Globe Photos; *center* Shooting Star International; *right* Adam Scull/Globe Photos. **142** *top* James McInnis; *bottom* Colin Cooke. **144** *top* Courtesy of the Gillette Company; *bottom* Marc Rosenthal. **145** Marc Rosenthal. **146** *both* The American Society for Aesthetic Plastic Surgery, Inc. **147** Myrleen Ferguson/Tony Stone Worldwide. **148** Private Collection. **150–151** *left* American Society of Aesthetic Plastic Surgery; *center* American Association of Facial Plastic and Reconstructive Surgery; *right* American Society of Aesthetic Plastic Surgery. **152** *all* American Association of Facial Plastic and Reconstructive Surgery. **153** Richard A. Mladick, M.D. **155** Courtesy of Jeanne Apple. **156–157** Colin Cooke. **158–159** *all* Comstock. **160** Aaron Rapoport/Onyx. **162–163** Marc Rosenthal. **164** *all* Courtesy of McAndrews Northern Dental Laboratories, Inc. **165** Courtesy of

Paul Slimak. **167** H. Armstrong Roberts. **168–169** *all* Marc Rosenthal. **172** Colin Cooke. **178** © Chip Simons 1992. **180** *left* New Choices; *right* U.S.News & World Report. **181** *top* Arthur Tilley/FPG; *bottom left* Marc Rosenthal; *bottom right* Susan Wood. **182** Marc Rosenthal. **187** *top* Rick Friedman/Black Star; *bottom* Nicole Bengiveno. **188** Peter Beck/The Stock Market, Inc. **192** Les Stone/Sygma. **195** Courtesy of Glenys Bittick. **198** Trix Rosen. **201** Pam O'Hara Smith. **202–203** Colin Cooke. **204** *top* M. Ruiz/Granata USA; *remainder* Jim Harrison/Elderhostel. **205** *top* E. Lee White; *bottom* Kevin Horan/Picture Group #9. **206** *left* Charles Gupton/The Stock Market, Inc.; *right* Joe Sohm/The Stock Market, Inc. **207** New Choices/Bill Stites. **209** *both* Photographics 2. **210–211** David Muench **212** Caroline Monaghan Pallat. **214** Colin Cooke. **216** Comstock. **218** *left* Kevin Horan; *right* Smithsonian Institution. **219** *left* Kevin Horan; *right* Malcolm S. Kirk. **221** Rick Friedman/Black Star; *inset* Jeffrey MacMillan/U.S. News & World Report. **223** Carlos Rene Perez. **224** Jan Cobb. **227** Marc Rosenthal. **230–231** William H. Helfand/Harry Abrams. **234** David A. Wagner/Phototake NYC. **235** Donald C. Johnson/The Stock Market, Inc. **238** Gideon Lewin. **239** John Barr/The Gamma Liaison Network. **240–241** *all* Memory Assessment Clinics, Inc., Bethesda, MD. **242** Colin Cooke. **243** *both* from *The Body Victorious* by Lennart Nilsson. Published by Dell Publishing Company, New York, ©Boehringer Ingelheim International GmbH. **245** Courtesy of William Boyd. **246** *both* Boehringer Ingelheim Limited. **248** Collection of Beverly A. Hamer. **251** Courtesy of Lupe Conway. **254–255** Jan Cobb. **256** Colin Cooke. **260–261** Jan Cobb. **262** Colin Cooke. **265** *all* The Skin Cancer Foundation, New York, NY. **267** Jan Cobb. **269** *both* Ira Wyman. **270** Courtesy of Juanita Watson. **271** Alex Webb/Magnum. **273** Education and Scientific Products Limited/photo by Colin Cooke. **274** Art Montes de Oca/FPG International. **276** Renée Comet/© Time-Life Books, Inc., from the series *Curious and Unusual Facts*. **277** Ira Wyman. **279** Stacy Pickerell/Tony Stone Worldwide. **282** Susan Lapides. **284** Colin Cooke/Collection of Rosemary Charlesworth. **285** Education and Scientific Products Limited/photo by Colin Cooke. **286** *left* Courtesy of Marie Herrick; *right* The Lighthouse, Inc./Photo by James McInnis. **287** The Lighthouse, Inc./Photo by James McInnis. **288** *top* American Academy of Ophthalmology; *bottom* Tim Street-Porter. **289** Tim Street-Porter. **291** *top left* Miracle Ear©; *remainder* Ensoniq Corp. **293** *right* Education and Scientific Products Limited/photo by Colin Cooke; *left* Colin Cooke. **294** Pulsair, Inc. **295** Brown Brothers. **297** *both* Education and Scientific Products Limited/photo by Colin Cooke. **299** Courtesy of Anatomical Chart Co. **300** Courtesy of Sarns™ Cardiovascular Systems, 3M Health Care. **302** Benn Mitchell/The Image Bank. **303** Colin Cooke. **304** *bottom* Mitchel P. Goldman, M.D./Dermatology Associates of San Diego County, Inc. **307** Lennart Nilsson © Boeringer Ingelheim GmbH. **309** Education and Scientific Products Limited/photo by Colin Cooke. **311** *left and inset* Custom Medical Stock Photo; *right* CNRI/SPL/Science Source/Photo Researchers, Inc. **314** Dianora Niccolini/Medical Images, Inc. **315** United States Surgical Corporation. **317** *top* Ulrike Welsch/Photo Researchers, Inc.; *bottom* Dan

McCoy/National Geographic Society. **319** Education and Scientific Products Limited/photo by Colin Cooke. **321** Education and Scientific Products Limited/photo by Colin Cooke. **324** Colin Cooke. **328** Colin Cooke. **330–331** Colin Cooke. **331** *top right* Amway Corporation; *bottom right* Ecowater Systems. **333** Colin Cooke. **338–339** Colin Cooke. **341** United States Department of Housing and Urban Development, Office of Lead-based Abatement and Poisoning Prevention. **342** *middle* Derek Fell; *remainder* Photo Researchers, Inc. **343** *bottom* The Center for Disease Control; *right* Courtesy of Hans Rennhard. **344** Anthony A. Boccaccio/The Image Bank. **345** *top* The Bilsom Group; *bottom* Colin Cooke. **346–347** Comstock, Inc. **348** Colin Cooke. **349** *top* Courtesy of Charlotte Cridland; *bottom* Colin Cooke. **351** Braun Corporation/Photo by Larry Gard.

Text

American Association of Retired Persons
YOUR HOME YOUR CHOICE. Copyright © 1991 American Association of Retired Persons. Reprinted by permission.

Memory Assessment Clinics Inc.
TEST YOUR OWN MEMORY – TESTS I AND II. Copyright © 1989 Memory Assessment Clinics Inc. Reprinted by permission.

RD Publications
THE FACTS ABOUT FOOD POISONING. *American Health*, June 1992. Copyright © 1992 by RD Publications. Reprinted by permission.

Scott, Foresman & Company
MEDICAL AND HEALTH GUIDE FOR PEOPLE OVER FIFTY by Eugene C. Nelson, D.Sc., Ellen Roberts, M.P.H., Jeannette Simmons, D.Sc., William A. Tisdale, M.D. Copyright © 1986 by Scott, Foresman and Company and American Association of Retired Persons. Reprinted by permission of Jeannette Simmons, D.Sc.

Special thanks to

John Wygand, Director of Adult Fitness Program
Adelphi University

Joan Gibala, Senior Specialist
Mike Seaton, Manager, Transportation
Rachel Weisman, Assistant Media Liaison, Public Affairs Department, Communications Division
American Association of Retired Persons

Stacey Charney, Media Relations Specialist, Media Office
American Cancer Society

American College of Sports Medicine

Dennis Bowman, Director, Communications
Steve Erickson, Vice President, Communications
Linda Ehrlich, Rheumatology Clinical Specialist
Arthritis Foundation

Starr Hope Ertel, Epidemiologist (Infectious Chronic Diseases)
Connecticut Department of Health and Addiction Services

Susan Johnson, Ed.D., Director of Continuing Education
Cooper Institute for Aerobics Research

League of American Wheelmen

Kevin McAndrews, Office Manager
McAndrews Northern Dental Laboratories, Inc.

Jacqueline Aker, Editorial Research Associate
National Crime Prevention Council

John W. Eberhard, Senior Research Psychologist
Timothy Hurd, Media Division Chief, Office of Public Affairs
National Highway Traffic Safety Administration

Jane Shure, Public Information Officer
National Institute on Aging

Allen Steere, M.D., Chief of Rheumatology/Immunology
Elise Taylor, Clinical Studies Researcher
New England Medical Center (affiliated with Tufts University)

Jerry Sanford, Press Officer
Department of Communications
New York City Fire Department

Debra A. Janes, Health Scientist
Occupational Safety and Health Administration

Arthur L. Rubin, M.D., Director
Bruce R. Gordon, M.D., Co-Director, Comprehensive Lipid Control Center
Stuart D. Saal, M.D., Co-Director, Comprehensive Lipid Control Center
Hedda Batwin, R.D., Senior Staff Nutritionist
The Rogosin Intitute at The New York Hospital–Cornell Medical Center

E. Stephen Wells, Market Development Manager
Sarns, 3M Health Care

Raymond J. Dattwyler, M.D., F.A.C.P., Associate Professor of Medicine
State University of New York at Stony Brook

C. Bruce Wenger, M.D., Ph.D., Research Pharmacologist
Andrew J. Young, Ph.D., Research Pharmacologist
Thermal Physiology and Medicine Division
U.S. Army Research Institute of Environmental Medicine

Tracy Lynn Bone, Environmental Scientist
Janice L. Canterbury, Environmental Scientist
Ken Feith, Senior Scientist
Lynne Gillette, Health Physicist, Office of Radiation and Indoor Air
Martin Halper, Radiation Studies Division
Charlene E. Shaw, National Drinking Water Advisory Council
U.S. Environmental Protection Agency

United States Swimming, Inc., International Center for Aquatics Research Division

Carol Jessop, R.N.
University Hospital, Sleep Disorders Center
University of New Mexico School of Medicine

Dixie Stanforth, Teaching Specialist, Department of Kinesiology
University of Texas

Arthur Weltman, Ph.D., Director of Exercise and Physiology
University of Virginia

Robert T. Schoen, M.D., F.A.C.P., Associate Clinical Professor of Medicine, Co-Director of the Lyme Disease Clinic
Yale University School of Medicine

Index

• • • • • • • • • •

A

Abdomen, 65, 256, 257, 310, **311**
  palpation of, 218
  plastic surgery on, 154, 155
Accidents, 20, 223, 225
  automobile, 255, 351
  bicycle, **129**
  falling, 270
Acetaminophen, 246, 249, 265, 271
Achilles tendinitis, 115
Acne, 140, 146
Acquired immune deficiency syndrome
   (AIDS), 194, 238, 294, 307
Acupuncture, 217, 271
Age spots, 146, 150
Aging, 10–33
  achievement and, 20-21, 28
  benefits and satisfactions of, 212,
   213
  emotional aspects of, 210–212
  genetic factors and, 22, **23, 24,**
   24–25, 28, 29
  health span and, 12–13, 20, 22
  hormonal clocks and, 22, 25
  independence and, 32, 187
  life expectancy and, 10–13, 19–20,
   185, 202
  longevity and, 10, 13, **13**, 26–33, **30**
  mental health and, 31–33
  of men vs. women, 19–20
  myths of, 17, 29
  physiological, 14–20, 22–33
  positive approaches to, 14, 211–212
  psychosocial, 14
Agoraphobia, 178
Agriculture Department, U.S., 36, 71, 76
Air conditioning, 146, 333
Air pollution, 102, 113, 346–347
  indoor, 332–335
  sources of, 333, 334–337, 346
Al-Anon, 199
Alcohol, 96, 112–113, 146, 247
  absorption of, 69
  brain damage and, 196, **197,** 241
  depressing effects of, 177, 182, 196
  driving and, 31, 199
  drug interaction with, 232, 235
  moderate use of, 20, 31, **37,** 51, 68,
   194, 196, 305

Alcohol (*contd.*)
  social drinking of, 196, 199
  withdrawal from, 198, 199
Alcoholics Anonymous (AA), 177, 198,
   199
Alcoholism, 196–199
  early vs. late onset of, 196, 198
  living with, 198–199
  physical effects of, 146, 196, **196,
   197,** 314
  recovery programs for, 198, **198,**
   199
  signs of, 196, 199
Alert bracelets, 232, **276,** 315
Alimony, 190
Allen, Gracie, 20
Allergies, 73, 75, 94, 144–145, 219, 342
  air pollution and, 333
  bee sting, 342
  food, 73, 75
  symptoms of, 75, 249, **249,** 292,
   332, 342
  vaccines for, 219
Alpha blockers, 296
Alpha hydroxy acids, 146
Alzheimer's disease, 226, 241, 276–277
American Association of Retired
   Persons (AARP), 202, 206, 207,
   350
American Cancer Society, 38, 51, 64,
   93, 226, 229, 244, 265, 323
American Diabetes Association, 280
American Heart Association, 50, 51, 63,
   226
American Hospital Association, 222
American Lung Association, 244
Amino acids, 42, 45
Amphetamines, 230, 233, 237
Ampicillin, **234**
Anal canal, **309, 321**
Analgesics, 220–221, **221,** 230, 233,
   265
Anaphylaxis, 75, 342
Anemia, 149, 232, 241, 306, 314
Anesthesia
  general, 148, 151, 153, 154, 221,
   222, 230
  local, 150, 151, 153, 222, 230, **317**
  regional, 222
  risks of, 148, 221
  side effects of, 222
Aneurysm, 305, **305,** 313

Anger, and stress, 63, 94, 175, 177,
   179, 183, 187
Angina pectoris, 38, 223, 230, 249, 297,
   299. *See also* Heart disease.
Angiotensin-converting (ACE) inhibitors,
   296
Animals
  bites of, 342
  pets, 133, **302**
  studies on, 27, 39, 45, 159, 302
Antacids, 256, 308
Antianginals, 230
Antiarrhythmics, 230
Antibiotics, 73, 147, 230, 234, 249, 265,
   294
Antibodies, 42, 230, 247, 280
Anticoagulants, 41, 232, 274, 275
Antidepressants, 178, 230, 233, 241,
   278
Antihistamines, 66, 232, 233, 235, 247,
   250, 291
Antihypertensives, 230, 296
Antioxidants, 25, 28, 38, 39, 55.
   See also Vitamins.
Antiserums, 230
Antivirals, 248, 265, 307
Anxiety, 45, 178, **178,** 226, 228, 230,
   239, 246
Appetite, loss of, 40, 41, 55, 194
Apple, Jeanne, 155, **155**
Aqueous humor, **285**
Arking, Robert, 24
Arm signals, when bicycling, 129
Arrhythmias, 67, 250, **297,** 304, **304.**
   See also Heart disease.
Arteries, 97
  blockage of, 38, 272, **272,** 297, 298,
   299, **299**
  carotid, 274, 275
  coronary, 280, 297, 299, **297,** 300,
   301
  pulmonary, **297**
  See also Blood vessels; Circulatory
   system; Heart disease.
Arthritis, 238, 247, 252, 266–269, **266,
   267,** 305
  exercise and, 93, 106, 125, 266,
   267, 268
  gout, 43, 267–268, **267**
  helping devices for, 268, **269**
  osteoarthritis, 247, 266, **266, 267**
  quack cures for, **219**
  rheumatoid, 266–267, **267**
  treatment of, 266, 267–269, 270

Asbestos, 333, 334
Aspartame, 45, 71
Aspirin, 230, 235, 246, 247, 249, 252, 265, 271, 275, 290, 303
Asthma, 67, 75, 232, 292, **292,** 303
Atherosclerosis, 38, 43, **297,** 299. *See also* Heart disease.
Athlete's foot, 260
AZT (zidovudine), 307

B

Backs, 252–255
    aches and pains of, 94, 103, 125, 154, 179, 183, 217, 252–253, 255, 271
    exercises for, 110, **136,** 253, **254–255**
    posture and, 103, 253
    stretches for, 100, **136, 254, 255**
Bacteria, 229
    in food, 71, 73, 74–75, 257
    killing of, 57, 230, 257
Baldness, 160–161, **160**
    genetic factors in, 156, 160
Balloon angioplasty, 300–301, **301,** 302
Baltimore Longitudinal Study of Aging, 17, 20, 28
Bandages, **144,** 153, 154, 155
Baruch, Bernard, 16
Basal cell carcinoma, 265, **265**
Basal metabolic rate (BMR), 60, 94
Bathing, **133,** 141, 146, 168, 221, 266, 267
Bathing caps, 127, 157, **157**
Beards, 144, 155
Beaton, Cecil, 168
Beds, **223,** 250
    raising heads of, 141, 256, 308
Bedsores, 222, 264, 274
Beer, 69, 71
Beef stew, 80
Benson, Herbert, **180**
Beta blockers, 246, 296
Beta carotene, 28, 38, 39, 53, 55. *See also* Vitamins.
Bicycles
    braking on, 128, **129**
    selection of, 128, 132
    shifting gears on, 128, **129**
    stationary, 101, 107, 128, 132, **132**

Bicycling, 28, 94, 97, 106, 107, 123, 128–129, 137, 195
    technique of, **128–129**
Bill of rights, patient's, 222
Biofeedback, 271, **271,** 291, 312
Biological clock, 348–349
Birthmarks, 150, 227
Bittick, Glenys, 195
Black bean chili, 84
Blackheads, **142,** 143
Bladder, 19, 228, **319, 321**
    cancer of, 67, 242, 316
Bleaching
    hair, 161
    skin, 166
    teeth, 164
Blisters, **117,** 166, 260, 265, 283
Blood
    chemistry of, 226, 228–229
    cholesterol in, 25, 38, 49, 50, 62, 116, 228–229, 298, **298**
    disorders of, 306
    drainage of, 153, **153**
    glucose in, 17, 226, 228–229, 241, 281–283, **282, 283**
    loss of, 15, 144, 148, **153, 197**
    occult, 226, 228–229, 312
    testing of, 18, 25, 220, 226, 228–229, 280, 282, **282**
    transfusions of, 220
    See also Circulatory system.
Blood pressure, 101, 296–297
    lowering of, 39
    measuring of, 101, 220, 221, **223,** 226, 228–229, 296–297
    raising of, 106, 137, 226, 230
    See also Hypertension.
Blood vessels, 95
    constriction of, 66, 140, 174, 183, 230
    dilation of, 113, 150, 230
    of eyes, 289
    of skin, 140, 141, **141,** 146, 150, **197**
    See also Arteries; Veins.
Body fat, 60–65, **61**
    drug accumulation in, 231–232
    of men vs. women, 62, **62**
    surgical removal of, 152, **153,** 154, 155
Boley, Helen, 25, **25**
Bones, 16, 217
    cancer of, 271
    dental, 162, 164, 165
    fractures of, 19, 114, 115, 130, 134, 223, **267,** 269, 270
    loss of mass in, 15, 20, 58, 94, 239, 269
    maintaining mass in, 16, 134, 239
    marrow of, 306, **307**

Bones (*contd.*)
    See also Calcium; Menopause; Osteoporosis.
Botulism, 75
Boyd, Bill, 245, **245**
Braces, dental, 165
Brain, 18, **18,** 240
    alcohol and, 196, **197,** 241
    damage and deterioration of, 16, 18–19, 196, **197,** 213, 222, 272–279, **272**
    intelligence and, 18, **273**
    monitoring of, **223,** 274
    neurons of, 16, 18
    stem of, **273**
    thrombosis in, **272**
    See also Nervous system.
Breast
    cancer of, 38, 39, 50, 154, 226, 228–229, 239, 322, **322**
    discharge from, **227**
    enlargement of, 154, 197
    examinations of, 154, 218, 227, **227,** 322
    fibrocystic, 67, 322
    lumps in, 227, **227,** 322
    pendulous, 146, 154
    surgery on, 154, 322, **322**
Breathing
    deep, 102, **102,** 174, 222
    difficulty with, **197,** 232, 235, 249, 250, 292–295
    exercise and, 102, 137
Bridges, dental, 163, 165
Brim, Gilbert, 184
Bronchitis, 242, 292, 295, 347
Bronchodilators, 292
Brynner, Yul, 161
Bunions, 260, **261**
Burglary, preventive measures against, 329
Burns, 223
Burns, George, 20, **20**
Bursitis, 115
Bush, Barbara, 280
Bush, George, 280

C

Cabbage and carrot soup with dill, 88
Caffeine, 59, 66–67, **66,** 96, 112–113, 247
Calcium, 43, 52, 54, 58–59, **58–59**
    absorption of, 58–59

Calcium (*contd.*)
cholesterol and, 59
dietary sources of, **58,** 59, **59,** 269
levels of in bones, 281
osteoporosis and, 58, 260, 269
supplements, 59, 269
See also Bones; Menopause;
Minerals; Osteoporosis.
Calcium channel blockers, 246, 296,
305
Calisthenics, 106, 110, 126
Calluses, 166, 261, 283
Calment, Jeanne, **19**
Calories
burning of, 60, 63, 94, 122, 124,
128, 245
extreme restriction of, 27, 28, 65
guidelines on, 36, 45, 51, 63, **77**
sources of, 49, 69
Cancer, 19, 20
causes of, 38, 39, 50, 239, 242
detection of, 227, **227,** 228
living with, 323
prevention of, 30, 38, 39, 76
survivors of, 137, 323
treatment of, 160, 218, 227, 295,
319, 322, 323
See also specific cancers.
Capsaicin, 75
Carbohydrates, **37,** 44–45, **44–46,** 69
complex, 44–45
dietary sources of, 44, 46
simple, 44
Carbon dioxide, 102, 346
Carbon monoxide, 334, 335, 346, 347
Cardiopulmonary resuscitation (CPR),
340
Cardiotonics, 230
Cardiovascular system. *See* Circulatory
system.
Carver, George Washington, 20
Casein, 57, 75
Cataracts, 16, 147, **285, 286**
surgery for, 286
Cellulite, 149, 155
Centenarians, 10, 13, **13,** 28, 29, **30**
Centers for Disease Control, 259
Cerebrovascular accident (CVA). *See*
Strokes.
Cervix, **321**
cancer of, 228–229, 242, 320
Chanel, Gabriel "Coco," 141
Chemical peels, 151, **151**
Chemotherapy, 160, 295, 319, 322, 323
Chest, 218
severe pain in, 38, 223, 230, 249,
297, 299
X-rays of, 228–229, 252, **301,** 304

Chewing gum
nicotine, 233, 243
sugarless, 162
Chicken, 82, 83, **83**
Chicken pox, 264–265
Children, 12, 191
adult, 191, 192, 209, 213
caring for, 185, 187, 188, 189, 190
death of, 12, 192
divorce and, 189, 190, 191
leaving home by, 184, 189
Chili, 84
Chiropractic, 217, 252
Cholesterol, 49, **49,** 67
calcium and, 59
fats and, 38, 48, 49–51
genetics and, 25, 50
heart disease and, 298
limiting of, 36, 49, 50, 51
testing of, 25, 298
See also Heart disease; High-
density lipoproteins; Low-density
lipoproteins; Very-low-density
lipoproteins.
Chunky pork and beans, 84
Circadian rhythms, 348, 349
Circulation problems, 304–305. *See
also specific conditions.*
Circulatory system, 15, 230, 239, 241
alcohol and, **197**
disorders of, 296–307
exercise and, 95, 96, 101, 102
See also Arteries; Blood; Heart;
Heart disease.
Cirrhosis, 39, **196, 197, 309,** 312, 314
Clarkson, Jane, **137**
Climbing
hills, 94, 122
stair climbing machine and,
132–133, **132**
stairs, 93, 97, 107
Clinics
independent, 149, 153, 223
pain, 271, **271**
sleep, 250
surgical procedures at, 149, 151,
153
Clothing
body shape and, 170–171, **170, 171**
cold weather, 113, 122
color of, 158, 169, **169**
exercise, 96, 113, 135
men's, 171, **171**
protective, 113, 120, 122, 146, 147
women's, 168, 169, 170, **170**
Cocaine, 233, 237

Coffee, 47, 66, **67,** 233
Cognitive-behavioral therapy, 178, 179,
278
Colds, 241, 248–249
prevention of, 248
symptoms of, 249, **249**
treatment of, 235, 249
Cold treatments (compresses, ice
packs), 154, 251, 252, 262, 265
Collagen, 140, **141,** 147
injections of, 151, **151**
Colon, 228–229, 257, **309, 319**
cancer of, 30, 38, 39, 46, 67, 303,
311, 312, 323
polyps of, 228, **309,** 312
spastic, 311–312
Colonoscopy, 310–311
Colostomies, 323
Community organizations, 31–32, 116,
123, 126, 200, 202, 203, 206
Computer imaging, **148,** 153, 252, 304,
313
Computerized axial tomography (CAT)
scan, 252, 304, 313
Condoms, latex, 238
Congestive heart failure, **297,** 302–303
Constipation, 41, 43, 45, 258, 312
Contact lenses, 285, 288–289
Conway, Lupe, 251, **251**
Cooldowns, 96, 104, 108, 109, 113,
114, 119, 126, 127, 128, 130,
135, 137
Cornea, **285**
Corns, 261, **261,** 283
Coronary artery disease (CAD), 297,
299, 300, 301, **301**
See also Heart disease.
Cortisone, 145, 265
Cosmetics
camouflaging, 155
hypoallergenic, 144, 155
ingredients in, 144, 145, 146
labeling of, 145
testing of, **144,** 145, 161, 166
Cough syrups, 233
Counseling
divorce, 190
family, 199
job, 200, 205–206
nutritional, 41
psychological, 177–179, 194, 195,
198, 221, 238, 241, 271,
278–279
retirement, 202, 205–206
Creams, 161, 167
antifungal, 166
bleaching, 166
cleansing, 142, 143, 155

Creams (*contd.*)
   concealing, 155
   foundation, 169
   shaving, 144
Cridland, Charlotte, 349
Crime, 120, 194, 201, 329, 351
Crohn's disease, 311
Cross-training, 106–107, 111
Crowns, dental, 164
Crustless potato and cheese pie, 89

D

Daily Values (DV's), 55, **77**
Dairy products, 13, 30, 36, 37, **37,** 42,
   43, 49, **49,** 50, **58,** 59
Dandruff, 156
Day care, 185
   adult, 187, **187,** 277
DDT, 72, 335
Death, 192–195
   childhood, 12, 192
   of family members, 174, **175,** 184,
      188, 192–194, 196
   fear of, 178
   mourning and, 192–194, **192,** 196
   practical considerations and, 193,
      195, 213
   religious and secular rituals of, **192,**
      193, 194
   sudden, 192, 195
Death rates, 12, 93, 205, 239
   heart disease and, 65, 93, 242
   weight and, 60, 65
Decongestants, 235, 247
Defibrillator, 302
   implants, 304, **304**
Dehydration, 43, 241, 249
Delirium tremens, 198
Dementia, 226, 240, 241, 272
   senile, 226, 241, 276–277
DeMille, Agnes, 275
Denmark, Leila, **15**
Dental care implements, **162,** 163, **163**
Dental floss, 162, **162, 163**
Dentists, 41, 162, 164, 165
Dentures, 41, 164–165
Deodorants, 141, 168
Deoxyribonucleic acid (DNA), 22, 28,
   55
Depilatories, 161

Depression, 196, 238, 246
   causes of, 278
   exercise and, 30, 93, **180**
   midlife, 184–185
   treatment of, 20, 230, 241, 246, 278,
      279
Dermabrasion, 150–151, **150**
Dermatitis, 144, 146
Dermatologists, 141–144, 149, 150,
   156, 160, 161, 166
Diabetes, 101, 238, 251, 281–283
   control of, 282–283
   diet and, 31, 41, 44, 45, 46, 62, 65,
      283
   exercise and, 93, 97, 282, 283
   testing for, 17, 228, 282, **282,** 283,
      283
   Type 1, 281, 282
   Type 2, 281, 282–283
Diabetic retinopathy, **288,** 289
Dialysis, kidney, 317, **317**
Diaphragm, 102, 293, 308
Diarrhea, 67, 72, 75, 233, 257, 258,
   311, 312
Dideoxyinosine (ddI), 307
Diets
   balanced, 30, 36–37
   changes in, 37, 63, 65
   disease and, 13, 31, 38–39, **39,** 48,
      49, 50, 51, 65
   government guidelines on, 36, 37,
      60
   low-fat, 31, 37, 38, 48–49, 51, 55,
      62, 63, 65, 256, 283
   weight control, 27–28, 31, 63, 65,
      149
   See also Food.
Digestive system, 15–16
   disorders of, 43, 45, 94, 183, **197,**
      256–258, 308–315
   examination of, 228–229, 310–311,
      311
   function of, 44–46, **309**
Digitalis, 303
Diphtheria, 219
Diseases
   alternative treatment of, 217
   autoimmune, 160, 266
   chronic, 13, 149, 196, 217, 225, 315,
      351
   diagnosis of, 17, 41, 220, 221, 222
   diet and, 13, 31, 38–39, **39,** 48, 49,
      50, 51, 65
   incurable, 195, 222, 225
   inoculations against, 219, 230, 248,
      259, 293
   mental incapacity and, 212, 213,
      226, 240, 241, 272, 276–277

prevention of, 11–12, 28, 38–39, **39,**
   217, 219, 238
   safe journeys with, 315
   sexual transmission of, 238,
      306–307, 312
   See also specific diseases.
Diuretics, 41, 47, 55, 112–113, 160,
   230, 274, 296, 303
Diverticulosis, 45, 310
Divorce
   adjustments to, 185, 189, 190–191
   children of, 189, 190, 191
   financial concerns and, 190, 191,
      191
   remarriage and, 189, 191, **191**
   stress of, 174, **175,** 189, 190–191
DNA, 22, **22**
Documents, 191
   safekeeping of, 193, 213
Dogs
   bites of, 342
   dealing with, 120
Dopamine, 275, 276
Driving
   drinking and, 31, 199
   drugs and, 235, 351
   posture and, **253**
   safety and, 277, 350–351
Drugs, 230–237
   absorption of, 15, 231–232, 234
   abuse of, **198,** 199, 230, 233, 237
   adverse interactions of, 196, 232,
      235
   alcohol and, 232, 235
   allergic reactions to, 232, 233, 235
   costs of, 224, 225, 232, 235
   dosage and administration of,
      220–221, **221,** 222, **223,** 232,
      236, 303
   generic, 225, 234
   mail-order, 218, 225, 235
   narcotic, 230, 233, 237
   overdoses of, 195, 232, 236, 278
   over-the-counter, 66, 232, 235, 250,
      251, 256, 257
   packaging and labeling of, **231, 234,**
      235, **235,** 236, 237
   quack, 29, 218
   records of, 216–217, 220, 232, 235
   safety of, 20, 218–19, 221, 230–233,
      236
   side effects of, 147, 149, 221,
      232–233, 235, **235,** 241, 303
   storing of, 236
Dryden, John, 133
Durable power of attorney, 186
Dyes
   food, 70, 71, 75
   cosmetic, 145

E

Ears, 270, 290–291
  hearing loss and, 18, 290–291, 344
  protection of, 344–345, **345**
  ringing in, 165, 291
  surgery on, 154
  See also Hearing aids.
Education, senior, 200, 202–204, **204**
Eggplant and mushroom lasagne, 86
Eggs, 36, 37, 40, 42, 43, 50, 74, 79, 145
  allergic reaction to, 219, 248
Elastin, 140, **141,** 146, 147
Elder Cottage Housing Opportunity
  (ECHO), 209
Elderhostel, 204, **204**
Electrocardiograms (EKG's), 101,
  228–229
Electrolysis, 161
Electrosurgery, 150
Emergency medical care, 135, 216
  advance directives and, 213, 222
  in hospitals, 222, 223, 274
Emphysema, 242, 294, 335, 347
Empty-nest syndrome, 184, 189
Emulsifiers, 70, 144, 145
Endocrine system, 16, 280–283, **281**
Endometrial cancer, 321
Endorphins, 93
Endoscopy, 225, 308, 311, **311,** 313,
  314, 315
Enemas, barium, 310, 311, **311**
Environmental Protection Agency (EPA),
  72, 242, 329, 330, 337
Enzymes, 15, 42, 69, 75, 231, 309
Esophagus, **197,** 256, **309, 311**
  cancer of, 39, 242
Estrogen, 20, 59, 68, 238
Estrogen replacement therapy (ERT),
  20, 238, 239, 269, 320, 321
Exercise, 92–137
  aerobic, 95–97, 101, 103, 106–111,
    116–133, 137, **180**
  aging and, 14, 92, 93, **93,** 96, 123,
    136–137
  benefits of, 31, 41, 92–95, **93,** 107,
    127, 136
  chair, 110, 136
  classes in, 108, 111, 121
  endurance, 96, 98, **98,** 99, **99,** 106,
    107, 134–135, 137
  flexibility, 96, 100, **100,** 104–105,
    106, 107, 136, 137
  home, 132–133, 136
  risks of, 96, 101, 111, 112–113,
    114–115, 125, 137

Exercise (*contd.*)
  safe levels of, 101, 109, 137
  social, **92,** 108, 116
  strength, 94, 98, **98,** 106, 107, 111,
    134–135, 136, 137
  stress and, 94, 127, 177, **180,** 182
  weather conditions and, 112–113
  weight control and, 31, 63, 93–94,
    116, 149
  weight training, 94, 106, 107, 110,
    134–135
  See also Cooldowns; Warmups.
Exercise equipment
  bicycling, 101, 107, 128, **129**
  cross-country skiing machines, 133,
    133
  hiking, 122
  home, 101, 107, 128, 132–133,
    132–133
  instruction with, 132, 134, **134,** 135
  rowing machines, 133, **133**
  stair-climbing machines, 132–133,
    132–133
  stationary bicycles, 132, **132**
  weight-training, 134–135, **134, 135**
Exercise programs, 50, **92, 93,** 101,
  106–111
  for beginners, 110–111, 119
  competition in, 109, 121, 123, 131,
    137
  cross-training, 106–107, 111
  customizing of, 106–111, 136
  for elderly, 136–137
  guidelines for, 109, 137
  physical examinations prior to, 31,
    101, 135, 137
  regularity of, 14, 30–31, 107, 109,
    111, 137, 182, 194
  support networks for, 109, 116
Eyeglasses, 147, 155, 171, 220, 285,
  286, 287, 288–289, **288–289,**
  350
Eyelid tucks, 153–154, **153,** 155
Eyes, 18, 141, 171, 284–289
  bags and circles under, 140–141,
    153, **153**
  "black," 154
  cosmetics for, 169
  crow's-feet around, 140, **146,** 151
  diseases of, 286–287, **286, 287,**
    288, 289
  floaters in, 284, 287
  injuries of, 148, 223
  irritation of, 141, 145, 285
  parts of, **285**
  tics of, 285
  vision problems and, 133, 147, 153,
    155, 171, 220, 284–289, **286,**
    287, 288, 350

F

Face lifts, 148, 152–153
  recovery from, **152,** 153, **153**
  risks and side effects of, 148, **152,**
    153, **153,** 154
Faces, 179
  cleansing of, 142, **142,** 143
  exercise of, 143–144
  men's, 144, **144,** 155
  skin of, 140–141, 142–146, **142,**
    150–154, **150, 151, 152, 153**
  treatment of, 142–144, **142, 144,**
    146, 148, 150–153, 155
  T-zone of, 142, **142**
  women's, 142, **142,** 155
Family histories, 212. *See also* Medical
  histories.
Fatigue, 67, 141, 182, 238, 280, 305
Fats, 13, 48–51, 49, **60–61**
  cholesterol and, 38, 48, 49–51
  cutting down on, 36, 37, **37,** 38, 49,
    50, 51, 62
  dietary sources of, 48–49
  disorders associated with, 36, 38,
    48, 49, 50–51, 76
  monounsaturated, 36, 38, 48, 49–50
  polyunsaturated, 36, 38, 48, 49–50
  saturated, 36, 38, 43, 48, 49, 51
Feet, 166–168
  diabetes and, 283
  problems with, 166–167, 260–261,
    260, 261, 283
Fettuccine with creamy broccoli sauce,
  86
Fever, 249, 255, 294, 311, 343
Fiber, dietary, 30, 38, 41, 43, 44, 257
  benefits of, 45–46, 51
"Fight or flight" syndrome, 174
Fingernails
  manicuring and polishing of, 166,
    167, **167**
  ridges on, 149, 166, 167
Fire, danger of, 326–328
First aid, 122, 340
Fish, 36, 37, **37,** 42, 43, 49, 55, 76
  cooking of, 73, 79
  fatty, 41, 51
  raw, 73, 74
Fitness tests
  aerobic, 97, 101, **101**
  body composition, 100, **100**
  flexibility, 100, **100**

Fitness tests (*contd.*)
 guidelines for, 96
 muscle, 98, **98,** 99, **99, 100**
 pinch, **100**
 stress, 101, **101,** 135, 137, 228
Flashlights, for safety, 120
Fluids, 46, 47, 112, 113, 114, 127, 249,
 257–258
Fluoride, 54
 in toothpaste, 163
 See also Minerals.
Food, 36–88
 additives in, 36, 70–73, 75
 allergic reactions to, 73, 75, 219,
 234, 235, 246, 247, 248
 appetite for, 40, 41, 55, 194
 contamination of, 57, 71, 72–75, 257
 cooking of, 36, 37, 38, 40, 49, 73,
 74, **78, 79,** 80–89
 drug interactions with, 41, 235
 genetically engineered, 72
 handling and preparation of, 72–75,
 79
 intolerances to, 75
 irradiation of, 73
 labeling of, 40, 55, 72, 73, 76–77, **77**
 meal planning and, 41, 80–89
 medicinal qualities in, 38–39, **39**
 nutrition and, 36–89, 220
 processed, 44, 45, 57, 70–73, 74
 pyramid, 36–37, **37**
 restaurant, 36, **40,** 57
 safety with, 71–75, **74**
 selection and storage of, 40, 74,
 78–79
 serving sizes of, 36, 64
 See also Diets; *specific foods and
 recipes.*
Food and Drug Administration (FDA),
 45, 55, 71, 72, 73, 76, **77,** 145,
 146, 151, 154, 219, 226, 232
Food poisoning, 57, 74–75, 256–257
Forehead lifts, **153,** 154
Formaldehyde, 334–335
401(k) plans, 202
Fragrances, 144–145, 168
Framingham Heart Study, 28, 65
Franklin, Benjamin, 20, 64
Free radicals, dangers of, 28, 38, 55
Friends
 loss of, 192, 193
 social life with, 14, 31, **31,** 182, 190,
 191, 212
 support of, 179, 190, 191, 202
Frostbite, 113
Fruits, 30, 36, 37, **37,** 38, 45, 49, 51, 76,
 78–79

Gallbladder, 15, **309, 315**
 diseases of, **309,** 314–315, **314**
Gallstones, 46, 63, **309,** 314, **314**
Gastritis, **197,** 308–309
Gastroenteritis, 257–258
Gastrointestinal tract. *See* Digestive
 system.
Gerontologists, 10–12, 14, 22, 212
Glands, 249
 adrenal, 16, **281**
 oil, 140, **141,** 150, 156
 parathyroid, **281**
 pituitary, 16, 26, **281**
 sweat, **141**
 thymus, 16
 See also Prostate gland; Thyroid
 gland.
Glaucoma, 287, **287,** 350
Gloves, 113, **129,** 146, 166
Glucose, 44, 45
 blood, 17, 226, 228–229, 241,
 281–283, **282, 283**
Glycerin, 145
Glycogen, 44, 63
Goals, 108, 176, 182, 188, 202, 205,
 212
Goiter, 280
Gout, 43, 267–268, **267**
 See also Arthritis.
Graham, Martha, 20–21, **20**
Grains, 30, 36, 37, **37,** 41, 42, 44–45,
 51, 85, 86–87
Grandchildren, 179, 184, 195, 211
Graves' disease, 183, 280
Grief, 174, **175,** 184, 188, 192–194
Grilled chicken with fruit chutney, 83
Gums, 162, 163, **163,** 164, 165

Hair
 analysis of, 41
 caring for, 146, 155, 156–160, **157,**
 168, **209**
 damage to, 156, 157, **157,** 159
 dyeing and tinting of, 157, 158–159,
 158

Hair (*contd.*)
 follicles of, 141, 158, 160, 161
 graying of, 156, 158–159, **158,** 171
 ingrown, 144
 loss of, 156, 160–161, **160,** 168
 men's, 159, 160–161
 permanent waving of, 157, 159
 pigmentation of, 156, 158, 159
 removal of, 161
 shaving of, 144, **144,** 155, 161; 168,
 222
 straightening of, 157
 styling of, 155, 156, 157, 160, 168
 sun exposure and, 157, **157,** 159
 women's, 157, 158–159, **158,** 160,
 161, 168
Hair dryers, 155, 157
Hairpieces, 161
Hallucinations, 198, 237
Hallucinogens, 230, 237
Hammertoes, 261, **261**
Hamstring, 100, 115, 126, 127, **134,**
 135, **254**
Hands, 147
 care of, 166, 167, 168
 tremors of, 275, 276
Hats, 113, 146, 147, 151, 155, **157**
Hayflick limit, 23
Headaches, 179, 183, 194, 233,
 246–247, **246,** 271, 343
 causes of, 246, 247
 chronic, 217
 cluster, 247
 migraine, 66, 246
 treatment of, 217, 246, 247
Health and Human Services
 Department, U.S., 228
Health care, 216–237
 alternative treatments and, 217, 225
 paying for, 149, 186, 187, 224–225
 preventive, 11, 28, 38–39, **39,** 217,
 219, 238
 self-education and, 220, 226
Health care proxies, 213, 222
Health clubs, 109, 134, 135
Health insurance, 149, 187
 deductibles and, 224, 225
 making claims on, 186, 225
 premiums for, 186, 225
 proof of, 216, 220
 supplemental, 186, 224
 types of, 224–225
 See also Medicaid; Medicare.
Health maintenance organizations
 (HMO's), 224–225
Hearing aids, 290, 291, **291**
Heart, 15, **297**
 enlargement of, **197**
 exercise and, 93, 95, 96–97

Heart (*contd.*)
  monitoring of, 97, 101, **101,**
    228–229, **223, 300–301**
  operations on, 300–301, **300-301**
  parts of, 15, **297**
  stress and, 175, 183
Heart attack, 101, 238, 299, 302
  causes of, 205, 242, 250, 299, 302
  symptoms of, 96, 111, 223, 299
  treatment of, 50, 223, 302
Heartburn, 232, 256
Heart disease, 19, 67, 101, 297–299
  alcohol and, **197**
  angina pectoris, 38, 223, 230, 249,
    297, 299
  arrhythmias, 67, 250, **297,** 304
  atherosclerosis, 38, 43, **297,** 299
  bypass surgery for, **301**
  cholesterol and, 298
  congestive heart failure, **297,**
    302–303
  coronary artery disease (CAD), 297,
    299, 300, 301, **301**
  death rates from, 65, 93, 242
  diet and, 13, 31, 38, 48, 49, 50, 51,
    65
  exercise and, 13, 93, 116, 125
  family history of, 101
  hypertension and, 30, 40, 57, 67, 94,
    101, 106, **197,** 228, 296–297,
    296
  prevention of, 13, 30, 239, 242, 297,
    299
  stress and, 19, 183
  symptoms of, 96, 111, 166, 223,
    228, 241, 299
  testing for, 228–229
  treatment of, 230, 300–301,
    300–301
  weight and, 62, 297
  *See also specific diseases and
    conditions.*
Heart-lung machine, **300–301**
Heart rate
  acceleration of, 126, 128, 137, 174,
    230, 304, **304**
  exercising, 15, 101, **101,** 228
  lowering of, 15, 183
  monitoring of, 97, **99,** 101, **101,** 112,
    226
  resting, 15, 101
  stress and, 183
  target rates for, 97, 126, 137, 228
  See also Heart disease.
Heat exhaustion, 112
Heatstroke, 112–113
Hemorrhages, **272,** 289, 299, 304
Hemorrhoids, 45, 228, 258

Hepatitis, **309,** 314
  A, 256–257, 312
  B, 312
  C, 312
Hepburn, Audrey, 140, **140**
Herbalism, 217
Herbs, 38, 40, 57
Hernias, 308
  hiatal, 308
Herrick, Marie, 286, **286**
High-density lipoproteins (HDL's), 25,
  62, 116, 228, 298
  benefits of, 38, 50, 68, **298**
  See also Cholesterol.
Hiking, **93,** 97, 116, 122–123
  See also Walking.
Hips, 62, 149
  joint replacement in, 268, **268,** 270
HMO's (health maintenance
  organizations), 224–225
Hodgkin's disease, 306–307
Holmes, Oliver Wendell, Jr., 21
Home health aides, 187
Homeopathy, 217
Home security, 328–329
Honey, 57, 75, 145
Hormone replacement therapy. *See*
  Estrogen replacement therapy
  (ERT).
Hormones, 42, 174, **180,** 230
  human growth, 26–27, **26,** 146
  imbalance of, **197,** 238
  menopausal changes in 20, 23, 161,
    238
  production of, 16, 23, 59, 146, **281**
  treatment with, 20, 26–27, 146, 238,
    239, 269, 320, 321, 322
Hospice care, 225
Hospitals, 213, 220–223
  admission to, 220
  advocacy in, 220, 221
  costs in, 220, 222, 224, 225
  emergency care in, 222, 223, 274
  extension facilities of, 223
  inpatient care in, 149, 154, 220–223,
    225
  intensive care units in, 223, **223**
  outpatient care in, 151, 153, 225
  physicians' affiliation with, 149, 216,
    220
  staff and facilities of, 220, 221, 222,
    223
  teaching, 220, 221
  technology in, 220, 223, **223**
  veterans, 220
  volunteering in, 32, 194, 206, **206,**
    221
Hot flashes, menopausal, 16, 20, 238,
  239

Housing, retirement options for,
  207–209
Human immunodeficiency virus (HIV),
  307, **307**
Human Nutrition Research Center on
  Aging, 93
Humor
  health benefits of, 127
  stress reduction and, 32, 127, 182
Hypertension, 30, 40, 57, 67, 94, 101,
  106, **197,** 228, 296–297, **296**
  treatment of, 160, 230, 232, 297
  weight and, 62, 297
  See also Blood pressure; Heart
    disease.
Hyperthyroidism, 280
Hypnosis, 271
Hypodermis, 141, **141**
Hypoglycemia, 282, 283
Hypothermia, 113
Hypothyroidism, 149, 280
Hysterectomy, 239

I

Ibuprofen, 246, 249, 252
Immune globulins, 230
Immune system, 25, 75, 306
  diseases of, 15, 160, 194, 238, 248,
    266, 294, 306–307, **307**
  stress and, 183, 194
Implants
  breast, 154
  defibrillator, 304
  dental, 165
  eye, 286
  pacemaker, 304
  penile, 238
Impotence, 238
Incontinence, 20, 238, 316, 320
  help for, 320
Indigestion, 232, 256–258, 308–309
Infections, 241
  bacterial, 229, 230
  fighting of, 38, 230, 260
  fungal, 166, 260
  postsurgical, 148, **152, 153,** 222
Inflammatory bowel disease, 311
Influenza, 248–249
  intestinal, 257–258
  spreading of, 248–249, **248**
  symptoms of, 249, **249,** 252, 257
  vaccine for, 219, 248, 293

Injuries
    common, 114–115
    prevention of, 94, 103, 104, 109,
        114, 115
    trauma, 114, 115, 223
    treatment of, 114–115, 125, 223
    See also specific injuries.
Insects, 73, 178, **178,** 259
    bites and stings of, 342–343
    repelling of, 72–73, 335, 339–340,
        347
Insomnia, 67, 194, 235, 250
Insulin, 281, 282, 283, **309**
Insurance, 32
    life, 195
    proof of, 216, 220
    See also Health insurance.
Intelligence, 18
Intensive care units (ICU's), 223, **223**
Intestines, 38, 46, 197, **309**
    diseases of, 257–258, 308,
        310–312
Iodine, 54
    added to salt, 70
    as therapy for hyperthyroidism, 280
    See also Minerals.
IRA's (individual retirement accounts),
    202
Iris, eye, **285**
Iron, 52, 54, 59
    adverse interactions with drugs,
        232
    iron-deficiency anemia, 305
    See also Minerals.
Irradiation, food, 73
Irritable bowel syndrome, 45, 311–312

J

Jaundice, **197, 309,** 314
Jaw pain, 247, 256, 276, 299
Jet lag, 259
Jobs
    changing of, 174, 185, 190,
        200–201, 202
    enjoyment of, **15,** 201, 207
    full-time, **205,** 207
    household, 28, 185, 190, 209
    loss of, 174, **175,** 189, 201

Jobs (*contd.*)
    part-time, 201, 202, 205, **205**
    placement in, 200, 205–206
    post-retirement, 185, 205–207, **205**
    seeking and starting of, 190,
        200–201, 202, 205–207
    stress of, 20, 174, 175, **175,** 179,
        184–185
    temporary, 201, 205
    time spent on, 182, 185
    women in, 185, 205
Jogging. *See* Running.
Joints, 114, 128, 167, 218
    range of motion in, 104, 266
    replacement of, 268, **268**
    soreness of, 137, 167, 217, 266,
        266, 267

K

Kegel exercises, 316, 320
Keogh accounts, 202
Keratoses, 146, 150
Kidneys, 19, 43, 148, 228
    dialysis of, 317, **317**
    diseases of, 225, 241, 251, 317
    failure of, 317
Kidney stones, 59, 317, **317**
Kinesiology, 135
Knees, 117
    arthritis of, 266, **266, 267,** 268
    joint replacement and, 268, **268**
    locking of, **103, 105**
    runner's, 115
Kobasa, Suzanne, 175

L

Laryngitis, 249
Larynx, 249
    cancer of, 242, 323
Lasagne, eggplant and mushroom, 86
Law, Jim, **137**
Lawyers, 190, 219
Lazarus, Richard, 175
L-dopa, 276

Lead, 59, 159, 329, 331, 341, **341**
Lean but hearty beef stew, 80
Lecithin, 39
Left atrium, **297**
Left ventricle, **297**
Legionnaires' disease, 294
Legumes, 36, 37, **37,** 42, 43, 45, 84
Lens, eye, **285,** 286
Leukemias, 306
Liddell, William, 207, **207**
Life Change Index Scale, **175**
Life expectancy, 10–13, 185, 202
    life span vs., 10–12
    of men, 12, 13, 19–20
    of women, 12, 13, 19–20
Life span, 10–13
    health span vs., 12–13, 20, 22
    life expectancy vs., 10–12
Lifestyle, 217
    change of, 13, 225, 232, 299
    French, 51
    healthy, 14, 210
    sedentary, **32,** 59, 101, 136, 211
Lightning, protection from, 329
Light therapy, 349
Linolenic acid, 39
Liposuction, 155
Lithium, 247, 278
Liver, 228, 241
    alcohol abuse and, 15, **196, 197,**
        314
    cancer of, 39
    cirrhosis of, 39, **196, 197, 309,** 312,
        314
    failure of, **196, 197,** 312
    function of, 15, 43, 231, **239, 309**
Liver spots, 147, 166
Living wills, 213, 222
Loneliness, 187, 194, 195, 205
Lotions, 141, 142, 143, 144, 145, 151,
    155, 161, 166
Low-density lipoproteins (LDL's), 25, 38,
    49, 50, 228, **298**
    See also Cholesterol.
Lucretius, 347
Lungs, **102,** 148, 222, **223**
    air flow in, 16, **17,** 95, 222, 292, **292**
    cancer of, 39, 242, 295, 334, 335
    diseases of, 39, 149, 228–229, 241,
        242, 292–295, **292, 294, 295,**
        334, 335
    smoking and, 242, **243,** 292, 293,
        295, 335
Lyme disease, 342–343
Lymphatic system, 218, 305, 306, **306**
Lymphomas, 306

M

Machines
massage, 160
testing, 226, 228, 282, **282,**
310–311, **311,** 313
See also Exercise equipment.
Macula, **285,** 287
Macular degeneration, 287, **287**
Magnesium, 54
supplements of for leg cramps, 251
See also Minerals.
Magnetic resonance imaging (MRI),
252, 313
Makeup. *See* Cosmetics.
Malignant melanoma, 265, **265**
Malnutrition, 41, **197**
Malpractice suits, 218–219, 222, 225
Mammograms, 154, 228–229, 322
Manicures, 166, 167
Marijuana, 237
Marriage, 174
changes in, 188, 189
financial concerns of, 191
maintaining health of, 188–189
remarriage, 189, 191, **191**
Masks, facial, **142,** 143
Massage, 114, **181**
facial, 143
foot, 166, 167
gum, 163
machines for, 160
Mastectomies, 154, 322, **322**
McClintock, Barbara, 21
Mead, Margaret, 184
Meal delivery programs, 187, **187**
Measles, 11
Meat, **37,** 42, 48
cooking of, 39, 49, 73, 74, 75, 79,
80–81
curing of, 38, 57, 71
lean cuts of, 36, 37, 49, 55
organ, 40, 50, 51, 73, 267
red, 43, 49, 50, 79
Meat loaf, 80
Medicaid, 186, 225
Medical histories, 216, 217, 218, 219,
226, 239
charting of, 31, 33
family, 33
Medical insurance. *See* Health
insurance.
Medical records, 218, 219, 220, 222

Medicare, 186, 187
applying for, 225
eligibility for, 225
Medigap insurance, 225
Meditation, **180,** 250
Melanin, 140
Memory, 240–241
dementia and, 240, 241, 277
long-term vs. short-term, 240, 277
loss of, 18–19, 196, 198, 240, 241,
277
reminiscence and, 212
testing of, 240, **240, 241**
Menopause
effects of, 16, 20, 161, 184, **184,** 238
estrogen replacement therapy (ERT)
for problems of, 15, 20, 238, 239,
269, 320, 321
hormonal changes during, 20, 161,
238
See also Bones; Calcium;
Osteoporosis.
Metabolism, 38, 40, 47, 60, 106, 136
of drugs, 15, 231, 234
Milk, 49, 57, **58,** 59, 75, 79, 145, 340
Minerals, 52–55, 70, 176
benefits of, 54
calcium. *See* Calcium.
chloride, 54
chromium, 54
copper, 54
dietary sources of, 54
Daily Values (DV's) for, 55, **77**
fluoride. *See* Fluoride.
iodine. *See* Iodine.
iron. *See* Iron.
magnesium. *See* Magnesium.
manganese, 54
molybdenum, 54
phosphorus. *See* Phosphorus.
potassium. *See* Potassium.
Recommended Dietary Allowances
(RDA's) for, 28, 40, 42, 43, 55, 58,
77
selenium, 54
sodium. *See* Sodium.
sulfur, 54
United States Recommended Daily
Allowances (USRDA's) for, 55, 77
zinc. *See* Zinc.
Mink oil, 145, 146
Minoxidol, 160
Mitosis, 23, **23**
Mnemonic devices, 241
Moisturizers, 141, 142, 143, 144, 145,
146, 151, 155
Moles, skin, 227
Monoamine oxidase (MAO) inhibitors,
278

Mononucleosis, 249
Monosodium glutamate (MSG), 70, 71
Moses, Grandma (Anna Mary), 21
Motion sickness, 259
Mouth, 161
cancer of, 165, 242
soreness or irritation of, 165, **197**
verticle lines around, **150,** 151, **151,**
169
Mouthwashes, 163
Muggeridge, Malcolm, 231
Muscles
contraction of, 98, 99, 114
cramping of, 114, 126, 251
deterioration of, 16, 94, **197,** 231
endurance of, 96, 98, **98,** 99, **99,**
106, 107, 134–135, 137
exercise of, 16, 41, 94, 98–99, 107,
110–111, 130, 134–137, 251,
255–256
flexibility of, 96, 100, **100,** 104–105,
106, 107, 136, 137
injuries to, 150, 114–115, 130
manipulation of, 217, 252
ratio of fat to, 100, 106, 107, 231
soreness and pain in, 103, 111,
114–115, **181,** 233, 252
strength of, 94, 98, **98,** 106, 107,
111, 134–135, 136, 137
tension of, 114, 179, **180, 181**

N

Nails
artificial, 167
caring for, 166, 167, **167**
infections of, 166, 167, 261
ingrown, 167, 261
ridges on, 149, 166, 167
split, 166, 167
See also Fingernails; Toenails.
National Academy of Sciences, 28, 42,
55, 56, 73
National Cancer Institute (NCI), 38, 46
National Heart, Lung and Blood
Institute, 25
National Institutes of Health (NIH), 21,
58, 65
Naturopathy, 217
Nausea, 45, 67, 222, 233, 246, 247,
255, 256, 323

Neck lifts, 152, **152,** 154
Necks, 151, 218
    pain in, 179, 252, 255
Nervous system, 16, 44, 66, 174
    breakdowns of, 272–279
    damage to, 16, 148, **152,** 153, **153,**
        182, 196
    treatment of, 230
    See also Brain.
Nicholson, Harold, 211
Nicotine, 233, 243, 245, 247, 251
Nitroglycerin, 299
Noise, dealing with, 344–345, **344**
Non-Hodgkin's lymphomas, 306
Nonsteroidal anti-inflammatory drugs
        (NSAID's), 267, 269
Northcutt, Robert C., M.D., 50
Nurses, 41, 200
    hospital, 220, 221, 222
    psychiatric, 279
    training and specialization of, 221
    visiting, 187
Nursing homes, 209, 213
    costs of, 225
    guidelines for, 186
    long-term care in, 225
Nutrition Education and Labeling Act
        (1990), 76

Oat bran, 51
Obesity, 43, 45, 57, 61, 64, 125
Oil
    hydrogenated, 48
    vegetable, 37, 41, 48, 49, 157
Ointments, 151, 154
    cortisone, 145
    titanium dioxide, 147
    zinc oxide, 147
Older Women's League (OWL), 187
Ombudsmen, 220
Omega-3 fatty acids, 41, 51
One-dish meat loaf dinner, 80
Ophthalmologists, 149, 154, 284, 286,
        287
Opium, **218,** 237
Optic nerve, 285, **285,** 287
Orienteering, 122–123, **123**
Orthodontia, 163, 165
Orthotic devices, 114
Osteoarthritis, 247, 266, **266, 267**
    See also Arthritis.

Osteopathy, 41, 217
Osteoporosis, 21, 43, 60, **267,** 269–270
    calcium and, 58, 269
    estrogen replacement therapy (ERT)
        for, 15, 20, 238, 239, 269
    exercise and, 93
    See also Bones; Calcium;
        Menopause.
Otolaryngology, 149, 290
Ovaries, **281, 321**
    cancer of, 67, 320
Oven-fried chicken, 82
Oxygen, 16, 95, 96, 101, 102, 230, 250,
        272
    supplemental, **223,** 247, **294,** 302,
        315
Ozone, 147, 347

Pacemakers, 304
Paige, Satchel, 258
Pain, 266–271
    chronic, 195, 196, 206, 233, 271
    exercise and, 96, 103, 104, 111,
        114, 115, **254–255**
    "phantom," 271
    postsurgical, 151, 153, 154, 155,
        220–221
    prevention of, 253, **254–255**
    severe, 220–221, **221,** 223, 230,
        246–247, **246,** 255, 271
    treatment of, 151, 153, 154,
        220–221, **221,** 230, 238, 246,
        247, 252, 267, 271
Painful heel syndrome, **260,** 261
Pancreas, 16, **281, 309**
    cancer of, 67, 242
Panic attacks, 178
Pap test, 218, 228–229, 320
Para-aminobenzoic acid (PABA), 145
Paranoia, 175, 233
Parents
    caring for, 174, 185, 186–187, **187**
    child care and, 185, 187, 188, 189,
        190
    death of, 184, 188, 192–193
    divorced, 189
Parkinson's disease, 272, 275–276
    therapy for, 275, 276
Parrish, John, **30**
Pastas, **37,** 43, 86–87

Pasta salad Niçoise, 87, **87**
Patient representatives, 220, 221
Pectin, 39
Pedicures, 166, 167
Pelvic examinations, 218, 229
Penis, 238, 318, **319**
Peroxide, 163, 164
Personal Earnings and Benefit Estimate
        Statement (PEBES), 202
Personality types, 175–176, 179
Perspiration, 47, 113, 127, 130, 141,
        144, 147, 198
Pesticides, 72–73, 335, 339–340, 347
Pests, dealing with, 339–340, 342–343
Pets, 133, **302**
Pharmacists, 235, **235,** 236
Phlebitis, 305
Phobias, 178, **178**
Phosphorous, 54, 58
    levels of in bones, 281
    See also Minerals.
Physical examinations
    exercise and, 101, 135, 137
    routine, 31, 218, 224, 226, 227, **227**
    self-administered, 154, 227, **227**
Physicians, 174–175
    certification and credentials of, 149,
        216, 217, 218, 219
    consultations with, **148,** 149,
        152–153, 154, 155, 216, 221, 225
    family, 149
    fees of, 224–225
    first visits to, 216–217, 233
    hospital privileges of, 149, 216, 220
    laboratory investments of, 228
    malpractice suits against, 218–219,
        222, 225
    primary care, 216, 221, 233
    questioning of, 216, **216,** 220, 225,
        232
    second opinions from, 218, 221
    specialization of, 149, 216, 218, 221
Picasso, Pablo, 21, **21**
Pizza, vegetable, 88–89, **88–89**
Plantar fasciitis, 115
Plants, 333
    poisonous, 342, **342**
Plaque
    arterial, 38, 272, **272,** 297, **298,** 299,
        299
    dental, 162, **162,** 163, **163**
Plastic surgery, 148–155
    computer imaging and, **148,** 153
    consultations prior to, **148,** 149,
        152–153, 154, 155
    effective duration of, **150, 151, 152,
        153,** 155

Plastic surgery (*contd.*)
  insurance coverage of, 149
  major, 152–155
  minor, 150–151
  pros and cons of, 148, 155
  recovery from, 148, **150,** 151, **151, 152,** 153, **153,** 154, 155
  risks of, 148, 149, **150, 151, 152, 153,** 154
  selecting surgeons for, 149
  side effects of, 148, **150, 151, 152, 153,** 154, 155
  See also specific procedures.
Pleurisy, 295
Pneumonia, 295
  mycoplasma, 294
  pneumococcal, 219, 294
  vaccine for, 219, 293
  viral, 294
Podiatrists, 166, 261
Poisons, 326
  emergency treatment for, 340
  food, 57, 74–75, 257
  household, 338–341
  plant, 342, **342**
Polyps, 228, **309,** 312
Ponce de Leon, Juan, 29
Pork and beans, 84
Pork chop and sweet potato bake, 81, **81**
Posture, 102, 103, **103,** 168
  back pain and, 103, 253
  running, 130
  walking, 118, **118**
Potassium, 52, 54, 55, 228
  increased need for, 41
  supplements of for leg cramps, 251
  See also Minerals.
Potato and cheese pie, 89
Poultry, 36, 37, **37,** 42, 43, 55
  cooking of, 49, 73, 74, 79, 82–83
Power of attorney, durable, 186
Prenuptial agreements, **191**
Presbyopia, 284, 288
Preservatives, 70, 71, 144, 145, 232, 234
Progesterone, 20, 239
Prostaglandins, 39
Prostate gland, 218, 238, **319**
  cancer of, 38, 318–319, 323
  enlargement of, 16, 318, **319**
Protein, 42–43, 151, 169
  dietary sources of, 42, 43, 46, 49
  guidelines for consumption of, 42, 43
  purified derivative of, used in test for tuberculosis, 228–229, 295
  serving sizes of, 42–43, **42–43**

PSA (prostate-specific antigen) test, 319
Psoriasis, 149
Psychiatrists, 177, 279
Psychologists, 175, 176, 177, 182, 184, 195, 196, 212, 279
Psychotherapy, 177, 179, 241, 278, 279, **279**
Pulmonary artery, **297**
Pupils, eye, 284, **285**

QR

Quackery, 29, 217, 218–219
Quinine, use of for leg cramps, 250
Rabies, 120, 230
Races, 109
  marathon, 131
  race walking, 121, **121,** 137
  10K road, 137
Race walking, 121, **121,** 137
Radiation, 336–337, **336**
Radiation therapy, 137, 160, 295, 319, 322, 323
Radiologists, 154, 310
Radon, 333, 337, **337**
Rashes, 144, 145, 146, 232, 233, 265, 343
Raynaud's phenomenon and disease, 305
Recommended Dietary Allowances (RDA's), 28, 40, 42, 43, 55, 58, 77
Records
  business and financial, 191, 193, 213
  drug, 216–217, 220, 232, 235
  medical, 218, 219, 220, 222
Rectum, 258, **309, 321**
  cancer of, 39
  examination of, 218, 228–229
Reflexes, 218, 252, 351
Relaxation, 127, 175, 291
  progressive, **181,** 250, 271
  techniques of, 32, 176, 180–181, **180, 181,** 238, 271
Remarriage, 189, 191, **191**
Rennhard, Hans, 343, **343**
Reproductive system, 16, 318–321
  female, 320–321, **321**
  male, 318–319, **319**
Respiratory system. *See* Lungs.

Rest, 31, 114, 115, 155, 247, 248
Restless leg syndrome, 251
Résumés, 201
Retina, **285**
  detached or torn, 284, 287, **287**
  diabetic damage of, **288,** 289
Retinoic acid (Retin-A)
  as part of hair growth treatment, 160
  derivation of, 146
  use of for skin rejuvenation, 146
  use of with chemical peels, 151
Retirement, 184, 202–209
  early, 185, 203, 205
  education and, 202–204, **204**
  financial planning for, 32, 202, 203
  goal setting for, 202
  housing and, 207–209, **209**
  stress of, **175,** 188, 189, 196, 200, 202, 205
  travel and, 202, **203,** 204, 205
  volunteering in, 206–207, **206**
  working after, 205–207, **205**
Reynolds, Momma Jo (Jo), 122, **122**
Rheumatoid arthritis, 266–267, 267
  See also Arthritis.
RICE (Rest, Ice, Compression, and Elevation) treatment, 114, 115
Right atrium, **297**
Right ventricle, **297**
Risotto, 85, **85**
Rosacea, 146
Rosen, John de, **32**
Rudman, Daniel, 25, 26–27
Runner's knee, 115
Running, 28, 94, 97, 106, 121, 124, 130–131
  benefits of, 107, 130
  competitive, 123, 131, 137
  form and posture in, 130
  injury risks and, 130–131

S

Saccharin, 45, 71
Safe-deposit boxes, 191, 213
Safety
  cosmetic, 144–145, 159
  with equipment and machines, 133, 326–327, 336, **336,** 350–351
  guidelines for, 326, 327
  home, 270, 326–341
  outdoor, 120, 122, 126, 128–129, 130, 342–343, 346–347

Safety (*contd.*)
  road, 120, 128–129, 350–351
  sports, 120, 122, 126, 128–129, 130
  weather conditions and, 112–113, 350
Salmonella, 73, 74, 79, 256–257
Salt, 40, 56–57, 141, 144
"Sandwich generation," 187
Saunas, 143, 305
Scalps, 156, 159, 160, 161, 168
Sciatica, 271
Seafood risotto with asparagus, 85, **85**
Seasonal affective disorder (SAD), 278, 349
Seaweed (kelp), 146
Sedatives, 151, 153, 230, 237
Self-awareness, 176, 179, 213
Self-esteem, 32, 179
Self-help groups, 177, 194, 195, 198, 199
Selye, Hans, 179
Senility, 226, 241, 276–277
Senior citizen centers, 123, 187, 202, 203, 206
Senior Games. *See* United States National Senior Sports Classic— The Senior Olympics.
Senses, 18
  decline of, 40, 55
Separation agreements, 190
Sex, 302, 320
  abstaining from, 307
  disease transmission and, 238, 306–307, 312
  pleasure and, 16
  problems with, 184, 188, 238
Seyle, Hans, 179
Shampoo
  antidandruff, 146, 156, 159
  types of, 156
Shaving, 144, **144,** 155, 161, 168, 222
Shingles, 264–265
Shin splints, 115
Shoes, 115, 135, 252
  components of, **116–117,** 260
  selection of, 166, 260, 261
  size of, 166, 261, 283
  sports, 122, **129,** 130, 260
Showering, **113,** 114, 146
Sigmoidoscopy, 228–229
Skiing, 245
  cross-country, 94, 97, 107, 123
  using cross-country ski machines, 133, **133**
Skin, 140–147
  aging, 140–141, **140,** 142, 145, 146, 150–155

Skin (*contd.*)
  allergic reactions of, 144–145, 159, 161, 167, 232
  benign growths on, 146, 150, 227
  bleaching of, 166
  blemishes of, 18, **142,** 143, 146, 150–151
  blood vessels of, 140, 141, **141,** 146, 150, **197**
  body, 141, 147, 154–155, 227
  bruising of, **197,** 264
  cancer of, 39, 147, 227, **227,** 265, **265**
  chemical peels of, 151, **151**
  cleansing of, 141, 142, **142,** 143
  color complementing of, 169
  dermabrasion of, 150–151, **150**
  diseases of, 146, 147, 149, 227, **227,** 264–265 **265**
  dryness of, 140, 141, **141,** 142, 143, 144, 166, 169
  examination of, 218, 227, **227,** 265, **265**
  facial, 140–141, 142–146, **142,** 150–154, **150, 151, 152, 153**
  freshening of, 142, 143
  genetic characteristics of, 140, 141, 147, 149
  hand, 147, 166
  hormone treatment of, 146
  irregular coloring of, 18, 146, 147, 148, 150, 155, 166, 227, 264
  layers of, 19, 140, **141**
  lesions of, **265**
  moisturizing of, 141, 142, 143, 144, 145, 146, 166
  moles and birthmarks on, 227
  nerve endings in, **141**
  oiliness of, 140, **141,** 142, **142,** 143, 144
  pigmentation of, 140, 147, 151, 155, 158, 166
  pores of, 141, **142,** 143, 149
  precancerous growths on, 146
  protection of, 140, 146, 147, 151, 155
  rashes of, 144, 145, 146, 232, 233, 265, 343
  rejuvenation of, 146, 148–155, **150, 151, 152, 153**
  sagging of, 19, 140–141, 152, **152,** 153, 154, 155
  scarring of, 148, **150,** 151, **151, 152, 153,** 154, 155, 161
  sensitive, 141, 143, 144, 145, 147
  sloughing of, 142, 143, 166, 167
  smoking and, 140, 146, 148
  sun exposure of, 140, 144, 146, 147, 166

Skin (*contd.*)
  surgery on. *See* Plastic surgery.
  tags, 146, 150
  thinning of, 140, **141,** 166
  toning of, 142, 143
  treatment of, 141–147, **142, 144, 146,** 149
  weather conditions and, 141, 146, 147, 166
  wrinkling of, 19, 140, **140, 141,** 144, 146, 147, 150–151, 152
Skin patches
  for delivery of medication, 231
  estrogen, **239**
  nicotine, 233, 243
Sleep, 250–251, **253**
  disturbances of, 31, 67, 179, 185, 194, 195, 233, 235, 250–251
  exercise and, 94, 130, 251
  inducing of, 31, 232, 235, 250
  need for, 141, 177, 233
Sleep apnea, 250
Sleeping pills, 31, 66, 232, 250
Slimak, Paul, 165, **165**
Smallpox, 11, 230
Smell, sense of, 40, 55
Smoke detectors, 327, 329
Smoking, 13, 51, 101, 109, 194, 242–245, 327
  cessation of, 20, 31, 50, 148, 242–245, **244,** 294, 308, 335
  lung disease and, 242, **243,** 292, 293, 295, 335
  per capita decrease in, 13
  relapses into, 244–245
  risks of, 18, 140, 146, 148, 242, **243**
  secondhand exposure to, 226, 242, **243,** 335
  withdrawal from, 243, 244, **244**
Snowshoeing, 121, **121**
Snyder, Virginia, 201, **201**
Soap, 144, 167
  facial, 142, 143, 151
  types of, 141, 143
Social Security, 186, 191, 202, 203, 206, 213, 225
Sodium, 54, 56–57, 72
  reducing intake of, 57
  See also Minerals.
Soup, cabbage and carrot, 88
Soybeans, 39, 42
Speech, 272
  impairment of, 233, 249, 274
  therapy for, 221, 274
Sphinx, 10, **10**

Spine, 252, **269,** 271
  epidural catheters in, **221,** 222
  herniated discs in, 252
  manipulation of, 217
Squamous cell carcinoma, 265, **265**
Stair climbing, 93, 97, 107
  stair-climbing machines, 132–133,
    132
Stepparenting, 189
Steroids, 247
Stethoscopes, 218
Stewart, Patrick, **160,** 161
Stokowski, Leopold, 28
Stomach, **309**
  cancer of, 39
  disorders of, 43, 45, 94, 179, 194,
    197, 231, 256–258, 308–310
  lining of, **197,** 308–309
Stool, 47, 258
  blood in, 226, 228–229, 312
  testing of, 218, 226, 228–229
Stress
  causes of, 174–175, **175, 176**
  chronic, 94, 174, 175
  dealing with, 14, 32, 94, 127,
    175–183, **176,** 194, 195, 238
  divorce and, 174, **175,** 189, 190–191
  effects of, 94, 146, 174–175, **174,**
    178, 183, 240
  emotional, 146, 174–176, 182, 183,
    184–185, 188, 192–195, 196
  exercise and, 94, 127, 177, **180,** 182
  "fight or flight" syndrome and, 174
  grief and, 174, **175,** 184, 188,
    192–194
  health risks and, 94, 146, 174–175,
    183, 194, 217
  heart and, 175, 183
  job-related, 20, 174, 175, **175,** 179,
    184–185
  measuring of, 174–175, **175**
  midlife, 174–185, 190–191
  personality types and, 175–176
  physical, 174, 176, 179, 182, 183,
    194
  relaxation techniques and, 32, 176,
    180–181, **180, 181**
  retirement and, **175,** 188, 189, 196,
    200, 202, 205
  self-awareness and, 176, 179
  severe, 146, 174, 183
  stimulation and, 174, **174**
  symptoms of, 166, 174, 179, 183
  therapeutic treatment of, 177–179
Stress fractures, 115, 130
Stress tests, 101, **101,** 135, 137, 228

Stretching exercises, 104–105, 109,
    114, 123, 251, **254, 255**
  in-seat, 110, 136
  safe, 104–105, 108
Strokes, 12, 20, 38, 93, 221, 241,
    272–275
  risk factors for, 272, 273–275
  therapy for, 221, 274, 275
  types of, **272**
  warning signs of, 273, 275
Study groups, 32, 203–204, **204**
Suction lipectomy, 155
Sugar, **37,** 44–45
  blood, 17, 226, 228–229, 241,
    281–283, **282, 282**
Suicide, 20, 192, 194, 195
Sulfite, 71, 75
Sun
  protection from, 151, 155, 157, **157**
  skin damage from, 140, 144, 146,
    147, 265
  ultraviolet rays of, 140, 147, 171, 286
Sunglasses, 147, 155, 171, 286, 289
Sunscreens, 113, 145, 146, 151, 155
  sun protection factor (SPF) in, 147,
    166
Support groups, 63, 177, 194, 198, 277
Suppositories, 231, 258
Surgery
  alternatives to, 225
  arthroscopic, 266, 267
  in clinics, 149, 151, 153
  cosmetic. *See* Plastic surgery.
  endoscopic, 225, 308, 310, 313,
    314, 315
  heart, 300–301, **300–301**
  laparoscopic, **315**
  laser, 150, 286, 287, **288,** 313, 317
  major, 149, 220–222, 223, 224
  preparation for, 220–222
  recovery from, 106, 176, 220–221,
    222
  stress of, 176, 222
  See also specific procedures.
Swallowing, 275, 276
Swimming, 97, 124–127, 147, 157
  beginning program of, 125, 126
  benefits of, 124–125
  classes in, 126, **127**
  safety and, 126
  techniques of, 94, 106–107,
    124–125, 125, 127
  warmup and cooldown for, 126–127
Syringes, disposal of, 236

Taste, sense of, 40, 55
Taxes, 32, 202
  estate, 193
  income, 193
  records of, 191, 213
Tea, 47, 58, **66,** 67
  green, 39
Teeth, 162–165
  artificial, 165
  bonding and laminating of, 164, **164**
  brushing and flossing of, 162–163,
    162
  capping of, 164
  chewing and, 41
  daily care of, 162–163, **162**
  decay of, 45, 162, 163, 164
  dentures for, 41, 164–165
  discoloration of, 164, **164**
  fillings in, 164
  loss of, 162
  polishing and bleaching of, 164
  professional care of, 164–165
  straightening of, 165
  tartar on, 162, 163
Temporomandibular joint syndrome
    (TMJ), 165
Tendinitis, 115
Testicles, **281, 319**
  cancer of, 227, 319
  examination of, 218, 227
  shrinking of, **197**
Testosterone, 20, 238, **319**
Tests, 226–229
  aging, 17
  anxiety about, 226, 228
  common types of, 228–229
  cosmetic, 144–145, 159
  costs of, 226
  criteria for, 226
  diagnostic, 41, 220, 221, 226, 227,
    228–229, 252
  drug, 20, 218–219, 221, 232
  fallibility of, 228, 233
  home, 226–227, 282, **282**
  hospital, 220, 221
  interpreting of, 226, 228
  preparation for, 226
  records of, 216–217, 220, 232, 235
  risks of, 226
  routine physical, 218, 227, **227**
  screening, 226, 228–229

Tests (*contd.*)
    stress, 101, **101,** 135, 137, 228
    technology for, 226, 228, 282, **282,**
        310–311, **311,** 313
    unnecessary, 216, 225, 226
Tetanus shots, 219, 230
Therapy
    alternative, 217, 271
    aquatic, 270, **274**
    light, 349
    physical, 187, 217, 221, 266, 270,
        271, 274, **274,** 275, 276
    psychological, 177–179, 198, 221,
        238, 241, 271, 278–279
    speech, 221, 274
Throat, 218, 233
    cancer of, 242
    soreness of, 222, 249
Thymus gland, 16
Thyroid gland, 16, 280, **281**
    disorders of, 149, 183, 241, 280
Tic douloureux, 276
Tinnitus, 165, 291
Toenails
    infections of, 166, 261
    ingrown, 167, 261, 283
Toes, 267, **267**
    caring for, 166, 167
    circulation in, 110
    exercising of, 110, 167
Toothbrushes, 162, **162**
Toothpaste, 163
    baking soda used as, 163
Toothpicks, 163, **163**
Toupees, 161
Tranquilizers, 178, 196, 230, 232, 233,
    246, 250
Transcutaneous electrical nerve
    stimulation (TENS), 271
Transient ischemic attack (TIA), 273,
    275
Transportation
    ambulance, 223
    discounts on, 202, **203**
Trauma centers, 222, 223
Travel, 195, 258, 329
    chronic disease and, 315
    exercise and, 110, 136
    immunizations required for, 219, 259
    retirement and, 202, **203,** 204, 205
Travel-study programs, 204, **204**
Treadmills, 101, **101,** 117
Tremors, 275, 276
Triathlon, 137
Triglycerides, 62, 228–229, 299
Truman, Harry S., 121

Tuberculosis, 11
    testing for, 228–229, 295
    treatment of, 295
"Tummy tucks," 154
Tumors, 228
    benign, 146, 150, 227
    malignant, 265, **265,** 317
    See also Cancer.
Turkey legs "osso bucco style," 82
Tutankhamen, 10, **10**
Tyramines, 75

U

Ulcerative colitis, 311
Ulcers, 67, 311
    peptic, 309–310
    stomach, **197**
Ultrasound scanning, 310, **311**
Uniform donor cards, 213
United States National Senior Sports
    Classic—The Senior Olympics,
    137
United States Recommended Daily
    Allowances (USRDA's), 55, **77**
Urea, 145
Uric acid, 43, 267, 269
Urinary system, 19
    problems with, 16, 20, 226,
        228–229, 281, 316–317, 320
    See also Incontinence.
Urinary tract infections, 226, 228–229,
    316
Urine, 47, 52, 231, 316–317
    testing of, 218, 226, 228–229
Uterus, **321**
    cancer of, 239, 321
    prolapse of, 320, **321**

V

Vaccines, 219, 230, 259
    annual, 248
    influenza, 219, 248, 293
Vagina, 316, **321**
    menopausal atrophy of, 16, 20, 238,
        320

Varicose veins, 31, 304–305, **304**
Vasodilators, 296, 302
Vegetable pizza, 88–89, **88–89**
Vegetables, 30, 36, 37 **37,** 38, 42, 43,
    45, 49, 51, 76, 78–79
    cruciferous, 39, 41, 78
    main course dishes of, 88–89
    organic, 73
Vegetarianism, 43
Veins, 166, 311
    enlarged, **197**
    spider, 150
    varicose, 304–305, **304**
Vertigo, 247, 291
Very-low-density lipoproteins (VLDL's),
    298
Video display terminals (VDT's), 336,
    337
Videotapes, 108, 121, 212
Villemez, Clyde J., 131, **131**
Viruses
    defense against, 219, 248–249
    influenza A, 248
    influenza B, 248
    viracella zoster, 264–265
Vitamins, 52–55, 176, 132
    A, 28, 38, 39, 41, 48, 53
        retinoic acid derived from, 146
    antioxidants, 38, 55
    B1, 53
    B2, 53
    B3, 53
    B5, 53
    B6, 40, 53
    B12, 40, 53
        adequate amounts of in vege-
            tarian diets, 43
    benefits of, 53
    beta carotene. *See* Beta carotene.
    biotin, 53
    C, 28, 38, 39, 53, 55
        interaction with drugs, 235
    D, 48, 53, 58
        milk fortified with, 70
    Daily Values (DV's) for, 55, **77**
    deficiencies of, 40
        and memory lapses, 241
    dietary sources of, 38, 52–55
    E, 28, 38, 39, 41, 48, 53, 55
        for relief of menopausal
            symptoms, 239
        studies on use of for reduction of
            women's risk of heart disease
            and cancer, 239

Vitamins (*contd.*)
  fat-soluble, 52, 53
  folic acid, 53, 55
  K, 41, 48, 53, 232
  megadoses of, 55
  Recommended Dietary Allowances
    (RDA's) for, 28, 40, 42, 43, 55, 58,
    77
  supplements of, 21, 28, 52, 55, 176
  United States Recommended Daily
    Allowances (USRDA's) for, 55, 77
  water-soluble, 52, 53
Vitreous humor, 284, **285,** 289
Volunteer organizations, 32, 186, 194,
  198, 205, 206–207, **206,** 213
Vomiting, 72, 75, 222, 236, 246, 247,
  255, 257–258, 340, 341

Walking, 94, 116–123, 137
  beginning programs of, 110, 119,
    121
  benefits of, 30–31, 63, 106, 107,
    116, 127
  classes in, 116, 121
  mall, 14, 123, **123**
  one-mile test of, 97

Walking (*contd.*)
  race, 121, **121,** 137
  safety in, 120, 122
  snowshoe, 121, **121**
  social, 116, 123
  technique of, 117, **157, 118,** 121, **121**
  treadmill, 101, **101,** 117
  variations of, 117–121
  See also Hiking.
Walking clubs, 121, 123
Warmups, 96, 104, 108, 109, 113, 114,
  119, 123, 126–127, 128, 130,
  135, 137
Water, 112, 113, 122, 330–331
  consumption of, 47
  contaminants in, 330
  treatment and filtering of, 331, **331**
  working out in, 126–127, **127,** 137,
    270, **274**
Watson, Juanita, 270, **270**
Weather, 278, 348–349
  cold, 113, 146, **157,** 166, 182,
    248–249, 348
  hot, 112–113, 146, 147, **157,** 166,
    348
Weight, 60–65
  aging and, 60–61, 93–94
  diet and, 27–28, 31, 63, 65, 149
  excessive, 63, 64, 101, 106, 109,
    125, 146, 154–155
  exercise and, 31, 63, 93–94, 116
  gaining of, 60–61, 62, 93–94, 245
  healthy, 60–61, **61,** 63
  loss of, 27–28, 44–45, 60, 62, 63,
    65, 69, 107–108, 250
  tests for body composition and, 62,
    100

Weight lifting, 93, 94, 97, 101, 134, 135,
  137
Whiteheads, **150, 151**
Wigs, 161
Wills, 32, 191, 193, 213, 222
Wine, 51, 68, 69, 71, 329
Women's Health Initiative, 21
Wright, Orville and Wilbur, 11, **11**

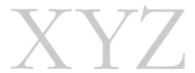

X-rays, 310, **311**
  chest, 228–229, 252, **301,** 304
  mammography, 154, 228–229, 322
Zidovudine (AZT), 307
Zinc, 52, 54, 59
  getting adequate amounts of, 40
  See also Minerals.